Clinical Cases in Cardiology

Clinical Cases in Cardiology

Editor: Tristian Jones

AMERICAN
MEDICAL PUBLISHERS
www.americanmedicalpublishers.com

AMERICAN
MEDICAL PUBLISHERS
www.americanmedicalpublishers.com

Cataloging-in-Publication Data

Clinical cases in cardiology / edited by Tristian Jones.
p. cm.
Includes bibliographical references and index.
ISBN 979-8-88740-626-8
1. Cardiology. 2. Heart--Diseases. I. Jones, Tristian.
RC667 .C55 2023
616.1--dc23

American Medical Publishers,
41 Flatbush Avenue,
1st Floor, New York,
NY 11217, USA

ISBN 979-8-88740-626-8 (Hardback)

Contents

Preface

Cardiology refers to the field of internal medicine that deals with the disorders of the cardiovascular system. It focuses on the diagnosis and treatment of heart-related conditions such as coronary artery disease, heart failure, congenital heart defects, valvular heart disease, and atheroma. High levels of low-density lipoprotein (LDL) cholesterol, obesity, high blood pressure, diabetes, physical inactivity, smoking, poor diet, and exposure to passive smoke are the major risk factors for cardiac diseases and strokes. Echocardiogram (ECHO), electrocardiogram (ECG), ambulatory ECG, and stress test are some of the most common diagnostic tests performed in cardiology. There are a variety of strategies for treating cardiovascular diseases including percutaneous coronary intervention, stenting, coronary artery bypass surgery, and percutaneous transluminal angioplasty. In order to manage heart health, people may also introduce certain lifestyle modifications such as consumption of balanced healthy diet (to lower cholesterol levels and blood pressure), regular exercise, taking prescribed medications, and maintaining a healthy body weight. In this book, using case studies, constant effort has been made to make the understanding of the difficult concepts of cardiology as easy and informative as possible. It is appropriate for students seeking detailed information in this area as well as for experts.

After months of intensive research and writing, this book is the end result of all who devoted their time and efforts in the initiation and progress of this book. It will surely be a source of reference in enhancing the required knowledge of the new developments in the area. During the course of developing this book, certain measures such as accuracy, authenticity and research focused analytical studies were given preference in order to produce a comprehensive book in the area of study.

This book would not have been possible without the efforts of the authors and the publisher. I extend my sincere thanks to them. Secondly, I express my gratitude to my family and well-wishers. And most importantly, I thank my students for constantly expressing their willingness and curiosity in enhancing their knowledge in the field, which encourages me to take up further research projects for the advancement of the area.

Editor

1

Coronary Embolism and Myocardial Infarction in a Transgender Male Undergoing Hormone Therapy

Sandesh Dinesh,[1,2] **Marcus Franz,**[2] **and Friedhelm Küthe**[1]

[1]*Ilmkreis-Kliniken, Clinic for Internal Medicine I, Bärwinkelstrasse 33, 99310 Arnstadt, Germany*
[2]*Department of Internal Medicine I, University Hospital Jena, Am Klinikum 1, 07747 Jena, Germany*

Correspondence should be addressed to Marcus Franz; marcus.franz@med.uni-jena.de

Academic Editor: Man-Hong Jim

Introduction. Due to the complex interaction between the underlying disease, psychosocial factors, and the high-dose hormonal therapy, transgender patients pose a therapeutic and diagnostic challenge, especially during emergencies. This case presents one such clinical dilemma using the example of a case of myocardial infarction. *Case.* A 35-year-old transgender male presented to our clinic with an acute inferior wall myocardial infarction. For the past 6 years, he was receiving high-dose testosterone therapy for the maintenance of hormone levels after female-to-male gender conversion. The emergency coronary angiography revealed a distal right coronary artery occlusion. Recanalization of the vessel was achieved by catheter-driven direct thrombectomy and subsequent intracardiac lysis. The appearance of the remaining coronary arteries bore no angiographic evidence of advanced coronary artery disease. We suspected a thromboembolic origin as the primary cause of the myocardial infarction. The presentation also fulfilled the proposed National Cerebral and Cardiovascular Center criteria for the clinical diagnosis of coronary embolism. In the diagnostic work-up, the most common causes of coronary embolism like atrial fibrillation, cardiomyopathies, endocarditis, and intracardiac tumors could be ruled out. The screening for hereditary thrombophilia was also negative. Likewise, the presence of a haemodynamically relevant right to left shunt could be excluded. In the end, the high-dose testosterone therapy seemed to be the most likely cause. *Conclusion.* Following major thromboembolic cardiovascular events, we believe that transgender males treated with high-dose testosterone therapy should receive oral anticoagulation, preferably with a DOAC, especially keeping in mind that the discontinuation of the hormone therapy is not always possible due to the various underlying psychosocial factors.

1. Case Presentation

A transsexual 35-year-old Caucasian male without known relevant medical history of cardiac disease presented to the emergency room with a sudden onset of typical anginal chest pain. Physical examination revealed a hemodynamically stable patient with resting pulse of 70/min and blood pressure of 110/70 mmHg, with no signs of acute cardiopulmonary decompensation. Cardiac examination was uneventful with normal heart sounds without pathological murmurs. Respiratory, abdomen, and neurological examinations remained normal. Active smoking accumulating to 20 pack years and a history of daily alcohol consumption were significant risk factors. Drug history revealed a hormonal therapy with intramuscular testosterone undecanoate for gender conversion over the past 6 years, with an initial dosage of 1000 mg per month over a period of 1 year from 2011 to 2012 and later at a dose of 1000 mg every 3 months to date. An electrocardiogram showed sinus rhythm with ST-Segment elevation in the inferior leads (Figure 1).

An emergency coronary angiography revealed normal coronary arteries with an occlusion of the distal right coronary artery (Figure 2(a)). The appearance of the remaining coronary arteries was smooth, not indicative of an advanced

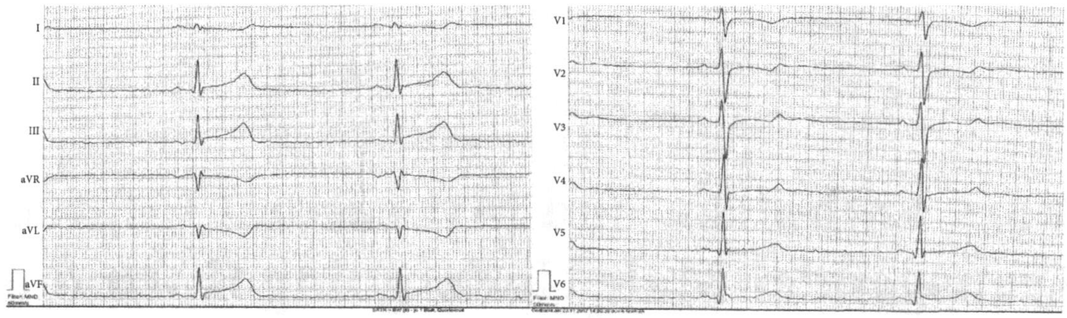

Figure 1: Electrocardiogram of the patient showing sinus rhythm with ST-Segment elevation in the inferior leads.

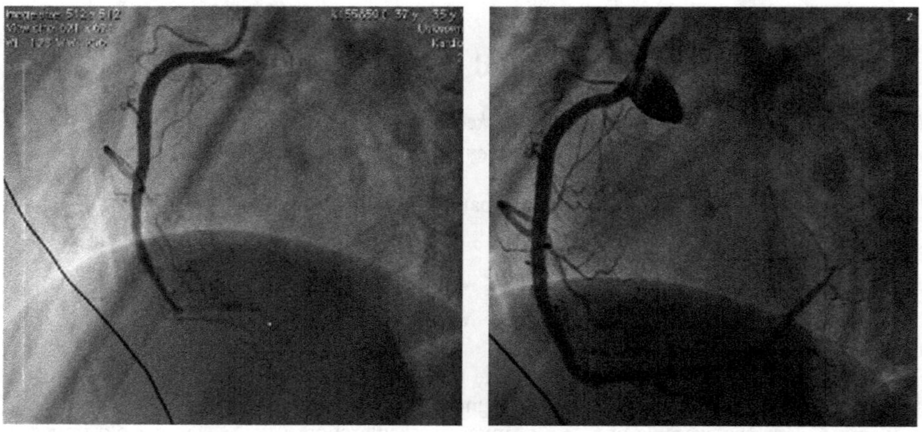

(a) (b)

Figure 2: Coronary angiography of the patient revealing normal coronary arteries with an occlusion of the distal right coronary artery (RCA) before (a) and after successful recanalization (b).

atherosclerotic coronary artery disease. We suspected a thromboembolic origin as the primary cause of the myocardial infarction by the appearance of the coronaries. Recanalization of the vessel was achieved by catheter-driven direct thrombectomy using an aspiration catheter. This was followed by intracardiac lysis with 20 mg tissue plasminogen activator, Alteplase, and subsequently the intravenous glycoprotein IIb/IIIa inhibitor Tirofiban. A short episode of reperfusion-related ventricular fibrillation and subsequent third-degree atrioventricular block (av-block) were overcome by defibrillation and intravenous administration of 2 mg Atropine, respectively. Finally, a successful recanalization was achieved with TIMI-3 flow (Figure 2(b)) with immediate resolution of the patient's symptoms. A stent implantation was not necessary. Cardiac biomarkers were subsequently elevated with Troponin I up to a maximum of 46.63 ng/ml (Reference range: 0.00–0.06 ng/ml). Echocardiography revealed a good systolic left ventricular function with postinfarct inferior wall hypokinesia. The patient remained haemodynamically stable without complications during the hospital stay.

Subsequently, investigations were conducted with the aim to identify an underlying cause for the suspected embolic myocardial infarction. The transthoracic echocardiography did not reveal intracardiac thrombus or valve vegetations as evidence for infective endocarditis. A deep venous thrombosis could also not be detected by ultrasonography, and the D-Dimer levels were negative.

The initially performed transoesophageal echocardiography under sedation (Midazolam) raised the suspicion of a possible small persisting foramen ovale (PFO). We performed a second contrast-enhanced TOE without sedation. No crossover of microbubbles over to the arterial circulation were observed even under Valsalva manoeuvre. Thus, a haemodynamically relevant right to left shunt could be ruled out.

No evidence of paroxysmal atrial fibrillation was reported in a 72 h Holter-ECG Monitoring. Cardiac embolic sources were thus deemed unlikely.

Other manifestations of atherosclerotic vessel diseases could not be seen in the colour-coded Doppler Ultrasound scans of the extracranial arteries or pelvic/lower limb arteries.

Laboratory tests for Antiphospholipid Syndrome (APS), Factor-V Leiden, Protein C and Protein S deficiency, Antithrombin III deficiency, and Hyperhomocysteinemia as possible causes for a hypercoagulable state were also negative.

In conclusion, the work-up for the definitive cause of the infarction remained inconclusive. The drug history of the patient with the use of high-dose hormonal therapy with testosterone for gender conversion was one of the significant factors in the patient's history.

This background of high-dose testosterone therapy for the purpose of gender conversion and its procoagulant associations led us believe this to be the factor leading to the coronary embolism.

A follow-up of the patient was performed at 3 months and 1 year. The echocardiography and ECG showed no signs of long-term detrimental effects following the myocardial infarction with resolution of the initial wall motion disturbances.

2. Discussion and Review of the Literature

Transgender patients undergoing sex change therapy pose a unique challenge with a complex interaction of underlying disease, psychosocial factors, and the additional high-dose hormone therapy. With the number of cases of gender conversion gradually increasing [1], the altered hormone milieu due to the hormone therapy in this patient group and its possible side effects like thromboembolism must be given special consideration.

In this case, we present one such diagnostic and therapeutic dilemma. At initial presentation, our patient met the diagnostic criteria for an acute inferior wall ST-elevation myocardial infarction (STEMI). Except for a significant smoking history accumulating to 20 pack years, there were no other known risk factors in the patient's past history. Due to the young age of the patient and the medical history, we thought of an alternative explanation rather than an atherosclerotic disease as the underlying cause for the acute myocardial infarction. The coronary angiogram supported our uncertainty with evidence of normal coronary arteries and with no evidence of underlying atherosclerosis. Other invasive coronary imaging modalities like optical coherence tomography or intravenous ultrasound were not performed in this patient, although these modalities would have helped in definitively ruling out significant atherosclerotic plaques. Other signs of systemic atherosclerotic vessel disease could also be ruled out in the subsequent colour-coded Doppler ultrasound scans of the extracranial arteries and pelvic/lower limb arteries.

The myocardial infarction was hypothesized to be of embolic origin, due to a coronary embolism. The subsequent successful treatment with catheter-directed thrombectomy and intracardiac lysis with Tirofiban, along with no evidence of plaque rupture, underlined the case for an embolic origin of the episode. The clinical case satisfying one major criteria with angiographic evidence of coronary embolism without atherosclerotic component and two minor criteria with <25% stenosis on angiography, except for the culprit lesion and the presence of an embolic risk in the form of hypercoagulable state in our case, of the proposed National Cerebral and Cardiovascular Center criteria for the clinical diagnosis of coronary embolism by Shibata and coworkers [2] also backed our clinical hypothesis.

Our further work-up was aimed at finding a causative link for the coronary embolism. Literature search showed the most common factors leading to coronary emboli in the order of descending significance to be (a) atrial fibrillation, (b) dilated cardiomyopathy, (c) endocarditis, and (d) intracardiac tumors [3]. Other systemic prothrombotic diseases like active malignancies or systemic autoimmune diseases are also found to be responsible for coronary embolism. Among the various causes, atrial fibrillation remained the most common cause in adults, including a subset of the patient population having new-onset AF, not on anticoagulation.

Given the known history of smoking and alcohol consumption of our patient [4], he possessed many of the risk factors associated with atrial fibrillation. Despite this, there was no documented evidence of atrial fibrillation. Nonetheless, repeated events of asymptomatic self-limiting paroxysmal AF occurring cannot completely be ruled out. An implantable cardiac loop recorder increases the chances of documentation of such episodes. Thus, at least in patients with cerebral embolism, the guideline for the management of atrial fibrillation published by the European society of cardiology in 2016 recommends the implantation as IIa indication with a level of evidence B [5]. For coronary embolism, a corresponding recommendation does not exist to our best knowledge. Therefore, after internal discussion, we decided against the implantation of a loop recorder. The other potential causes for coronary embolism mentioned above could be ruled out through further work-up as described. Among others, since cases of venous thromboembolism presenting as coronary embolism due to paradoxical embolization over a PFO have been well documented in the literature [6], special emphasis was given on the exclusion of this constellation in our patient by ruling out lower limb deep venous thrombosis and a PFO or a atrial septal defect.

Finally, the search for the cause for the coronary embolism failed to clearly identify the underlying aetiology of the event. An important factor at this point seemed to be the high-dose testosterone therapy for gender conversion causing the activation of the thrombotic cascade in the arterial circulation, leading to formation of thrombotic material (white clots).

Recent published reports have suggested an increased cardiovascular mortality associated with testosterone therapy. The effects of testosterone and its association with increased myocardial infarction and stroke in cisgender men under testosterone therapy for age-related hypogonadism were issued recently as an FDA Warning in accordance with recent studies [7]. It was advised to weigh the potential increased risk of major adverse cardiovascular outcomes against the potential benefits of treating hypogonadism, after FDA review of five observational studies and two meta-analyses.

On the other hand, these evidences and risks associated have also been widely disputed with contrasting evidence. Morgentaler and colleagues found no convincing evidence of increased CV risk with testosterone therapy in hypogonadism [8].

In contrast, patients on testosterone therapy for gender conversion, like the one in our case, receive significantly higher doses in comparison to that used in hypogonadism. There have been reports of increasing risk of venous thromboembolism under testosterone therapy used for gender conversion [9]. A worsening of CVD risk factors like blood pressure, insulin resistance, and lipid derangement have been reported during hormone therapy in transgender males (female to male) [10]. A direct increase in cardiovascular disease or morbidity and mortality have however not been observed [11]. The relatively young age of patients taking gender conversion therapy and short follow up durations are the limiting factors in these studies. In view of the growing transgender population, there is a need for adequately powered prospective studies with focus on the side effects of the therapy and its association with cardiovascular disease.

These factors led us to believe that testosterone therapy for gender conversion might have led to a general hypercoagulable state favoring intraarterial thrombus formation. Our patient in this case had a history of hormonal therapy with intramuscular testosterone undecanoate for gender conversion over the past 6 years. An interaction of factors like (a) vascular stasis due to episodes of paroxysmal AF, along with the (b) procoagulant tendency under high-dose testosterone therapy, and (c) endothelial injury due to the excessive smoking could also have led to the intraarterial activation of the clotting cascade leading to thrombus formation, possibly in the left atrial appendage. This is in accordance to the Virchow's triad of factors contributing to thrombus formation. The embolization of this thrombus into the coronaries could have been the cause for the acute myocardial infarction.

We believe this subpopulation of patients demand an individualized approach to further therapy. A guideline-based approach is not available here due to the very low research base. A generalized approach to therapy with the otherwise conventional CHA_2DS_2-VASc-Score for risk stratification in cases of paroxysmal atrial fibrillation in this subpopulation might be misleading.

Due to the high risk of recurrence of coronary embolism after the first episode, consideration was given to treating the patient with an oral anticoagulant. Despite the increased risk of recurrence, stopping of the testosterone therapy is a very delicate decision and is almost always not acceptable to the patient due to the various psychosocial factors bound with this decision.

The risk of major bleeding episodes under DOAC therapy increases with age. We believe that the risks associated with major bleeding episodes in a younger patient, like the one in this case, are tolerable compared to the risk of recurrence of the coronary embolism. Keeping all this in mind and after discussion with the patient about the potential risks, we decided to treat the patient with an oral anticoagulation—in this case with Apixaban. Regular follow-ups were advised due to the increased risk of recurrence. After 3 months and 1 year, the patient remained asymptomatic with no evidence of similar episodes under continuing testosterone therapy, as well as no major bleeding complications. However, if the patient would have reliably stopped smoking and one could manage to optimally address cardiovascular risk factors, it could have also been justifiable to omit anticoagulation or to replace it by antiplatelet therapy. But, again, evidence is low, and the decision has to be reached individually.

References

[1] J. K. Canner, O. Harfouch, L. M. Kodadek et al., "Temporal trends in gender-affirming surgery among transgender patients in the United States," *JAMA Surgery*, vol. 153, no. 7, pp. 609–616, 2018.

[2] T. Shibata, S. Kawakami, T. Noguchi et al., "Prevalence, clinical features, and prognosis of acute myocardial infarction attributable to coronary artery embolism," *Circulation*, vol. 132, no. 4, pp. 241–250, 2015.

[3] B. Popovic, N. Agrinier, N. Bouchahda et al., "Coronary embolism among ST-segment-elevation myocardial infarction patients: mechanisms and management," *Circulation. Cardiovascular Interventions*, vol. 11, no. 1, article e005587, 2018.

[4] P. O. Ettinger, C. F. Wu, C. de la Cruz Jr., A. B. Weisse, S. S. Ahmed, and T. J. Regan, "Arrhythmias and the "Holiday Heart": alcohol-associated cardiac rhythm disorders," *American Heart Journal*, vol. 95, no. 5, pp. 555–562, 1978.

[5] P. Kirchhof, S. Benussi, D. Kotecha et al., "2016 ESC guidelines for the management of atrial fibrillation developed in collaboration with EACTS," *European Heart Journal*, vol. 37, no. 38, pp. 2893–2962, 2016.

[6] U. Neisius, D. B. Northridge, N. L. Cruden, and M. A. Denvir, "Myocardial infarction associated with patent foramen ovale and paradoxical embolism: a case series," *International Journal of Cardiology*, vol. 180, pp. 34–37, 2015.

[7] FDA Drug Safety Communication, "FDA cautions about using testosterone products for low testosterone due to aging; requires labeling change to inform of possible increased risk of heart attack and stroke with use," https://www.fda.gov/Drugs/DrugSafety/ucm436259.html.

[8] A. Morgentaler, M. M. Miner, M. Caliber, A. T. Guay, M. Khera, and A. M. Traish, "Testosterone therapy and cardiovascular risk: advances and controversies," *Mayo Clinic Proceedings*, vol. 90, no. 2, pp. 224–251, 2015.

[9] K. Stanley and J. Cooper, "Hormone therapy and venous thromboembolism in a transgender adolescent," *Journal of Pediatric Hematology/Oncology*, vol. 40, no. 1, pp. e38–e40, 2018.

[10] C. G. Streed Jr., O. Harfouch, F. Marvel, R. S. Blumenthal, S. S. Martin, and M. Mukherjee, "Cardiovascular disease among transgender adults receiving hormone therapy: a narrative review," *Annals of Internal Medicine*, vol. 167, no. 4, pp. 256–267, 2017.

[11] L. J. Gooren, "Management of female-to-male transgender persons," *Current Opinion in Endocrinology, Diabetes, and Obesity*, vol. 21, no. 3, pp. 233–238, 2014.

2

Coronary Artery Fistula Diagnosed by Echocardiography during NSTEMI

Angelo Acitelli,[1] Sabrina Bencivenga,[1] Maria B. Giannico,[2] Chiara Lanzillo,[2] Luciano Maresca,[2] Renata Petroni,[1] Maria Penco,[1] Leonardo Calò,[2] and Silvio Romano[1]

[1]*Cardiology, Department of Life, Health & Environmental Sciences, University of L'Aquila, Italy*
[2]*Division of Cardiology, Policlinico Casilino, Rome, Italy*

Correspondence should be addressed to Silvio Romano; silvio.romano@cc.univaq.it

Academic Editor: Hajime Kataoka

Coronary artery fistulas are rare abnormal connections between a coronary artery and a cardiac chamber or a major vessel. Often, they are asymptomatic and the diagnosis is accidental. The case we present is the incidental finding of a fistula displayed with echocardiography during acute coronary syndrome (ACS). A 73-year-old man presented in the emergency room for non-ST-elevation ACS. Echocardiogram showed in a parasternal short axis view an abnormal diastolic flow inside the ventricular inferior wall. Angiography and CT confirmed the diagnosis of coronary fistula from the right coronary into the left ventricular cavity. A literature analysis with discussion about coronary fistulas classification and management was also performed.

1. Introduction

Coronary artery fistulas are rare abnormal connections between a coronary artery and a cardiac chamber or a major vessel. They are often asymptomatic and the diagnosis is accidental. The case we present is the accidental finding of a fistula displayed with echocardiography during acute coronary syndrome (ACS).

2. Case Presentation

A 73-year-old man, with a history of hypertension, diabetes mellitus, and hypercholesterolemia, presented in the emergency room because of sudden onset of chest pain at rest. ECG abnormalities associated with an increase of cardiac enzymes (hs troponin 70 pg/ml and CK-MB 8 ng/ml) were suggestive of an ACS (non-ST-elevation myocardial infarction). The patient was admitted to the Coronary Care Unit. Echocardiogram showed left ventricular hypertrophy (septum 14 mm), end-diastolic diameter (53 mm), and mild hypokinesia of the basal segment of the inferior wall with normal systolic function (EF 55%). In the parasternal short axis view, we noticed an abnormal diastolic flow inside the ventricular inferior wall. This flow was directed from the basal segment of the inferior wall into the left ventricular cavity. In the apical two-chamber view, we could follow its entire intramural course, from the apex to the basal portion of the left ventricle, under the mitral valve posterior leaflet, where it was thrown into the ventricular cavity during diastole. Pulsed Doppler sample volume positioned at the level of the flow into the left ventricle confirmed that it was a diastolic flow (Figure 1). The echocardiographic data were suggestive for coronary fistula.

According to ESC guidelines, the GRACE (Global Registry of Acute Coronary Events) risk score of the patient was 146 and early invasive strategy of myocardial revascularization (within the first 24 hours from admission) was indicated. The patient underwent coronary angiography, which revealed 90% stenosis in the middle portion and 70% stenosis in the distal portion of the left anterior descending artery, a double 70% stenosis in the proximal and the middle portion of the circumflex artery and the right coronary artery, dominant, with stenosis of 50% at the end of the proximal portion. Angiography confirmed the presence of a

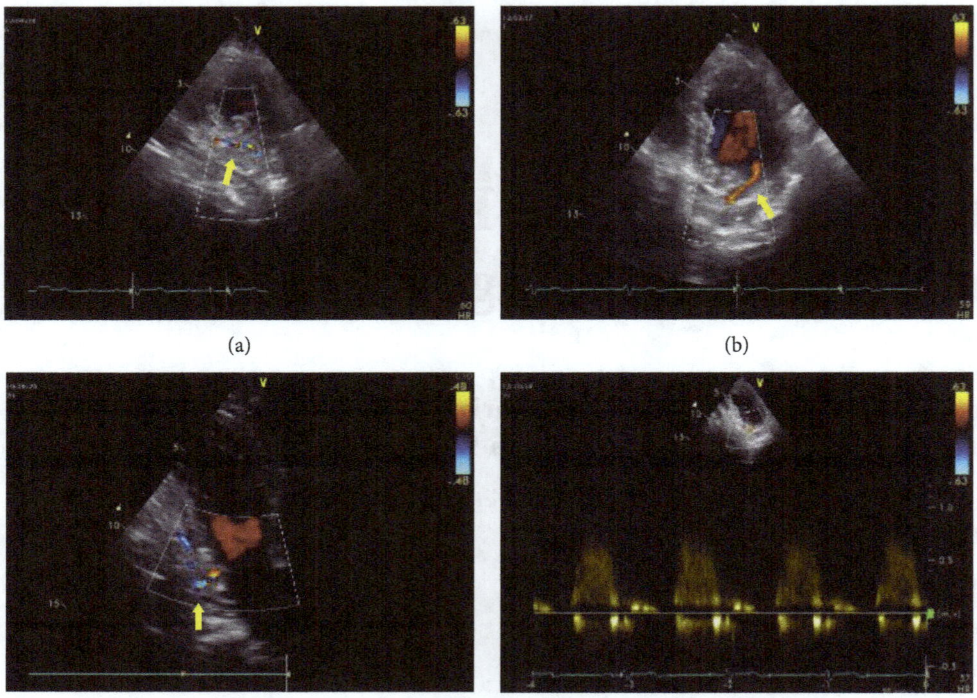

FIGURE 1: Midventricular (a) and basal (b) short axis view and 2-chamber (c) with color Doppler, showing fistula's course in the left ventricle inferoposterior wall (arrows). (d) PW-Doppler recording fistula flow that is predominantly diastolic.

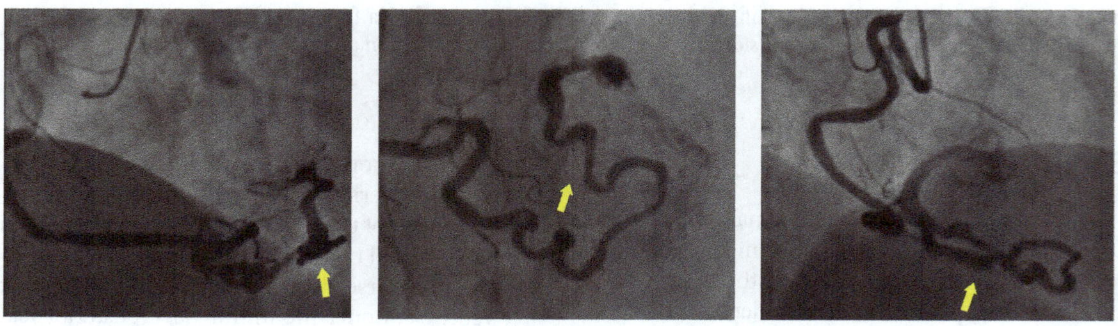

FIGURE 2: Coronary angiography: right coronary artery stenosis of 50% at the end of the proximal portion. Presence of a tortuous voluminous coronary fistula (arrow).

tortuous voluminous coronary fistula: it originated from the interventricular posterior artery and coursed along the posterior interventricular sulcus from the apex to the base of the left ventricle. The terminal portion of the fistula (approximately two-millimeter vessel diameter) crossed the inferoposterior wall of the left ventricle under the mitral annulus, and with a phasic flow, typically diastolic, it went into the ventricular cavity (Figure 2). The patient underwent percutaneous coronary angioplasty with the placement of two drug-eluting stents in the left anterior descending artery (2.5×18 mm in the distal tract and 2.75×28 mm in the middle tract) and a single drug-eluting stent (2.75×33 mm) in the circumflex artery.

To complete evaluation, cardiac CT was performed to detect coronary fistula anatomy, its relationships with cardiac structures and its course. CT images documented that coronary fistula originated from the distal portion of the right coronary artery, ran into the left ventricular inferior wall, and drained into the left ventricular chamber under the mitral valve, with a final tract with an intramyocardial course (Figure 3). Because the coronary artery fistula did not determine a hemodynamic overload, it was not treated by angioplasty or surgery. At 24-month follow-up, the patient was asymptomatic.

3. Review of Literature and Discussion

Coronary fistulas are defined as an abnormal communication between a coronary artery and a cardiac chamber ("coronary-room fistula"), bypassing the capillary bed or any part of the systemic or pulmonary circulation. The first description was by Krause in 1865 and the first surgical treatment

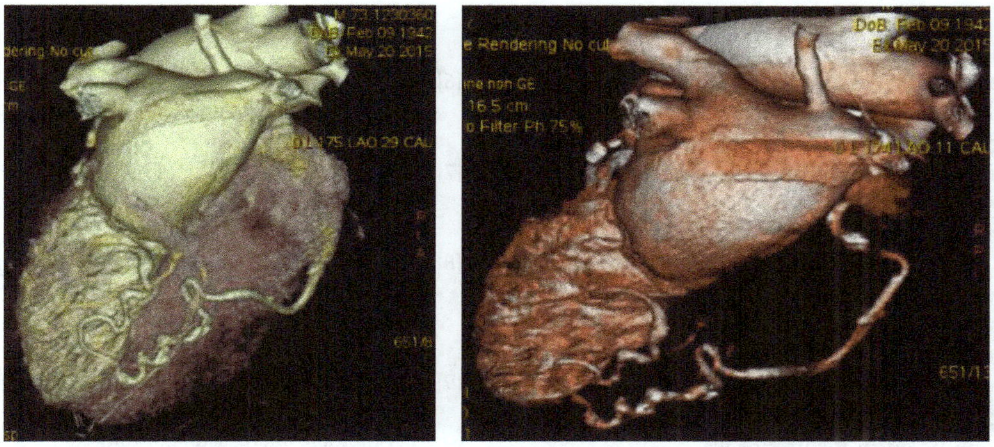

(a) (b)

FIGURE 3: Three-dimensional (3D) reconstruction of the right coronary artery and fistula using computed tomography angiography.

was reported by Bjork and Crafoord in 1947 [1]. Fistulas are rare anomalies. They are present in 0.002% of the general population, and they are found in 0.25% of patients undergoing coronary angiography [2]. In an autoptic series of 18950 autopsies, Alexander and Griffith found 54 coronary anomalies (0.3%) [3]. They are often asymptomatic, so their diagnosis is often incidental. Epidemiological data and their incidence may be underestimated in literature. Coronary fistulas may be congenital or acquired. Most of the fistulas are congenital, and their embryological origin appears to be due to the persistence of sinusoidal connections between the lumens of the primitive tubular heart. The acquired forms may be further divided into iatrogenic (during percutaneous coronary intervention, cardiac surgery, myocardial biopsy, and septal myectomy), traumatic, or related to a disease (such as myocardial infarction, Takayasu arteritis, and cardiomyopathies) [4, 5]. Several classifications have been proposed. The first one was by Ogden in 1970, placing coronary fistulas between major coronary anomalies [2]. In 1999, Angelini proposed a new classification of congenital coronary anomalies, identifying anomalies of origin and course, intrinsic coronary anomalies (myocardial bridging, aneurisms > 1.5 mm) and termination anomalies. According to this scheme, fistulas are anomalies of termination [4].

Fistulas are also classified, according to the scheme of Sakakibara et al., into two types: type A, which presents proximal vessel dilation from which originates the fistula, and type B, with the expansion of the entire vessel [6]. Most originates from the right coronary artery and the left anterior descending, less frequently from the circumflex artery. The origin of fistula is rarely bilateral, involving both right and left coronary arteries. In more than 90% of cases, fistulas drain to venous system (in order of frequency: right ventricle, right atrium, pulmonary artery, and coronary sinus), rarely in the left chambers [7] or in the pericardium [8]. Said described the fistulas according to the number of vessels (single channel or multiple channels) and their course (linear or serpentine). Single fistulas are much more frequent than multiple ones [9].

From the pathophysiological point of view, the main problem is shunt entity. It is determined by the size of the fistula and the pressure difference between the coronary artery and the chamber into which the fistula drains. The fistulas that drain into the right-sided chambers (low resistance system) may cause volume overload with hemodynamic impairment, while drainage into the left chambers (high resistance system) leads to a lower overload but may cause an arterial runoff with dilatation of native vessel. In general, small fistulas do not cause symptoms. Larger fistulas can lead to the "steal phenomenon," which is the reduction of myocardial blood flow distal to the site of the fistula, resulting in myocardial ischemia, more evident in combination with increased demand of oxygen, such as during exercise [10].

Natural history is variable: some close spontaneously, while others persist. It may happen that the coronary artery which originates fistula gradually dilated up to frank aneurysm, while the fistula may be complicated by ulceration of the intima, degeneration of the media, atherosclerotic plaques, calcification, mural thrombus, and rarely rupture [1]. The clinical manifestations increase with age. The most frequent symptoms are dyspnea on exertion, angina, fatigue, palpitations, and paroxysmal nocturnal dyspnea. The gold standard for the detection of coronary fistulas remains coronary angiography. Other imaging techniques such as MRI and CT may provide additional diagnostic elements thanks to 3D reconstructions. Transthoracic and transesophageal echocardiography is useful especially in the evaluation of the hemodynamic effects of the fistula on cardiac chambers [11].

The closure of the fistula is recommended when it is symptomatic, while the treatment in asymptomatic patients remains controversial. Large coronary fistulas should be closed by transcatheter or surgical treatment, regardless of symptoms, while small to moderate size fistulas should be treated only if they cause symptoms [12]. The surgical approach is ligation of epicardial fistula, less frequently intraluminal endarterectomy. Transcatheter closure may be performed with various types of devices (stents, umbrellas, balloons, coils, etc.) but requires favorable anatomy, i.e., not tortuous artery with single fistula and accessibility of the distal portion to closure device [12].

The peculiarity of our case, compared to others reported in the literature [13], is the echocardiographic diagnosis during an acute coronary syndrome. The suspicion of coronary fistula draining in the left ventricle was given by the finding of an abnormal color flow in the ventricular cavity and its route in the wall. Our deductions were then confirmed by coronary angiography and CT. As reported in the literature, fistulas draining into the left ventricle are extremely rare [7]. Echocardiography can give a suspicious diagnosis when there is a hemodynamic impairment, but in our case, it happened during a routine examination by the detection of an abnormal coronary flow in the myocardial wall. The patient's angina was not determined by the fistula but by the presence of atherosclerotic plaques on the left anterior descending and circumflex artery. In fact, the fistula drained into the left ventricle without making any hemodynamic impairment. Therefore, no indication was given for its closure.

4. Conclusions

Coronary artery fistulas are described as a direct connection between a coronary artery and one of the cardiac chambers, large vessels, or other vascular structures. They are usually congenital or acquired in rare cases. Most of them are asymptomatic; in fact, small fistulas do not cause any hemodynamic impairment. Some patients, typically with larger fistulas, present symptoms such as fatigue, dyspnea, angina, heart failure, pulmonary hypertension, or infective endocarditis. Often, signs of ventricular overload may be observed by echocardiography. Sometimes, an abnormal flow is observed in the drainage chamber. More rarely, the course in the ventricular wall may be followed with the echocardiogram. The peculiarity of this case is the echocardiographic description of a fistula draining into the left ventricle. In fact, the echocardiographic visualization of a fistula is a rare event. Our patient showed no signs of left ventricular overload, so the fistula was an occasional finding that occurred during ACS. Its closure was not indicated because it did not cause any hemodynamic overload or any symptom, so conservative treatment was preferred.

References

[1] Y. Ata, T. Turk, M. Bicer, M. Yalcin, F. Ata, and S. Yavuz, "Coronary arteriovenous fistulas in the adults: natural history and management strategies," *Journal of Cardiothoracic Surgery*, vol. 4, no. 1, p. 62, 2009.

[2] D. Challoumas, A. Pericleous, I. A. Dimitrakaki, C. Danelatos, and G. Dimitrakakis, "Coronary arteriovenous fistulae: a review," *International Journal of Angiology*, vol. 23, pp. 1–10, 2014.

[3] R. W. Alexander and G. C. Griffith, "Anomalies of the coronary arteries and their clinical significance," *Circulation*, vol. 14, no. 5, pp. 800–805, 1956.

[4] P. Angelini, "Coronary artery anomalies – current clinical issues. Definitions, classification, incidence, clinical relevance, and treatment guidelines," *Texas Heart Institute Journal*, vol. 29, no. 4, pp. 271–278, 2002.

[5] Y. Rozenman, A. Weiss, C. Lotan, and M. S. Gotsman, ""Congenital" coronary arteriovenous malformations: are they truly congenital?," *Catheterization and Cardiovascular Diagnosis*, vol. 37, no. 2, pp. 166-167, 1996.

[6] S. Sakakibara, M. Yokoyama, A. Takao, M. Nogi, and H. Gomi, "Coronary arteriovenous fistula: nine operated cases," *American Heart Journal*, vol. 72, no. 3, pp. 307–314, 1966.

[7] D. Sagar, A. Hernandez, and T. Heimowitz, "Coronary artery-left ventricle fistula: a case report of a rare connection error!," *Cureus*, vol. 7, no. 4, article e266, 2015.

[8] M. Nagiub, D. Mahadin, S. Gowda, and S. Aggarwal, "Prenatal diagnosis of coronary artery fistula: a case report and review of literature," *American Journal of Perinatology Reports*, vol. 4, no. 2, pp. e83–e86, 2014.

[9] S. A. M. Said and T. Van der Werf, "Dutch survey of congenital coronary artery fistulas in adults: coronary artery-left ventricular multiple micro-fistulas. Multi-center observational survey in the Netherlands," *International Journal of Cardiology*, vol. 110, no. 1, pp. 33–39, 2006.

[10] J. Koneru, A. Samuel, M. Joshi, A. Hamden, F. E. Shamoon, and M. Bikkina, "Coronary anomaly and coronary artery fistula as cause of angina pectoris with literature review," *Case Reports in Vascular Medicine*, vol. 2011, Article ID 486187, 5 pages, 2011.

[11] M. Kimura, J. Shiraishi, D. Ito et al., "Usefulness and limitation of transthoracic echocardiography in the diagnosis of large coronary artery fistula," *Echocardiography*, vol. 27, no. 10, pp. 1291–1295, 2010.

[12] D. Buccheri, P. R. Chirco, S. Geraci, G. Caramanno, and B. Cortese, "Coronary artery fistulae: anatomy, diagnosis and management strategies," *Heart, Lung and Circulation*, vol. 27, no. 8, pp. 940–951, 2018.

[13] S. Maragkoudakis, A. Patrianakos, E. Kallergis, F. Parthenakis, and P. Vardas, "Echocardiographic demonstration of coronary artery to left ventricle fistulas: case report and review of the literature," *Hellenic Journal of Cardiology*, vol. 55, pp. 171–173, 2014.

3

A Case of Transcatheter Aortic Valve Implantation in a Centenarian Patient

Salem Badr,[1] Daniel O. Johnsrud,[1] Charnai D. Sherry,[1] Suhail Q. Allaqaband,[1,2] Eric S. Weiss,[1] and Tanvir K. Bajwa[1,2]

[1]*Aurora Cardiovascular and Thoracic Services, Aurora Sinai/Aurora St. Luke's Medical Centers, 2801 W. Kinnickinnic River Parkway, Ste. 880, Milwaukee, WI 53215, USA*
[2]*University of Wisconsin School of Medicine and Public Health, 750 Highland Ave., Madison, WI 53726, USA*

Correspondence should be addressed to Tanvir K. Bajwa; publishing2@aurora.org

Academic Editor: Assad Movahed

Calcified aortic stenosis has become the most common form of acquired valvular heart disease in very old patients. Despite this fact, a majority of these patients were turned down by surgery owing to a risk of mortality > 10% in patients older than 90 years. In recent years, transcatheter aortic valve implantation (TAVI) has emerged as a therapeutic option for severe aortic stenosis. However, there is a paucity of data regarding the outcomes of TAVI in patients older than 100 years. We present the oldest patient who has undergone successful TAVI reported in the current literature.

1. Introduction

As the population continues to age, calcified aortic stenosis has become the most common form of acquired valvular heart disease in older adults [1]. Although centenarians are still rare in the world population, the United Nations World Population Prospects 2019 report projects that the number of centenarians will increase from 573,000 in 2020 to more than 19 million in 2100 [2]. Both the prevalence and severity of aortic stenosis increase with extreme age, so it is anticipated that the number of centenarians presenting with severe symptomatic aortic stenosis will increase. Without aortic valve replacement, severe symptomatic aortic stenosis drastically reduces quality of life and increases mortality risks. Surgical aortic valve replacement is associated with 10% perioperative mortality in patients who are more than 90 years old [3]. In recent years, transcatheter aortic valve implantation (TAVI) has emerged as a therapeutic option for severe symptomatic aortic stenosis in patients at high surgical risk [4]. Data regarding the effectiveness of TAVI in centenarians are scarce. Here, we present the case of the oldest patient to successfully undergo TAVI reported in the literature.

2. Case Presentation

A 103-year-and-9-month-old female patient with a past medical history significant for moderate aortic stenosis since five years prior, hypertension, chronic kidney disease, and hyperlipidemia presented to an outside hospital with 2 weeks of progressive shortness of breath, lower-leg swelling, and hematuria that had started the day before the admission. The patient was independent at baseline and lived by herself. Her blood pressure was 161/72 mmHg, her heart rate was 59 beats per minute, and her respiration rate was 15 breaths per minute. Auscultation of the heart revealed the classic murmur of aortic valve stenosis: a loud, late-peaking ejection murmur with single S2 radiating to the carotid arteries. Lung auscultation revealed diminished air entry and bibasilar rales. She had bilateral lower-extremity edema that was 1+ and nonpitting. The electrocardiogram revealed sinus rhythm with second-degree Mobitz type 1 heart block and the right bundle branch block that had been noted beginning five years prior (Figure 1(a)). A transthoracic echocardiogram revealed severe calcified aortic valve stenosis with an area of $0.78\,cm^2$ (normal is $3\text{-}4\,cm^2$) and a mean transvalvular gradient of 48 mmHg.

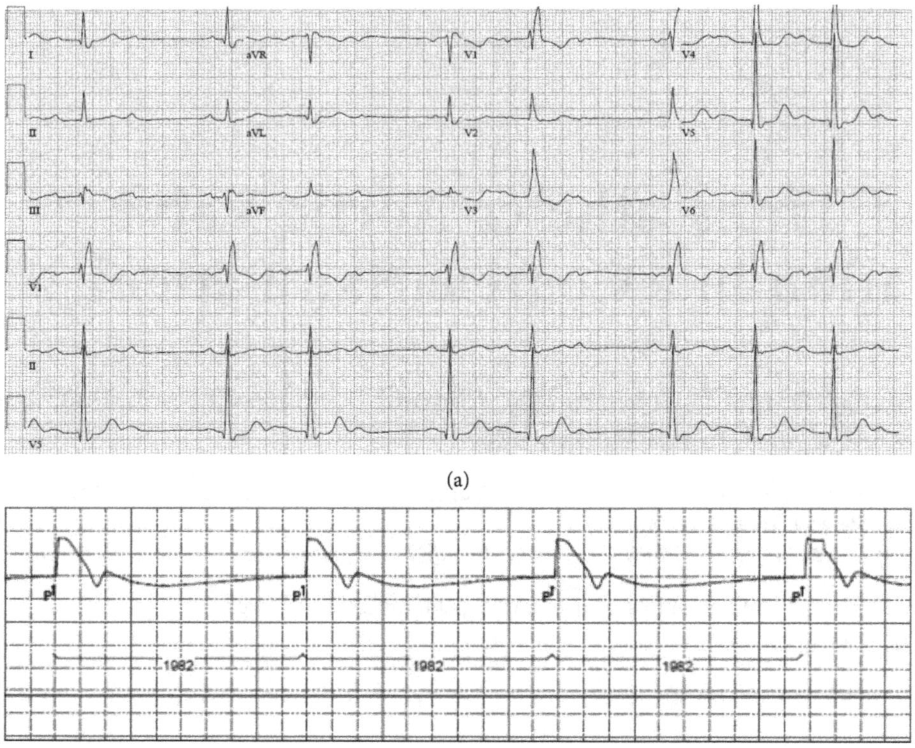

(a)

(b)

Figure 1: (a) An electrocardiogram performed before transcatheter aortic valve implantation (TAVI) shows sinus rhythm with second-degree AV block (Mobitz type 1), right bundle branch block, and left ventricular hypertrophy with repolarization abnormalities. (b) Post TAVI, a pacemaker check showed sinus rhythm with complete heart block.

Mild-to-moderate aortic valve regurgitation (Figure 2) also was seen.

2.1. Preoperative Evaluation for TAVI. Subsequently, the patient was transferred to our tertiary care center and evaluated by the heart team. Her preoperative risk assessment for 30-day mortality was intermediate, with a Society of Thoracic Surgeons score of 5.7%. Her frailty score was 4, which means vulnerable (although not reliant on others for daily help, symptoms often limit activities). Multiple tests were performed to assess the feasibility of the TAVI procedure; these included a coronary angiogram that showed diffuse calcification of the coronary arteries without significant stenosis and computed tomographic angiograms of the thorax, abdomen, and pelvis that demonstrated a trileaflet aortic valve with severe valvular calcification (aortic valve calcium score of 1,859 Agatston units) and mild left ventricle outflow calcification. Computed tomography measurements were annulus perimeter, 68 mm; sinus of Valsalva, 27.9 × 29.1 mm; right coronary artery height, 11.8 mm; and left coronary artery height, 12.1 mm. Patent ilio-femoral arteries suitable for a transfemoral TAVI approach were noted. Based on high surgical risk scores, age, frailty, and patient comorbidities, the heart team decided to proceed with TAVI using a transfemoral approach.

2.2. Performance of TAVI. Under monitored anesthesia care, the right internal jugular vein and the right femoral artery were each accessed with 6-French sheaths. A temporary pacemaker was placed in the right ventricle through a 6-French sheath in the right internal jugular vein. Two Perclose ProGlide (Abbott Vascular Devices, Santa Clara, CA, USA) suture-mediated devices were employed using the preclosure technique while exchanging the 6-French sheath with a 14-French sheath in the right femoral artery. A 20-mm Z-MED II balloon (Braun International Systems, Melsungen, Germany) was used for predilation of the aortic valve. Subsequently, a self-expanding TAVI 26-mm Evolut PRO+ (Medtronic, Minneapolis, MN, USA) was deployed during rapid pacing at a depth of 3 mm in the aortic valve (Figure 3). This led to a marked improvement of the transvalvular gradient with only mild paravalvular aortic regurgitation. Successful hemostasis was achieved in the right femoral artery using the preclosure technique. There were no intraoperative complications.

2.3. Postoperative Course. A 2D echocardiogram performed on the first postoperative day showed that the prosthetic aortic valve was well seated, with a mean transvalvular gradient of 4 mmHg and trace paravalvular regurgitation. No transvalvular regurgitation was seen. A temporary pacemaker check revealed ventricular paced rhythm (99.4%) with underlying sinus rhythm and complete heart block (Figure 1(b)). Subsequently, the patient underwent dual-chamber pacemaker implantation, which she tolerated well without complication. Urology was consulted for intermittent hematuria and recommended observation while she was in the hospital. She was discharged home four days after the TAVI procedure. The patient was seen in the clinic for a 6-month follow-up; she

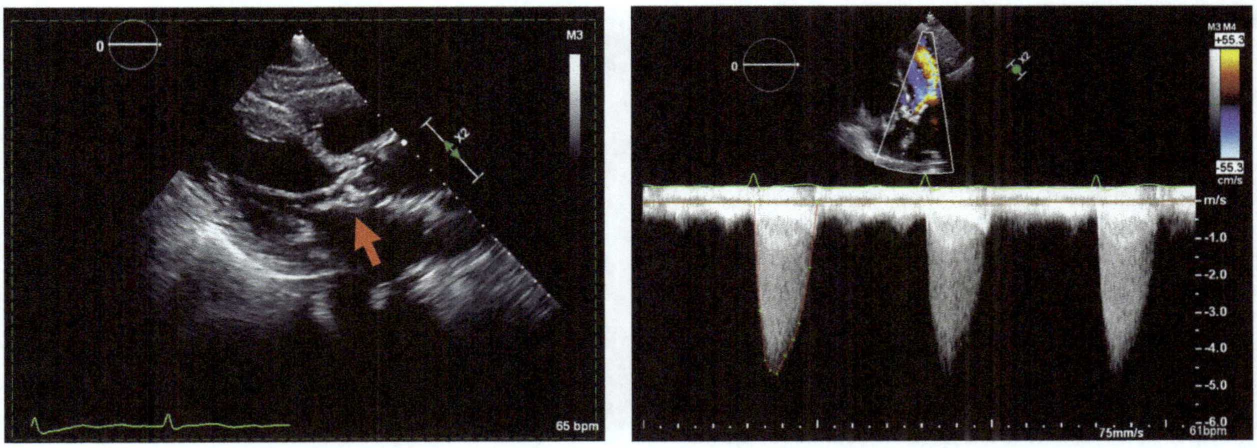

(a) (b)

FIGURE 2: (a) The parasternal long-axis view on transthoracic echocardiography shows bulky calcification of the aortic valve (arrow). (b) The apical five-chamber view on transthoracic continuous-wave Doppler analysis shows a mean gradient of 48 mmHg.

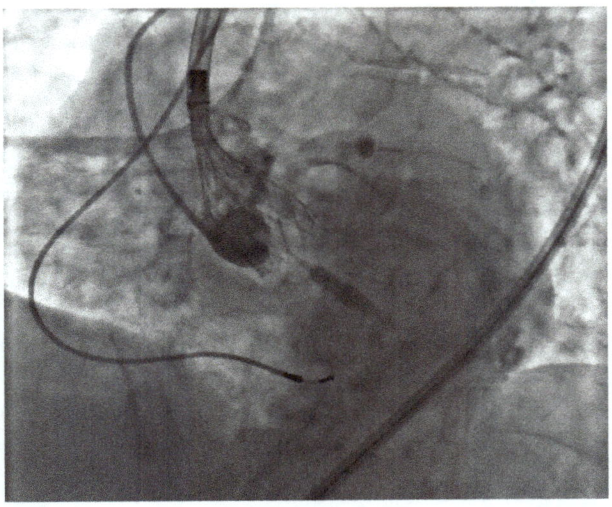

FIGURE 3: This periprocedural fluoroscopic image shows deployment of a self-expanding TAVI Evolut PRO+ (Medtronic, Minneapolis, MN, USA) device at a depth of 3 mm in the aortic valve during rapid pacing.

had turned 104 years old and was still doing well. Repeat echocardiography revealed a well-seated and expanded valve with a mean gradient across of 6 mmHg and trace paravalvular regurgitation.

3. Discussion

Although centenarians are still rare, the number of centenarians worldwide has grown rapidly over the past 30 years and is projected to increase sixfold by 2050 [2]. Therefore, physicians are expected to encounter more centenarians with severe symptomatic aortic stenosis. TAVI is an attractive treatment modality for centenarians who are not a candidate for surgery due to advanced age and comorbidities [4]. Furthermore, centenarians can paradoxically have greater resilience and fewer comorbidities than younger patients. They can tolerate the TAVI procedure quite well, with low in-hospital and 1-year adverse event rates; however, we acknowledge that this group of patients is underrepresented in the literature and evidence stems only from scarce data that include observational data and one case report [5]. Arsalan et al. reported outcomes for an exceedingly small cohort of centenarians undergoing TAVI. Overall, 24 centenarians who were treated were included in the Society of Thoracic Surgeons/American College of Cardiology Transcatheter Valve Therapy Registry; in this cohort, there was no mortality at 30 days, and an incredibly low 1-year mortality (6.7%) considering the 1-year death probability of centenarians is more than 30% [6]. From the current literature, the oldest patient known to have had TAVI was a 102-year-old woman. In this patient, a 23-mm Edwards Sapien XT valve (Edwards Lifesciences, Irvine, CA, USA) was successfully deployed under general anesthesia using a transfemoral approach. Post TAVI, aortic valve area improved from 0.5 cm^2 to 1.7 cm^2, and the patient was discharged about 2 weeks later without any complications. Four years later, a transthoracic echocardiogram revealed the bioprosthetic valve was functioning well, and she was able to perform her daily living activities without support [7].

4. Conclusions

We present the oldest patient, to the best of our knowledge, who has undergone successful TAVI. A transfemoral approach was employed under monitored anesthesia care. We believe that in the current TAVI era, age alone should not be a factor in refusing access to this advanced technology. Ultimately, the process of shared decision-making is paramount to ensuring that the course of action is patient-centered and balances the expected risks and benefits of the procedure with the centenarian's preference and values.

References

[1] B. Iung and A. Vahanian, "Epidemiology of acquired valvular heart disease," *The Canadian Journal of Cardiology*, vol. 30, no. 9, pp. 962–970, 2014.

[2] United Nations and Department of Economic and Social Affairs, Population Division, "World Population Prospects 2019, custom data acquired via website," July 2021, https://population.un.org/wpp/DataQuery/.

[3] M. C. Mack, M. Szerlip, M. A. Herbert et al., "Outcomes of treatment of nonagenarians with severe aortic stenosis," *The Annals of Thoracic Surgery*, vol. 100, no. 1, pp. 74–80, 2015.

[4] M. B. Leon, C. R. Smith, M. Mack et al., "Transcatheter aortic-valve implantation for aortic stenosis in patients who cannot undergo surgery," *The New England Journal of Medicine*, vol. 363, no. 17, pp. 1597–1607, 2010.

[5] C. Galatas and J. Afilalo, "Transcatheter aortic valve replacement over age 90: risks vs benefits," *Clinical Cardiology*, vol. 43, no. 2, pp. 156–162, 2020.

[6] M. Arsalan, M. Szerlip, S. Vemulapalli et al., "Should transcatheter aortic valve replacement be performed in nonagenarians?: insights from the STS/ACC TVT Registry," *Journal of the American College of Cardiology*, vol. 67, no. 12, pp. 1387–1395, 2016.

[7] A. N. Aslan, H. Ayhan, E. Özdemir, and E. Bozkurt, "A centenarian transcatheter aortic valve implantation case," *Journal of Geriatric Cardiology*, vol. 13, pp. 869–871, 2016.

4

Anomalous Left Coronary Artery Connected to the Pulmonary Artery in a 15-Year-Old Girl: Case Report and Discussion on Secondary Prevention of Sudden Death

Jérémy Laïk,[1] Virginie Fouilloux,[2] Philippe Aldebert,[3] Linda Koutbi,[3] Jérôme Hourdain,[3] Philippe De Swardt,[4] Fabrice Tiger,[4] Anne Bellemain-Appaix,[1] François Bernasconi,[1] and Laurent Jacq[1]

[1]*Department of Cardiology, Antibes Juan-les-Pins Hospital, France*
[2]*Department of Cardiac Surgery, La Timone Children Hospital, France*
[3]*Department of Cardiology, La Timone Children Hospital, France*
[4]*Department of Reanimation, Antibes Juan-les-Pins Hospital, France*

Correspondence should be addressed to Jérémy Laïk; jeremy.laik@hotmail.fr

Academic Editor: Ertugurul Ercan

Background. Anomalous left coronary artery connected to the pulmonary artery (ALCAPA) is a rare congenital heart disease. Adaptive development of sufficient heterocoronary collaterality in the newborn may allow survival to a later age. In older children or adults, malignant ventricular arrhythmias can reveal the disease. *Case Report.* A 15-year-old girl was referred to the local hospital after a resuscitated out-of-hospital cardiac arrest. CT scan and coronary angiography revealed an ALCAPA. Direct aortic reimplantation of the left coronary artery was performed. Postoperative ECG monitoring showed short episodes of nonsustained ventricular tachycardia. Transthoracic echocardiography and cardiac MRI revealed subendocardial fibrosis of the anterolateral papillary muscle. Beta-blockade therapy was initiated at first intention. After hospital discharge, the patient reported several fainting without loss of consciousness. Considering sudden death nonrelated to effort, episodes of nonsustained ventricular tachycardia, and areas of myocardial fibrosis, the patient underwent subcutaneous cardioverter-defibrillator implantation. 6-month follow-up is satisfactory without clinical or rhythmic abnormalities. *Discussion.* Indication for surgical correction of ALCAPA is well defined, but rhythmic secondary prevention after resuscitated cardiac arrest is less consensual. Cardiac MRI is an essential tool in the identification of a potential rhythmic substrate and should be taken into account in the discussion of a preventive cardioverter-defibrillator implantation.

1. Introduction

Anomalous left coronary artery connected to the pulmonary artery (ALCAPA) syndrome is a rare congenital coronary anomaly with an incidence of 1 in 300000 live births [1] and accounts for approximately 0.25–0.5% of all congenital heart diseases [2]. The high pulmonary vascular resistance at birth explains the conserved antegrade perfusion in the abnormally connected left coronary artery and therefore the absence of early neonatal symptoms. As pulmonary vascular resistance declines, the left coronary blood flow becomes retrograde and may result in myocardial infarction with heart failure. Without surgery, prognosis is appalling with a mortality rate of 90% within the first year of life [3]. More rarely, adaptive development of sufficient collaterality from the right coronary artery may allow survival to a later age and sometimes to adulthood. Clinical manifestations may then include subclinical ischemia or sudden death due to ventricular arrhythmias.

2. Case Presentation

A 15-year-old girl was referred to the local hospital following an out-of-hospital cardiac arrest. She was sitting by a

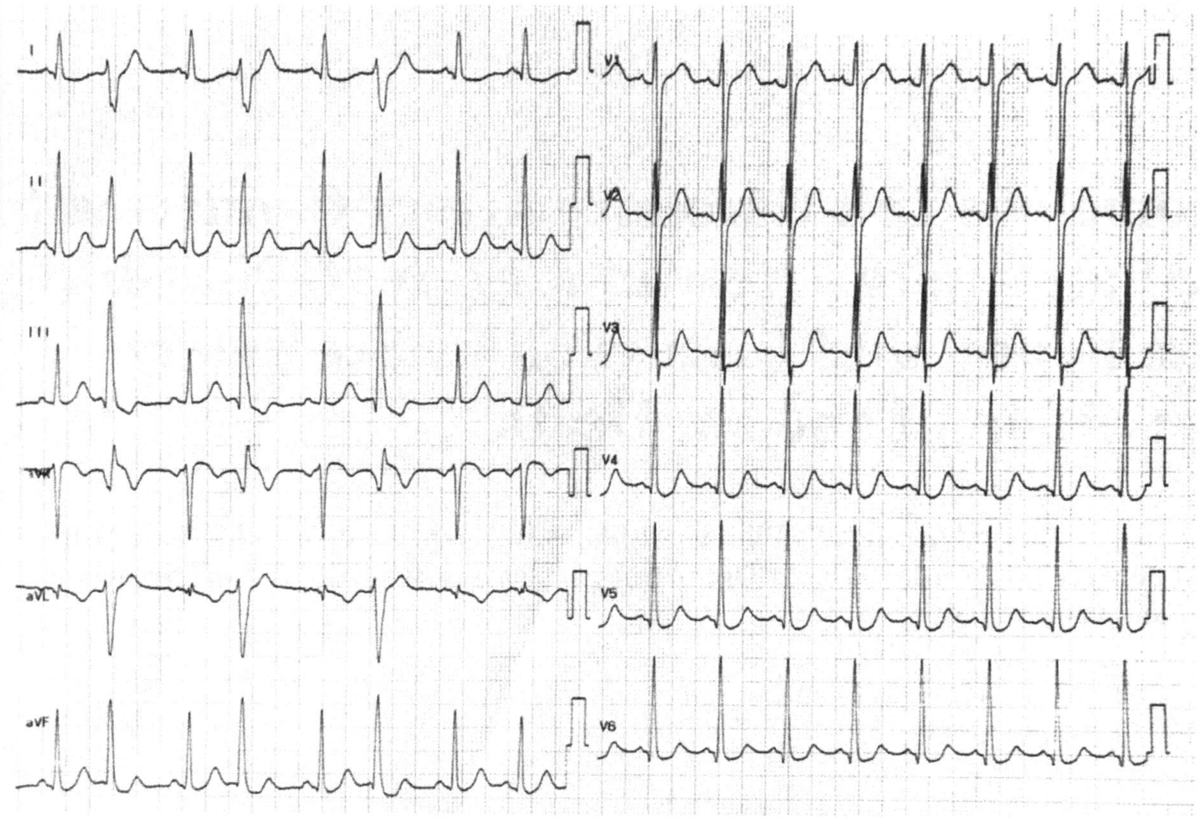

FIGURE 1: Post-resuscitation electrocardiogram.

swimming pool when she passed out. Resuscitation maneuvers were initiated immediately, and two external electric shocks were delivered by the semiautomatic defibrillator on ventricular fibrillation. She had no history of heart disease, but her parents had noticed exertional dyspnea.

In the intensive care unit, hemodynamics was stable without inotropic support. High-sensitivity troponin T was 240 ng/L (reference value < 14 ng/L) with no evidence for acute myocardial ischemia. 12-lead electrocardiogram (ECG) showed apicolateral ST depression with negative T-waves and ventricular bigeminy (Figure 1). Transthoracic echocardiography revealed an undilated left ventricle with moderately impaired systolic function and mild mitral regurgitation. The left coronary artery was not seen at the left aortic sinus. Increased echodensity of the anterolateral papillary muscle and the chordae tendineae was noticed. Chest CT scan showed the presence of an ALCAPA with a compensatory dilated right coronary artery (RCA) (Figure 2). Coronary angiography demonstrated the left-to-right shunt, from the normally implanted RCA towards the left coronary artery and into the pulmonary trunk, through an important network of collaterals (Figure 3). The patient was transferred to the referral center for urgent corrective surgery.

Direct aortic reimplantation of the left coronary artery to the aorta was successfully performed. 24 h electrocardiographic monitoring revealed episodes of nonsustained ventricular tachycardia. Postoperative cardiac MRI showed an undilated left ventricle (end-diastolic left ventricular volume 82 mL/m^2) with preserved systolic function (ejection fraction 63%). Morphological analysis and phase-sensitive inversion recovery sequences found hypertrophy of the anterolateral papillary muscle with late gadolinium enhancement, suggesting areas of subendocardial cicatricial fibrosis (Figure 4). The patient was discharged home twenty days after surgery on bisoprolol 2.5 mg once daily.

One month after hospital discharge, the patient reported several fainting without loss of consciousness. Control coronary angiography revealed a satisfactory operative result with no anastomotic stenosis of the left coronary artery. Given the sudden death at rest, episodes of nonsustained ventricular tachycardia, presence of myocardial fibrosis, and persistent fainting, the patient underwent subcutaneous cardioverter-defibrillator (S-ICD) implantation. Six-month follow-up is satisfactory without clinical or rhythmic abnormalities.

3. Discussion

Surgical correction of ALCAPA is the rule and is one of the main emergencies in congenital heart surgery. Different technical approaches have been suggested. Currently, restoration of 2-coronary circulation is considered the gold standard, via direct aortic reimplantation of the left coronary with its pulmonary artery button [3, 4]. Most recent surgical series demonstrated a good postoperative course with low early mortality and a 20-year survival of almost 98% [5]. If the anatomical anomaly has been correctly corrected, long-

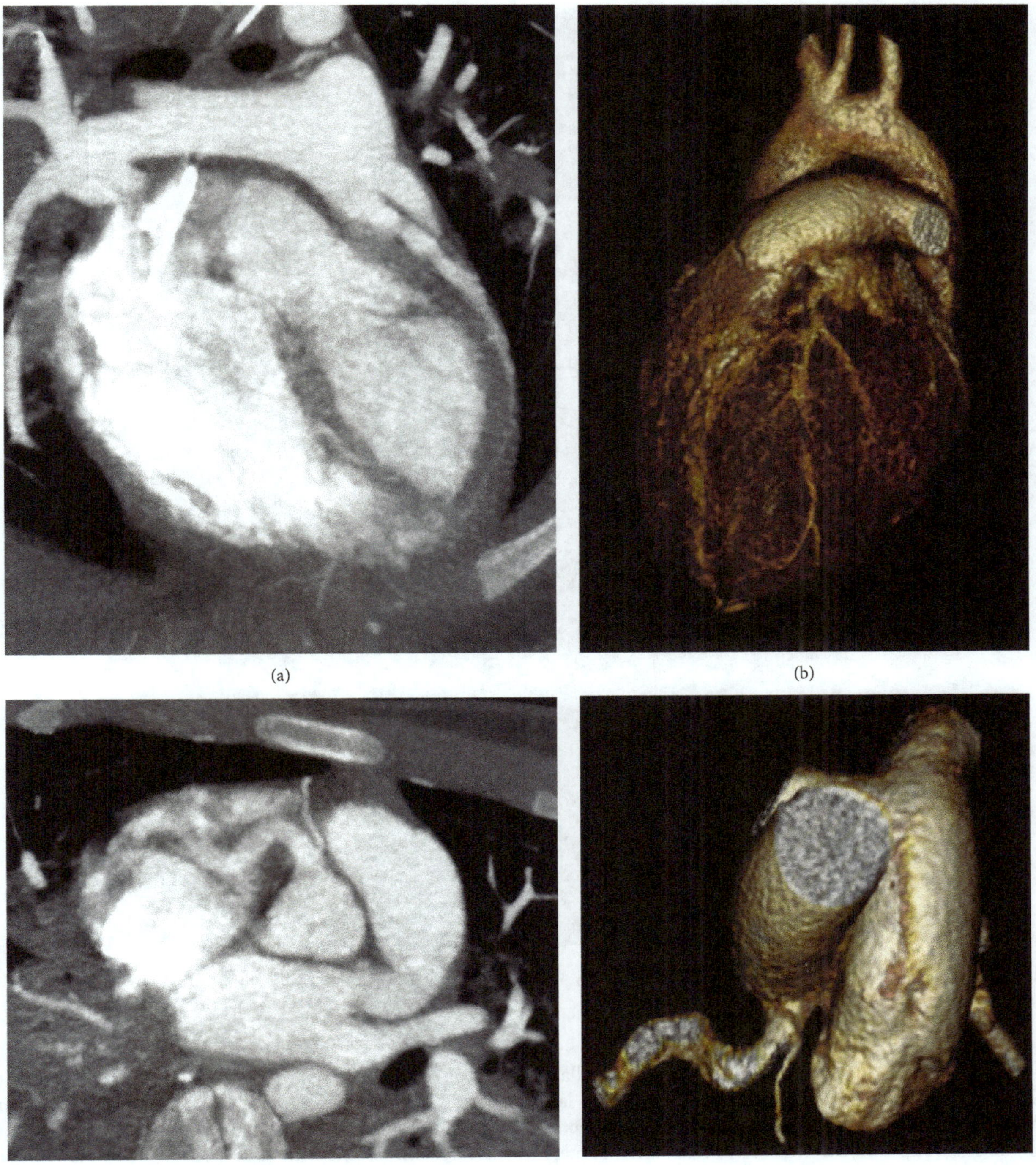

(a) (b) (c) (d)

FIGURE 2: Computed tomography. Three-dimensional multiplanar and volume rendering reconstructions. (a, b) Left coronary artery connected to the pulmonary trunk; (c, d) right coronary artery (and its marginal branch) connected to the aorta.

term ischemia may be responsible for persistent myocardial reshuffle that could be arrhythmogenic. If so, this substrate deserves to be identified and taken into account in the secondary prevention approach, especially if the clinical presentation was a cardiorespiratory arrest.

Shivalkar et al. showed on intraoperative samples that the chronically hypoperfused myocardium is remodeled but theoretically viable, with a postoperative recovery potential [6]. However, histological analysis shows up to 50% cellular fibrosis and there are no published studies after surgery, which raises the question of true reversibility. Current cardiac imaging modalities allow routine noninvasive assessment of myocardial fibrosis. Transthoracic echocardiography is the first-line examination and guides the diagnosis by showing an increased echodensity of the endocardium [7]. Localization is variable and can involve the papillary muscles that may appear hypertrophied [8, 9]. Cardiac MRI is the reference test and looks for late gadolinium

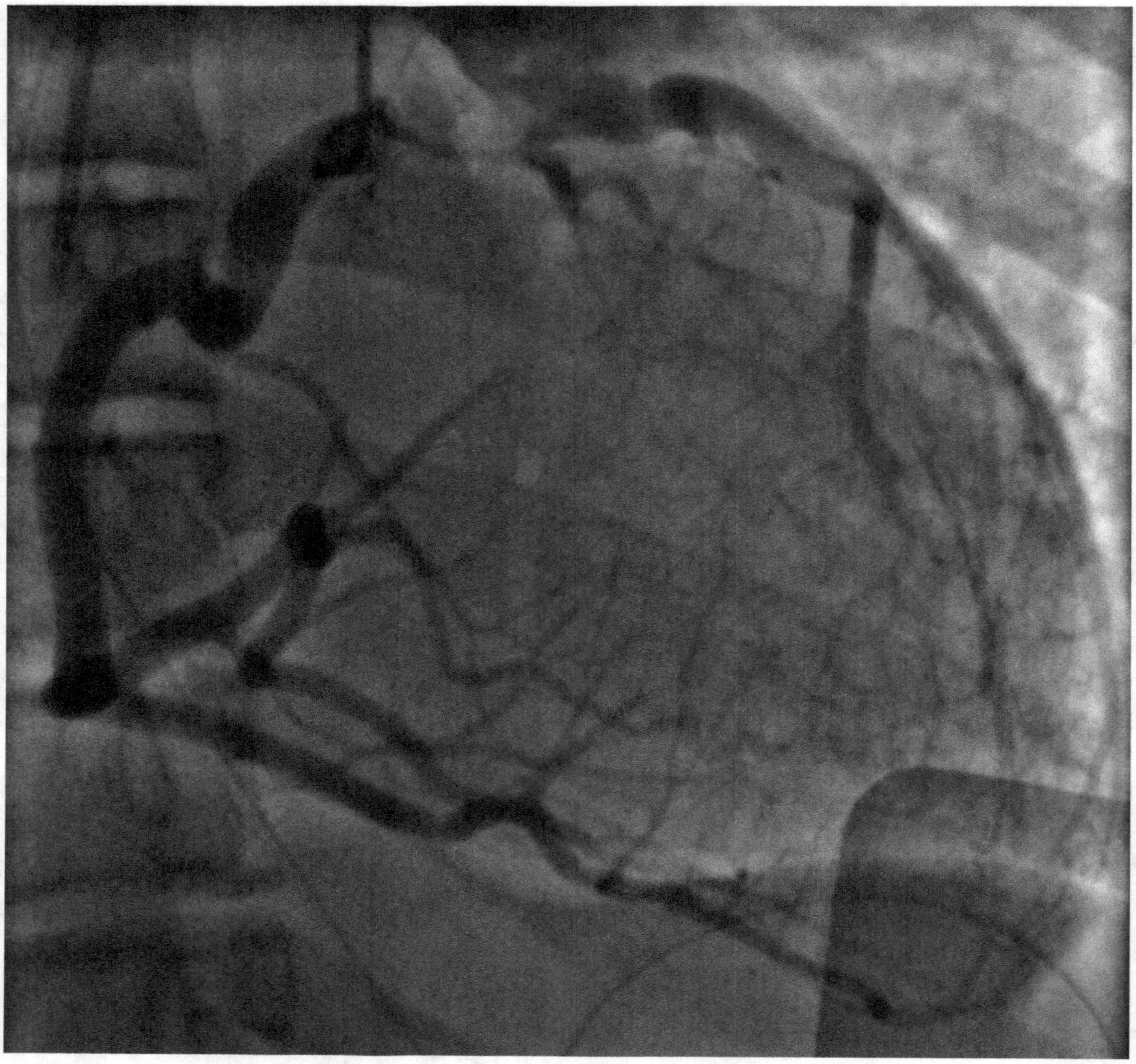

Figure 3: Coronary angiogram. Dilated right coronary artery with left-to-right shunt towards the left coronary artery connected to the pulmonary trunk; note the important collateral network.

enhancement that may also involve the mitral papillary muscle [10, 11]. Browne et al. showed that areas of late enhancement in ALCAPA correspond to areas of microscopic fibrosis [12]. 10-year MRI follow-up after surgery shows that between 65% and 71% of patients keep an abnormal enhancement which, even if generally not very extensive, suggests incomplete myocardial recovery [13, 14].

The long-term clinical significance of these enhancement zones in ALCAPA is not clearly defined, but it is reasonable to believe that they are a potential arrhythmogenic substrate. Indeed, the presence of a myocardial scar is known to serve as a substrate for malignant ventricular arrhythmias. From an electrophysiological point of view, fibrosis promotes the formation of reentry circuits at risk of degenerating into ventricular fibrillation but also creates electrical heterogeneity and automaticity changes that induce fatal arrhythmias [15, 16]. In ALCAPA, ventricular arrhythmias can be secondary to acute local ischemia induced by the coronary steal, but also to a reentry circuit around an infarcted area or to electrical instability due to endocardial fibrosis [17]. In our patient, the occurrence of sudden death at rest argued for a scar-related mechanism and was an additional argument for a preventive implantable cardioverter-defibrillator (ICD).

To date, indication of an ICD for secondary prevention of sudden death in ALCAPA is not consensual. Not all reported cases of cardiac arrest secondary to ALCAPA have been implanted [18]. Nevertheless, implantations have often been motivated by MRI identification of myocardial fibrosis [19–22]. In addition to an identified myocardial scar, the decision-making process should look for other risk factors for sudden death such as severe left ventricular systolic dysfunction, episodes of nonsustained ventricular tachycardia in Holter-ECG or on exertion, or a inducible ventricular arrhythmia at programmed ventricular stimulation if this was performed [23]. Indication for implantation must be

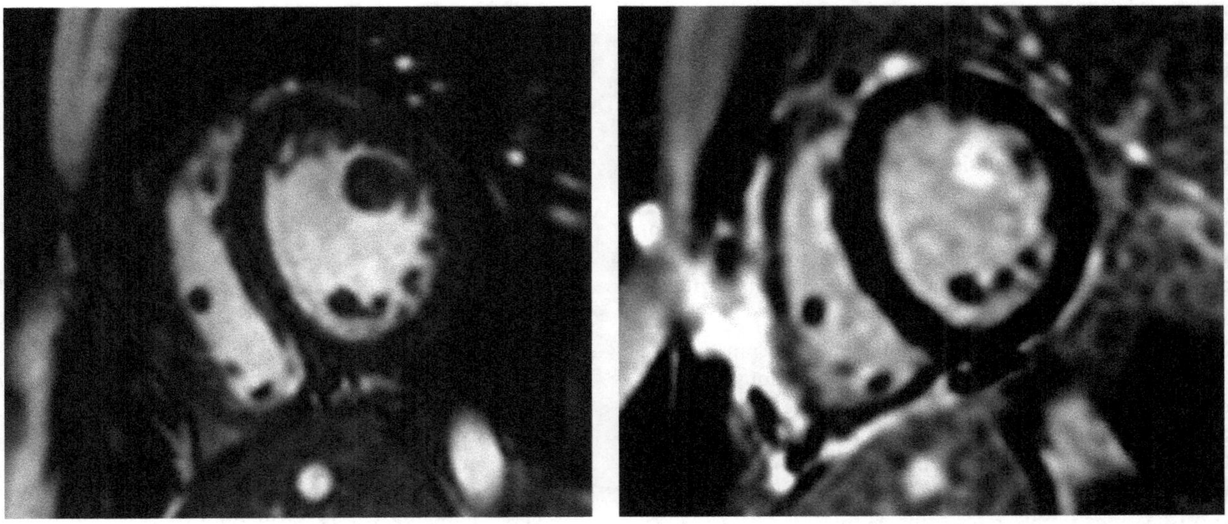

(a) (b)

Figure 4: Cardiac MRI—short-axis views. (a) Cine acquisition: note the hypertrophy of the anterolateral papillary muscle; (b) phase-sensitive inversion recovery (PSIR) sequence: late gadolinium enhancement (LGE) of the anterolateral papillary muscle.

balanced against the absence of reported appropriated shocks on implanted ICDs, the necessary risk of complications after ICD implantation in young people regardless of the approach, and the absence of established causality between fibrosis in ALCAPA and long-term rhythmic risk.

Subcutaneous ICD provides an attractive approach in the prevention of sudden death in young patients with congenital heart disease. This technology avoids the frequent lead-related complications of the epicardial or endocavitary material [24, 25]. The infection rate is comparable to endocavitary system but remains low and at lower risk of causing extraction surgery [26]. Inappropriate shocks represent the main complication and are often related to T-wave oversensing [25, 26]. The pre-implantation process must therefore ensure that the patient does not require pacing, and that ventricular sensing is performed correctly in one of the device vectors. Due to the absence of antitachycardia pacing for termination of ventricular tachycardia, management may include antiarrhythmic therapy and possible ablation procedures to treat organized arrhythmias. Recent studies suggest efficacy and complications comparable to the transvenous device in congenital heart disease [26]. Long-term data will confirm whether this approach remains safe and reliable in this very specific population.

4. Conclusion

The management of ALCAPA is first and foremost surgical but must also consider the electrophysiological consequences and the potential arrhythmogenic substrate. MRI identification of scar fibrosis is an important element to take into account in the decision-making process for secondary prevention. The S-ICD is an interesting approach in young subjects with congenital heart disease, but preliminary screening has to be rigorous. Scarcity of the pathology makes hardly imaginable comparative studies of prevention strategies, so the successive description of cases may help to enhance the literature on this subject. In the meantime, the discussion of secondary prevention should be taken on a case-by-case basis within a tertiary congenital cardiology center.

Abbreviations

ALCAPA: Anomalous left coronary artery connected to the pulmonary artery
ECG: Electrocardiogram
RCA: Right coronary artery
MRI: Magnetic resonance imaging
S-ICD: Subcutaneous implantable cardioverter-defibrillator.

References

[1] J. D. Keith, "The anomalous origin of the left coronary artery from the pulmonary artery," *British Heart Journal*, vol. 21, no. 2, pp. 149–161, 1959.

[2] J. Pfannschmidt, H. Ruskowski, and E. R. de Vivie, "Das Bland-White-Garland-Syndrom (BWGS)," *Klinische Pädiatrie*, vol. 204, no. 5, pp. 328–334, 1992.

[3] W. H. Neches, R. A. Mathews, S. C. Park et al., "Anomalous origin of the left coronary artery from the pulmonary artery. A new method of surgical repair," *Circulation*, vol. 50, no. 3, pp. 582–587, 1974.

[4] P. R. Vouhé, F. Baillot-Vernant, F. Trinquet et al., "Anomalous left coronary artery from the pulmonary artery in infants: which operation? When?," *The Journal of Thoracic and Cardiovascular Surgery*, vol. 94, no. 2, pp. 192–199, 1987.

[5] P. S. Naimo, T. A. Fricke, Y. d'Udekem et al., "Surgical intervention for anomalous origin of left coronary artery from the pulmonary artery in children: a long-term follow-up," *The Annals of Thoracic Surgery*, vol. 101, no. 5, pp. 1842–1848, 2016.

[6] B. Shivalkar, M. Borgers, W. Daenen, M. Gewillig, and W. Flameng, "ALCAPA syndrome: an example of chronic myocardial hypoperfusion?," *Journal of the American College of Cardiology*, vol. 23, no. 3, pp. 772–778, 1994.

[7] T. W. Riggs, T. E. Berry, and M. H. Paul, "Two-dimensional echocardiographic recognition of papillary muscle fibrosis in pediatric patients," *Chest*, vol. 83, no. 1, pp. 98–101, 1983.

[8] Y.-L. Yang, N. C. Nanda, X.-F. Wang et al., "Echocardiographic diagnosis of anomalous origin of the left coronary artery from the pulmonary artery," *Echocardiography*, vol. 24, no. 4, pp. 405–411, 2007.

[9] M. Li, Y. Wang, W. Zhu, C. Zhang, and H. Fei, "Transthoracic echocardiography features of adult-type anomalous left coronary artery from the pulmonary artery before and after surgery: highlights from observational study in a single center of China," *The International Journal of Cardiovascular Imaging*, vol. 36, no. 8, pp. 1477–1487, 2020.

[10] N. Mewton, C. Y. Liu, P. Croisille, D. Bluemke, and J. A. C. Lima, "Assessment of myocardial fibrosis with cardiovascular magnetic resonance," *Journal of the American College of Cardiology*, vol. 57, no. 8, pp. 891–903, 2011.

[11] A. Secinaro, H. Ntsinjana, O. Tann et al., "Cardiovascular magnetic resonance findings in repaired anomalous left coronary artery to pulmonary artery connection (ALCAPA)," *Journal of Cardiovascular Magnetic Resonance*, vol. 13, no. 1, p. 27, 2011.

[12] L. P. Browne, D. Kearney, M. D. Taylor et al., "ALCAPA: the role of myocardial viability studies in determining prognosis," *Pediatric Radiology*, vol. 40, no. 2, pp. 163–167, 2010.

[13] S. Fratz, A. Hager, C. Schreiber, M. Schwaiger, J. Hess, and H. C. Stern, "Long-term myocardial scarring after operation for anomalous left coronary artery from the pulmonary artery," *The Annals of Thoracic Surgery*, vol. 92, no. 5, pp. 1761–1765, 2011.

[14] B. Schmitt, S. Bauer, S. Kutty et al., "Myocardial perfusion, scarring, and function in anomalous left coronary artery from the pulmonary artery syndrome: a long-term analysis using magnetic resonance imaging," *The Annals of Thoracic Surgery*, vol. 98, no. 4, pp. 1425–1436, 2014.

[15] J. M. de Bakker, F. J. van Capelle, M. J. Janse et al., "Slow conduction in the infarcted human heart. 'Zigzag' course of activation," *Circulation*, vol. 88, no. 3, pp. 915–926, 1993.

[16] T. P. Nguyen, Z. Qu, and J. N. Weiss, "Cardiac fibrosis and arrhythmogenesis: the road to repair is paved with perils," *Journal of Molecular and Cellular Cardiology*, vol. 70, pp. 83–91, 2014.

[17] U. Kreutzer, J. Krülls-Münch, M. Angres, and A. Schiessler, "Successful resuscitation of a patient with ventricular fibrillation in Bland-White-Garland syndrome in adulthood. A case report," *Zeitschrift für Kardiologie*, vol. 87, no. 7, pp. 560–565, 1998.

[18] O. Alsara, J. K. Kalavakunta, V. Hajjar, A. Alsarah, N. Cho, and G. Dhar, "Surviving sudden cardiac death secondary to anomalous left coronary artery from the pulmonary artery: a case report and literature review," *Heart & Lung*, vol. 43, no. 5, pp. 476–480, 2014.

[19] J. X. Quah, L. Hofmeyr, H. Haqqani et al., "The management of the older adult patient with anomalous left coronary artery from the pulmonary artery syndrome: a presentation of two cases and review of the literature," *Congenital Heart Disease*, vol. 9, no. 6, pp. E185–E194, 2014.

[20] P. Dilaveris, I. Koutagiar, N. Alexopoulos, D. Tsiachris, and K. Gatzoulis, "Secondary prevention of sudden cardiac death in a 65 year untreated ALCAPA patient," *International Journal of Cardiology*, vol. 176, no. 2, pp. e73–e74, 2014.

[21] H. Kubota, H. Endo, H. Ishii et al., "Adult ALCAPA: from histological picture to clinical features," *Journal of Cardiothoracic Surgery*, vol. 15, no. 1, p. 14, 2020.

[22] M. V. Regeer, O. Bondarenko, K. Zeppenfeld, and A. D. Egorova, "Anomalous left coronary artery from the pulmonary artery: a rare cause of an out-of-hospital cardiac arrest in an adult-a case report," *European Heart Journal-Case Reports*, vol. 4, no. 3, pp. 1–5, 2020.

[23] P. Parizek, L. Haman, J. Harrer et al., "Bland-White-Garland syndrome in adults: sudden cardiac death as a first symptom and long-term follow-up after successful resuscitation and surgery," *Europace*, vol. 12, no. 9, pp. 1338–1340, 2010.

[24] P. Bordachar, C. Marquié, T. Pospiech et al., "Subcutaneous implantable cardioverter defibrillators in children, young adults and patients with congenital heart disease," *International Journal of Cardiology*, vol. 203, pp. 251–258, 2016.

[25] N. Bogush, R. E. Espinosa, B. C. Cannon et al., "Selecting the right defibrillator in the younger patient: transvenous, epicardial or subcutaneous?," *International Journal of Cardiology*, vol. 250, pp. 133–138, 2018.

[26] J. C. von Alvensleben, B. Dechert, D. J. Bradley et al., "Subcutaneous implantable cardioverter-defibrillators in pediatrics and congenital heart disease: a pediatric and congenital electrophysiology society multicenter review," *Clinical Electrophysiology*, vol. 6, no. 14, pp. 1752–1761, 2020.

5

A Case of Severe Mitral Valve Regurgitation in a Patient with Leadless Pacemaker

Srikala R. Gumireddy, Minako Katayama, and Hari P. Chaliki

Division of Cardiovascular Diseases, Mayo Clinic, Scottsdale, Arizona, USA

Correspondence should be addressed to Hari P. Chaliki; chaliki.hari@mayo.edu

Academic Editor: Alfredo E. Rodriguez

An 85-year-old man with cardiac history notable for atrial fibrillation diagnosed 10 years ago which was being treated with atenolol and warfarin presented to our institution with persistent atrial fibrillation. His echocardiogram showed ejection fraction (EF) of 56%, no regional wall motion abnormalities, mild mitral and pulmonary regurgitation, and trivial tricuspid regurgitation. Despite this treatment, he had recurrent episodes of paroxysmal symptomatic atrial fibrillation with a rapid rate requiring multiple emergency department visits and hospital admissions. Given difficulty to control the rate, he underwent atrioventricular (AV) nodal ablation and leadless pacemaker insertion. Fifteen days after the procedure, he was found to have a severe mitral regurgitation murmur.

1. Introduction

Leadless pacemakers have been shown to have lesser risk of complications such as pocket infections, endocarditis, pacemaker-induced tricuspid regurgitation, and tamponade. However, this newer technology can lead to significant mitral regurgitation due to iatrogenic LBBB and left ventricular (LV) dyssynchrony.

2. Case Presentation

An 85-year-old man presented to our institution complaining of recurrent fever and a mitral regurgitation murmur. He has a past history significant for atrial fibrillation being treated with apixaban status post leadless pacemaker implantation and AV nodal ablation 15 days ago, hypertension, hyperlipidemia, obstructive sleep apnea on continuous positive airway pressure, diverticulosis and diverticulitis, dental caries, melanoma in situ, and persistent pulmonary coccidioidomycosis on fluconazole.

He underwent a transthoracic echocardiogram which showed normal left ventricular size and no wall motion abnormalities, LVEF of 56%, severe mitral regurgitation due to incomplete coaptation of the mitral valve leaflets (Figures 1(a) and 1(b)), mild right ventricular enlargement, systolic dysfunction with visible apical right ventricular lead, mild tricuspid regurgitation, and no pericardial effusion. A transesophageal echocardiogram confirmed restricted mitral valve leaflets resulting in incomplete coaptation and severe mitral regurgitation (Figures 1(c) and 1(d)). No vegetations were seen. Blood cultures ruled out endocarditis as the cause of fever, and he was later found to have non-Hodgkin's lymphoma.

His cardiac history is notable for atrial fibrillation diagnosed 10 years ago which was treated with atenolol and warfarin. Despite this treatment, he had recurrent episodes of paroxysmal symptomatic atrial fibrillation with a rapid rate requiring multiple emergency department visits and hospital admissions (Figure 2). Given difficulty to control the rate, he underwent AV nodal ablation and leadless pacemaker insertion 15 days prior to current presentation with resultant LBBB on his electrocardiogram (ECG) post implantation (Figure 3). His echocardiogram days before pacemaker insertion revealed only mild mitral regurgitation and normal coaptation of the mitral valve leaflets (Figure 4).

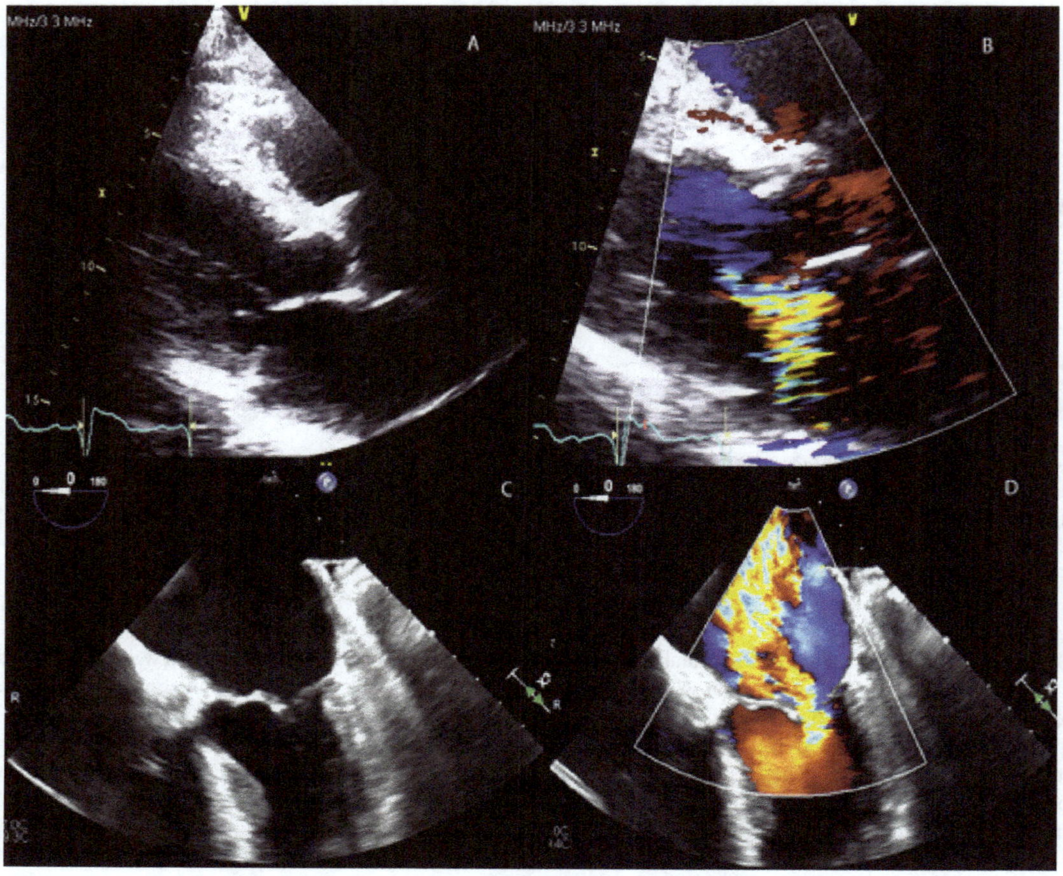

FIGURE 1: Transthoracic and transesophageal echocardiograms after leadless pacemaker insertion. (a) A transthoracic echocardiogram (parasternal long) taken after insertion of the leadless pacemaker showing incomplete coaptation of mitral valve leaflets. (b) A transthoracic echocardiogram with color (parasternal long) showing severe mitral regurgitation (effective regurgitant orifice area of 0.51 cm^2 and regurgitant volume of 52 ml) after leadless pacemaker insertion. (c) A transesophageal echocardiogram showing incomplete coaptation of mitral valve leaflets following leadless pacemaker implantation. (d) A transesophageal echocardiogram with color showing severe mitral regurgitation following leadless pacemaker implantation.

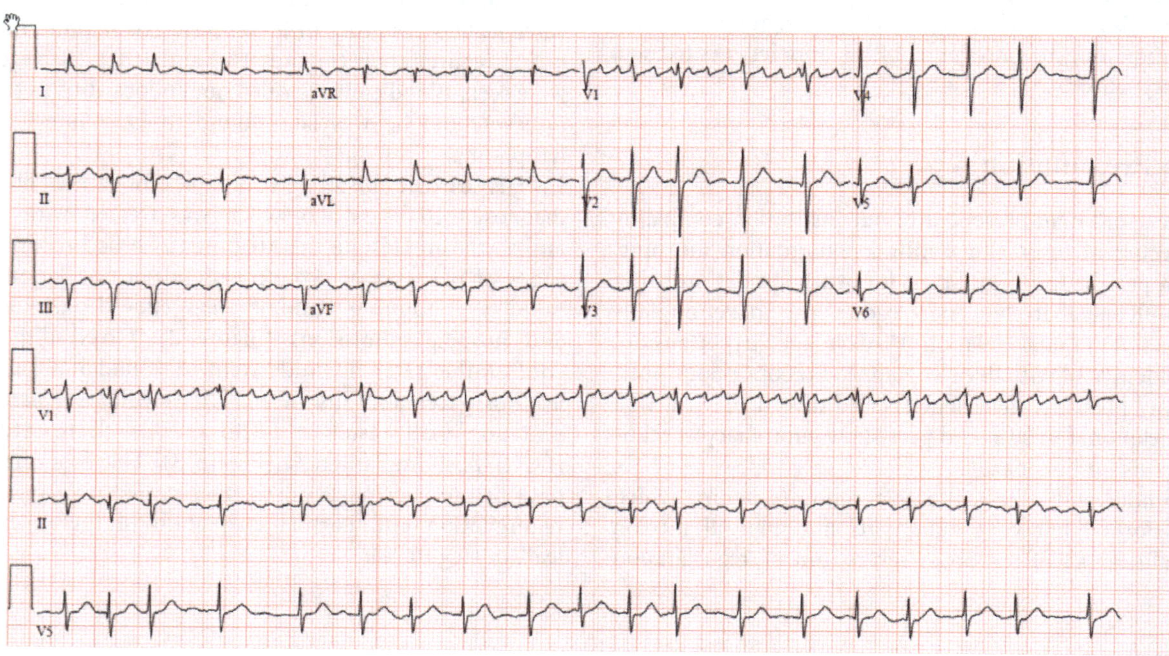

FIGURE 2: ECG prior to leadless pacemaker insertion. An ECG demonstrating atrial fibrillation with a rapid ventricular rate prior to insertion of the leadless pacemaker.

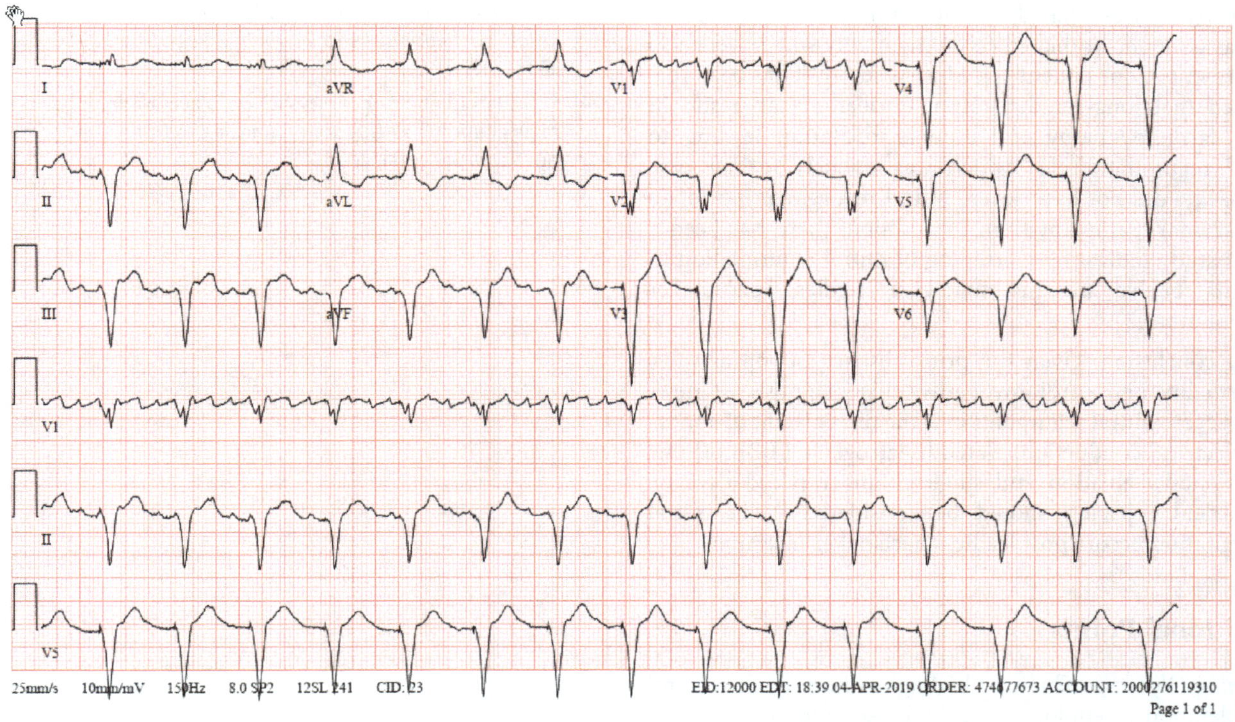

FIGURE 3: ECG after leadless pacemaker insertion. An ECG taken after insertion of the leadless pacemaker that demonstrates LBBB.

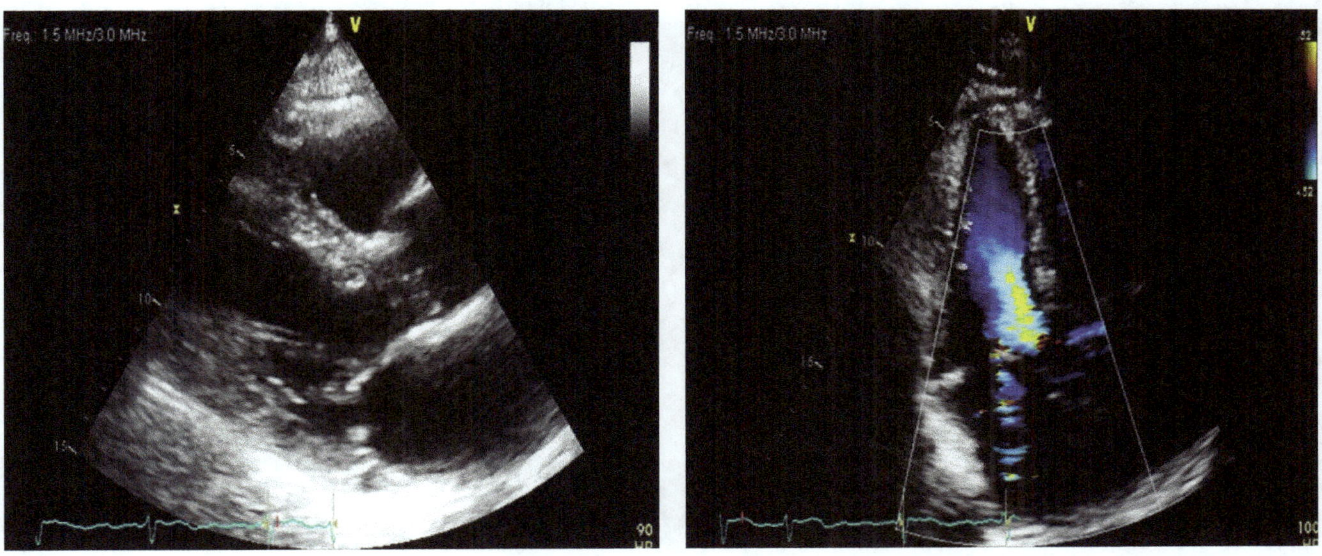

(a)

(b)

FIGURE 4: Echocardiograms 25 days prior to leadless pacemaker insertion. (a) A transthoracic echocardiogram (parasternal long) prior to leadless pacemaker insertion showing normal coaptation of mitral valve leaflets. (b) An apical 4-chamber view taken prior to leadless pacemaker insertion showing only mild mitral regurgitation.

Given the absence of degenerative mitral valve abnormality and no evidence of cardiomyopathy, his diagnosis of new-onset severe mitral regurgitation is the direct result of abnormal electrical conduction related to iatrogenic LBBB due to AV nodal ablation and single-chamber paced rhythm.

3. Discussion

Mitral regurgitation in majority of cases is related to primary mitral valve diseases such as mitral valve prolapse, endocarditis, or rheumatic heart disease which was not the case in our patient [1]. Mitral regurgitation can also occur due to secondary causes related to left ventricular abnormalities such as ischemic or dilated cardiomyopathy which were also not present in our patient [1]. More recently, it has been recognized that long-standing atrial fibrillation can result in atrial cardiomyopathy and annular dilatation leading to mitral regurgitation [2] which was unlikely in our case because he did not have severe mitral regurgitation prior to his pacemaker implantation. In addition, there has been a recent study indicating worsening of mitral regurgitation in patients twelve months following leadless pacemaker implantation [3].

In conclusion, given the prior absence of mitral valve abnormality and cardiomyopathy, this diagnosis of new-onset severe mitral regurgitation is the direct result of abnormal electrical conduction related to iatrogenic LBBB [4] due to AV nodal ablation and single-chamber paced rhythm. Biventricular pacing should be considered when mitral regurgitation occurs post leadless pacemaker insertion.

Additional Points

Learning Objective. This case highlights the need for careful consideration of etiology for mitral regurgitation following leadless pacemaker implantation. Our patient's severe mitral regurgitation is the direct result of abnormal electrical conduction related to iatrogenic left bundle branch block (LBBB) due to AV nodal ablation and single-chamber paced rhythm. It is important to recognize this entity as such patients will benefit from biventricular pacing rather than surgery or mitral clip.

Disclosure

The content of this publication is solely the responsibility of the authors and does not necessarily represent the official views of the MCA CV CRC.

Acknowledgments

This publication was supported by Mayo Clinic Arizona Cardiovascular Clinical Research Center (MCA CV CRC). We are thankful for their generous support.

References

[1] W. A. Zoghbi, D. Adams, R. O. Bonow et al., "Recommendations for noninvasive evaluation of native valvular regurgitation: a report from the American Society of Echocardiography developed in collaboration with the Society for Cardiovascular Magnetic Resonance," *Journal of the American Society of Echocardiography*, vol. 30, no. 4, pp. 303–371, 2017.

[2] J. J. Liang and F. E. Silvestry, "Mechanistic insights into mitral regurgitation due to atrial fibrillation: "atrial functional mitral regurgitation"," *Trends in Cardiovascular Medicine*, vol. 26, no. 8, pp. 681–689, 2016.

[3] N. E. G. Beurskens, F. V. Y. Tjong, R. H. A. de Bruin-Bon et al., "Impact of leadless pacemaker therapy on cardiac and atrioventricular valve function through 12 months of follow-up," *Circulation. Arrhythmia and Electrophysiology*, vol. 12, no. 5, article e007124, 2019.

[4] S. S. Barold and I. E. Ovsyshcher, "Pacemaker-induced mitral regurgitation," *Pacing and Clinical Electrophysiology*, vol. 28, no. 5, pp. 357–360, 2005.

6

Severe Chest Pain in a Young Patient with Behçet's Disease: A Rare Manifestation

Steen Reed,[1] **Michael McGee**,[2,3,4,5,6] **and Shanathan Sritharan**[5]

[1]*Department of Medicine, John Hunter Hospital, Australia*
[2]*Hunter Medical Research Institute, Australia*
[3]*The University of Newcastle, Australia*
[4]*The University of New England, Australia*
[5]*Department of Medicine, Tamworth Hospital, Australia*
[6]*Department of Cardiology, John Hunter Hospital, Australia*

Correspondence should be addressed to Steen Reed; steen.reed@gmail.com

Academic Editor: Christopher S. Snyder

A 32-year-old man with a background of Behçet's disease developed severe chest pain. The onset coincided with an episode of sacroiliitis. The patient was diagnosed with pericarditis and was successfully treated with a combination of anti-inflammatory agents. Pericarditis is a rare manifestation of Behçet's disease.

1. Case Presentation

1.1. History of Presentation. A 32-year-old man with no prior history of cardiovascular disease presented to the emergency department with a 24 hour history of retrosternal chest pain. The pain was described as sharp, pleuritic with some radiation to the left shoulder. The onset of pain was gradual and occurred after an episode of exercise. Serial troponins, electrocardiogram, and chest X-ray were performed and deemed normal. He was commenced on simple analgesia and discharged following a diagnosis of atypical chest pain with a recommendation of outpatient cardiology review.

The patient represented the following day with increasing chest pain despite analgesia. His temperature was 37.9°C, the heart rate 110 bpm, the blood pressure 109/78 mmHg, respiratory rate 16 breaths/min, and oxygen saturation 98% on air. On examination, there were multiple oral aphthous ulcers (Figure 1). There was reproducible tenderness bilaterally on the sacroiliac distraction test. The jugular venous pulse was not elevated. The pulse was regular. Heart sounds were dual with no murmurs and no pericardial rub on auscultation. The lung fields were clear on auscultation. The chest wall was not tender to palpation. There was no peripheral pitting oedema, and there were no clinical signs of deep vein thrombosis.

The patient had never experienced chest pain of this nature before. There was no recent history of either respiratory or gastrointestinal viral symptoms. Two days prior to the onset of pain, he was commenced on colchicine 500 μg twice daily for lumbosacral pain attributed to sacroiliitis (Figure 2).

1.2. Past Medical History. The patient was diagnosed with Behçet's disease (BD) a year prior to presentation. This was following a history of recurrent oral and scrotal ulcers, associated with self-limiting episodes of colitis. More recently, the patient had been suffering from episodes of large joint polyarthritis and sacroiliitis. Aside from the recent prescription of colchicine for sacroiliitis, the patient's only other medication was paracetamol. The patient had received short courses of oral prednisone to manage symptoms of oral ulcers and arthralgias associated with BD in the recent past. Other past medical history included alpha-thalassemia trait. The patient was of Indian descent. The

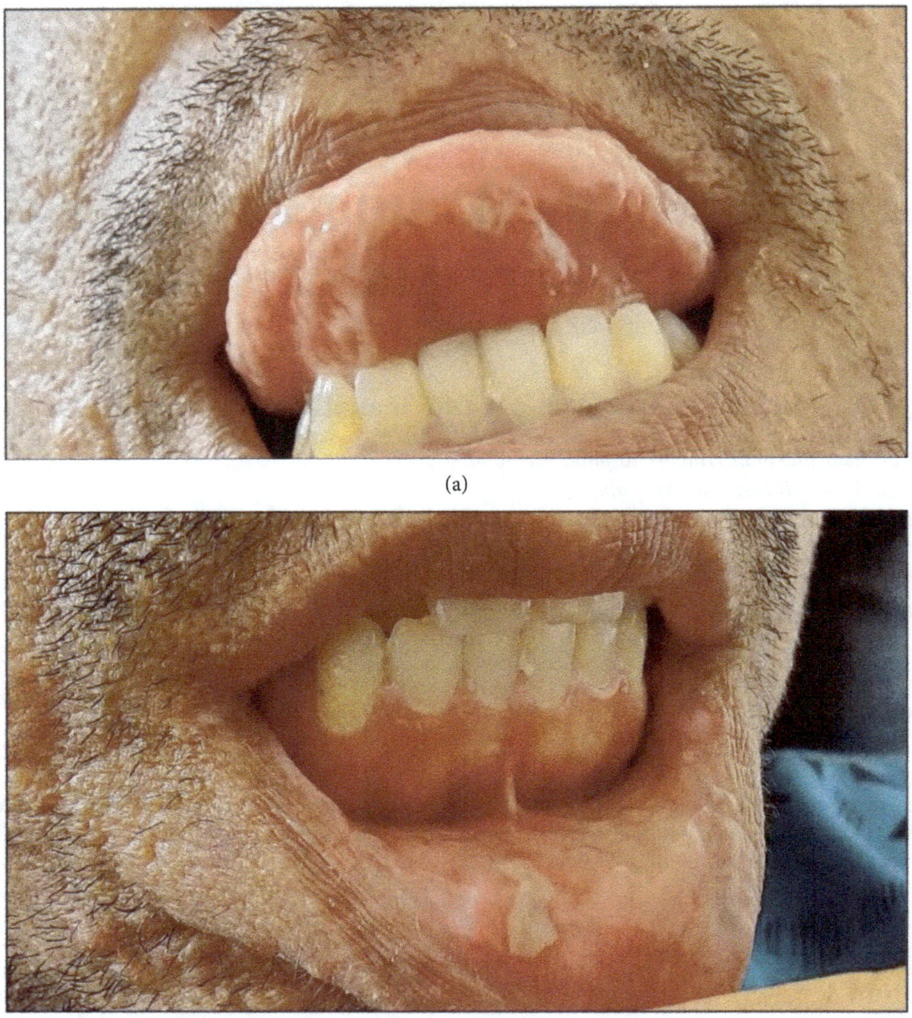

(a)

(b)

FIGURE 1: Photographs of the patient. Photographs of the patient's oral mucosa demonstrating aphthous ulcers of the tongue (a) and the lower lip (b).

patient had no personal or family history of tuberculosis and had completed full health screening on immigration to Australia. His family history was significant for cardiovascular disease with his father dying from myocardial infarction at the age of 50.

1.3. Investigations. Full blood count revealed white blood cell count 16.7 10^9/L (range 4.0-11.0 10^9/L), neutrophil count 12.9 10^9/L (range 2.0-8.0 10^9/L), haemoglobin 129 g/L (range 130-180 g/L), C-reactive protein (CRP) 179 mg/L (range < 5 mg/L), and erythrocyte sedimentation rate 71 mm/hr (range 0-15 mm/hr) (Table 1). D-dimer was 0.76 mg/L (range < 50 mg/L). 3 sets of blood cultures were taken and were negative for growth. On the first presentation to the emergency department, serial troponin I was measured at 8 ng/L (normal range < 26 ng/L) and 15 ng/L, respectively. On the subsequent presentation, troponin I was measured at 64 ng/L, then 63 ng/L on 2 hour repeat. Electrocardiography (ECG) revealed ST-segment elevations and associated PR-segment depression in leads I, II, aVF, aVL, and V2-V6 (Figure 3). Transthoracic echocardiogram showed normal ventricular size and systolic function. The left ventricular ejection fraction was 56%. There was no pericardial effusion or restrictive physiology. Computed tomography pulmonary angiogram (CTPA) showed no evidence of pulmonary embolism and no significant airspace consolidation. Computed tomography coronary angiogram (CTCA) and cardiac magnetic resonance imaging (cMRI) were performed a month following discharge from hospital. CTCA revealed plaque within the mid left anterior descending artery involving the origin of the first diagonal branch, resulting in mild stenosis. The pericardium was noted to be unremarkable with normal contour and no effusion. On cMRI, the pericardium was normal in thickness, and no effusion was seen. No abnormality was detected in the pericardial space. There was no increased myocardial signal on T2 imaging and no postgadolinium contrast enhancement on T1 imaging to suggest myocardial involvement.

1.4. Differential Diagnosis. The differential diagnosis for this patient included acute coronary syndrome, pulmonary embolism, atypical infection, and pericarditis.

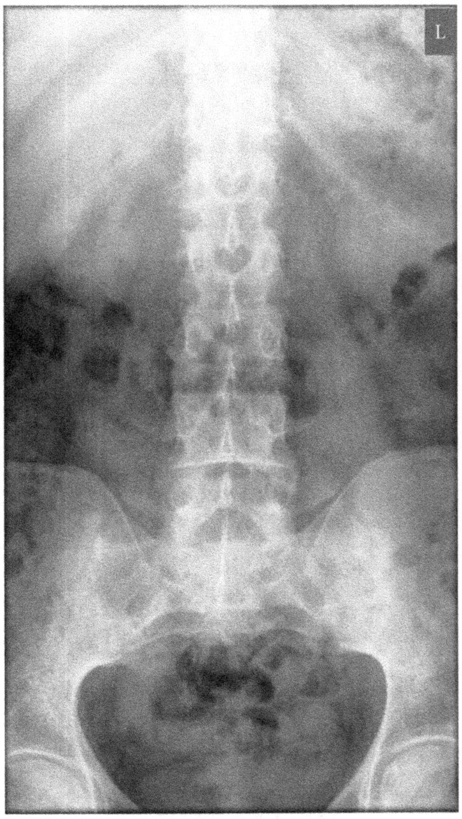

FIGURE 2: Plain film radiograph of the patient. Anteroposterior plain-film radiograph of the patient performed prior to his initial presentation. Significant sacroiliitis is seen with sclerosis and partial ankylosis of the sacroiliac joints demonstrated bilaterally.

Given the features of low-grade fever, raised inflammatory markers, and widespread ST-segment changes on ECG presenting in a patient with a background of autoimmune disease, a working diagnosis of pericarditis with possible myocardial involvement was made. Important alternative diagnoses were ruled out following CTCA and CTPA. Whilst the echocardiogram showed no evidence of pericardial effusion, this does not rule out a diagnosis of pericarditis. Given that effusion reflects the degree of inflammation in the pericardial space, it is possible that the development of an effusion may have been suppressed by the commencement of colchicine 2 day prior to onset of symptoms.

1.5. Management. On admission, the patient was commenced on aspirin 900 mg three times daily; colchicine was continued at 500ug twice daily. The patient was admitted to the coronary care unit and placed on cardiac monitoring. Despite this, the patient's pain remained severe; 50 mg oral prednisone once daily was therefore commenced in addition to the above regimen. The patient was commenced on bisoprolol 2.5 mg once daily and candesartan 4 mg once daily due to the initial suspicion of myocardial involvement. After 3 days of anti-inflammatory treatment, his chest pain subsided. He was discharged home on colchicine and prednisone. The prednisone was weaned slowly under supervision of the patient's rheumatologist. Thiopurine methyltransferase genotyping, hepatitis serology, and Quantiferon Gold assay were performed in case the patient's treatment needed to be escalated to either azathioprine or biological therapy.

2. Discussion

BD is a multisystem inflammatory vasculitis of unclear aetiology. Disease is strongly associated with the presence of the HLA-B51 allele. Whilst BD has a global distribution, cases are seen most frequently in populations around the ancient silk road (Turkey has the highest prevalence) and is rare amongst western populations [1].

The most frequent manifestations of BD are oral and genital aphthous ulcers, ocular lesions, and skin lesions. Others include gastrointestinal inflammation, central nervous system lesions, and arthritis. Whilst not fully understood, the underlying pathophysiology of BD is thought to relate to vasculitis, which can affect both large and small vessels [1].

Cardiac manifestations are rare but important to recognise amongst BD sufferers, as mortality is increased in these patients [2, 3]. In one series, cardiac manifestations were seen in 6% of patients (pericarditis accounting for 38.5% of these). Death was observed in 15.4% of these patients, compared with 5.4% of those without cardiac involvement [3]. In the same series, cardiac manifestations occurred more frequently in male patients and less frequently in patients of European descent [3]. Other cardiac manifestations include valvular insufficiency, intracardiac thrombosis, and myocardial infarction [4].

Treatment is empirical and aimed at reducing inflammation. Suitable agents include nonsteroidal anti-inflammatory drugs, colchicine, and corticosteroids [2, 5]. In this case, the patient received a combination of aspirin, colchicine, and prednisone, which led to resolution of symptoms. In severe or resistant disease, immunosuppressant agents such as cyclophosphamide and azathioprine may be considered [6]. Antitumor necrosis factor alpha (TNFa) agents are emerging as a therapeutic option in severe and life-threatening BD. High-quality randomised controlled trials are sparse, and data generally relates to noncardiac manifestations of BD; however, initial data is promising, and this may represent an important treatment option in the event of life-threatening disease resistant to conventional therapies [7, 8].

3. Follow-Up

The patient was followed up by both rheumatology and cardiology in the outpatient setting. The previously noted ECG changes resolved on repeat testing (Figure 4). The patient was continued on regular colchicine, whilst the prednisone was weaned under the supervision of his rheumatologist. The dose of prednisone was weaned to 7.5 mg daily over a period of 8 weeks. Whilst there was no recurrence of symptoms of pericarditis during this time, the patient was suffering from recurrent oral ulcers. Azathioprine was therefore commenced as a steroid sparing therapy.

After cMRI revealed no evidence of myocardial involvement or reduced left ventricular ejection fraction, the

Table 1: Table summarising the key investigations of the patient.

Investigation	Reference range	1st episode of pericarditis	1 month of anti-inflammatory treatment	2nd episode of pericarditis
CRP	<5 mg/L	179	5	128
ESR	0-15 mm/hr	71	13	51
Troponin I peak	<26 mg/L	64	11	16
WCC	4.0-11.0 10^9/L	16.7	10.5	13.3
Neutrophil	2.0-8.0 10^9/L	12.9	6.0	11.2

CRP: C-reactive protein; ESR: erythrocyte sedimentation rate; WCC: white blood cell count.

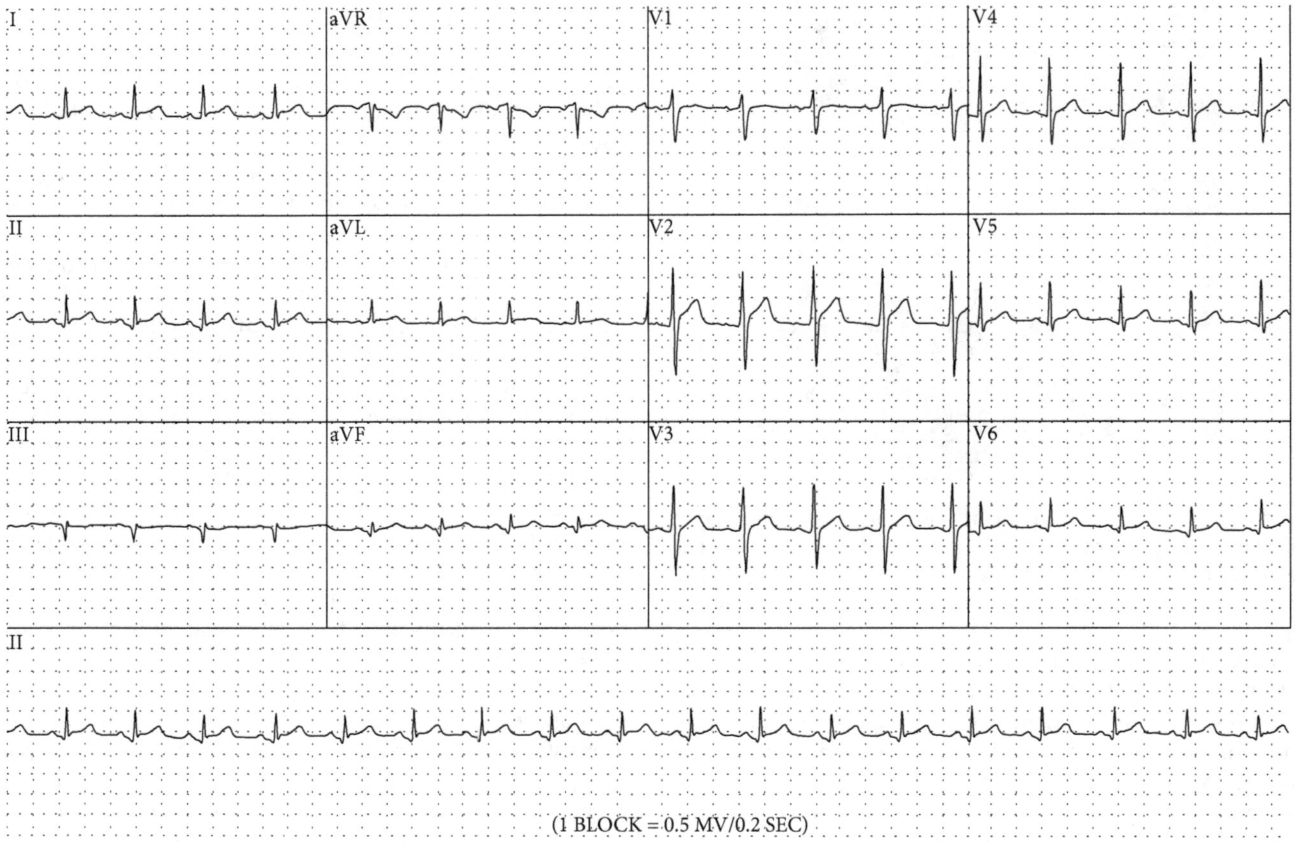

Figure 3: Electrocardiogram of the patient. Electrocardiograph (ECG) recorded during the patient's initial presentation. PR segment depression and ST segment elevation in leads I, II, aVF, aVL, and V2-V6 and demonstrated.

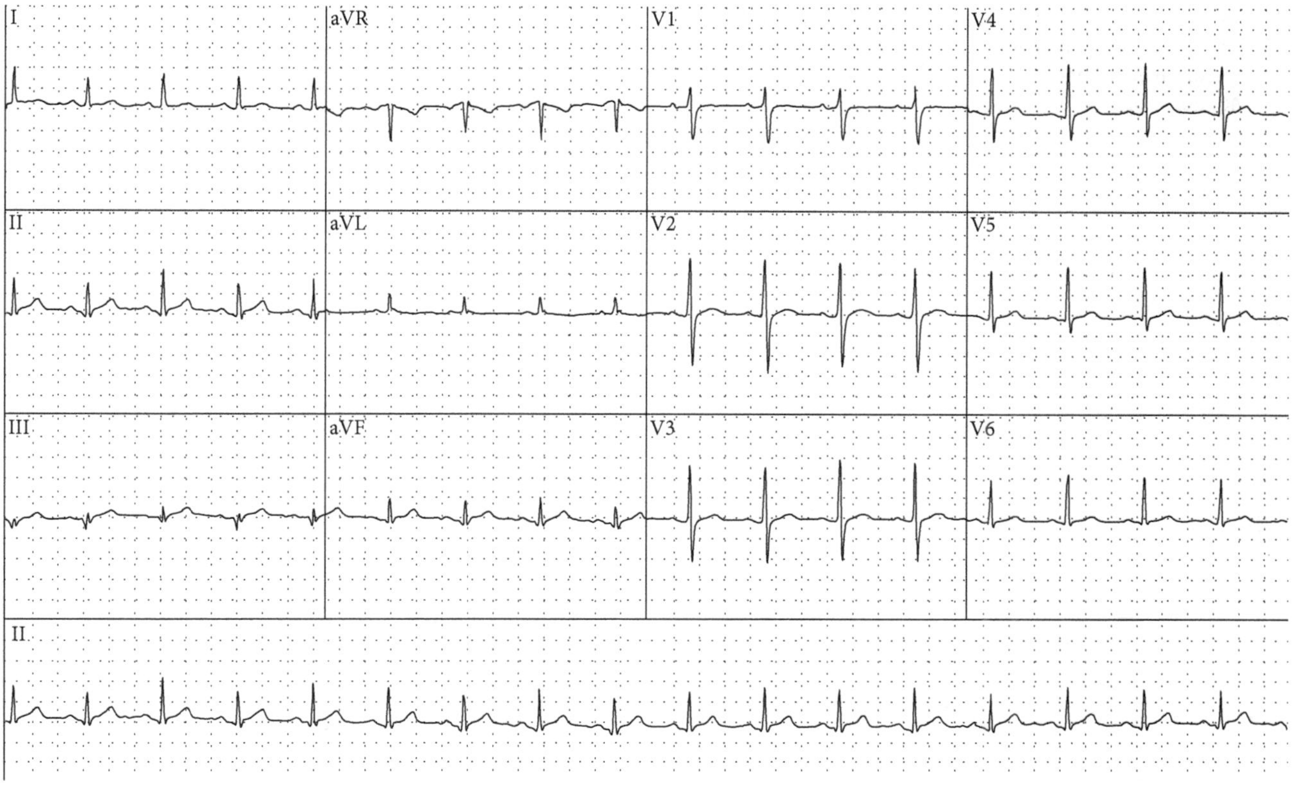

FIGURE 4: Electrocardiogram of the patient. Electrocardiogram (ECG) recorded during outpatient follow-up in cardiology clinic. This ECG shows resolution of widespread ST-segment elevation following the initial admission with pericarditis.

candesartan and bisoprolol were ceased. He was commenced on statin therapy due to his family history of ischaemic heart disease and coronary artery atherosclerosis evident on CTCA.

9 weeks after discharge, the patient represented to the hospital with pleuritic chest pain. This occurred 15 days following his second dose of Comirnaty (Pfizer) COVID-19 vaccine. Investigations revealed a CRP of 128 mg/L, normal serial troponin I, and mild ST elevation in inferior and lateral leads on ECG (Table 1). The patient was treated for a recurrence of pericarditis. Prednisone was increased to 25 mg daily with resolution of symptoms. The CRP normalised on repeat testing 2 weeks following this, and the prednisone dose was weaned once more.

4. Conclusion

Pericarditis is a rare manifestation of BD. It is important to recognise cardiac manifestations in BD as increased mortality is seen amongst these patients. Pericarditis can be successfully treated with anti-inflammatory agents though immunosuppressants can also be considered. Biological therapy, such as anti-TNFa agents, is a possible treatment option in severe and refractory cases.

Consent

Written informed consent was provided by the patient to publish the case, data, and photos contained within the manuscript.

Acknowledgments

The manuscript was completed during employment by Hunter New England Local Health District, New South Wales Health, Australia.

References

[1] T. Sakane, M. Takeno, N. Suzuki, and G. Inaba, "Behçet's disease," *NEJM*, vol. 341, no. 17, pp. 1284–1291, 1999.

[2] S. Demirelli, H. Degirmenci, S. Inci, and A. Arisoy, "Cardiac manifestations in Behçet's disease," *Intractable & rare diseases research*, vol. 4, no. 2, pp. 70–75, 2015.

[3] G. Geri, B. Wechsler, D. L. Thi Huong et al., "Spectrum of cardiac lesions in Behçet disease: a series of 52 patients and review of the literature," *Medicine (Baltimore)*, vol. 91, no. 1, pp. 25–34, 2012.

[4] S. Morelli, C. Perrone, L. Ferrante et al., "Cardiac involvement in Behçet's disease," *Cardiology*, vol. 88, no. 6, pp. 513–517, 1997.

[5] J. G. Chiabrando, A. Bonaventura, A. Vecchié et al., "Management of acute and recurrent pericarditis: JACC state-of-the-art review," *Journal of the American College of Cardiology*, vol. 75, no. 1, pp. 76–92, 2020.

[6] T. Tahir, "A case of acute constrictive pericarditis associated with Behçet's disease," *International Journal of Rheumatic Diseases*, vol. 14, no. 4, pp. e51–e53, 2011.

[7] A. Arida, K. Fragiadaki, E. Giavri, and P. P. Sfikakis, "Anti-TNF agents for Behçet's disease: analysis of published data on 369 patients," *Seminars in Arthritis and Rheumatism*, vol. 41, no. 1, pp. 61–70, 2011.

[8] P. P. Sfikakis, N. Markomichelakis, E. Alpsoy et al., "Anti-TNF therapy in the management of Behcet's disease–review and basis for recommendations," *Rheumatology (Oxford, England)*, vol. 46, no. 5, pp. 736–741, 2007.

7

Coronary Artery Fistula and Pectus Excavatum Paradox

Mohammad Hashim Jilani,[1] **Hina Khawar Jamali**,[2] **Fahad Waqar**,[2] **and Mohamed Effat**[2]

[1]*Department of Medicine, Carle Foundation Hospital, Urbana IL, USA*
[2]*Division of Cardiovascular Health and Disease, University of Cincinnati College of Medicine, Cincinnati OH, USA*

Correspondence should be addressed to Fahad Waqar; fahad.waqar@uc.edu

Academic Editor: Assad Movahed

Pectus excavatum is the most common congenital chest wall deformity. Its effects on cardiopulmonary function, exercise capacity, and body image are variable across affected patients. Management practices for pectus deformity vary considerably, but most authors agree on the need for surgical correction if pectus index is >3.0 and there is evidence of cardiac compression on imaging. We encountered a case of a middle-aged man with severe pectus deformity and a coincidental large coronary artery to right atrium fistula. Despite a pectus index of 4.8 and severe right heart compression on thoracic imaging, he had not developed any symptoms or hemodynamic complication from this pectus deformity. Additionally, hemodynamic studies revealed normal left and right heart function, normal pulmonary artery pressures, and absence of any evidence of myocardial ischemia or significant left-to-right shunt. These abnormalities would have been expected with a coronary fistula of this size. His pectus deformity and coronary fistula had opposing hemodynamic effects, thus protecting him from severe complications of either. Presently, an association between congenital coronary fistulae and pectus excavatum is not known, and this is one of the very first reported cases of these two congenital abnormalities coexisting in a patient. Additionally, concurrence of these two conditions poses a unique therapeutic challenge due to their opposing hemodynamic effects.

1. Introduction

Pectus excavatum is a common congenital deformity which, in its severe form, can cause significant cardiac dysfunction via right heart compression. Coronary fistulae are rare congenital malformations, and large size fistulae are associated with significant shunt physiology as well as cardiac ischemia. These two congenital deformities have not been reported to coexist in the current literature.

2. Case Presentation

A 35-year-old man with known atrial fibrillation, severe uncorrected congenital pectus excavatum (pectus index 4.8), and congenital left main coronary artery to right atrium fistula with a prior unsuccessful coil embolization presented with an accidental two-story fall. Preoperative risk assessment for trauma surgery prompted a coronary angiogram and right heart catheterization.

Coronary angiography was performed via right radial artery approach showing a short left main coronary artery bifurcating into an intermediate size left anterior descending artery and left circumflex artery, along with filling of an expected coronary artery fistula seen as a large caliber tortuous vessel originating from left main coronary artery near bifurcation and draining into the right atrium. A previously deployed coil within the fistula was also seen but did not appear to offer any meaningful impedance to the fistula flow (Figure 1). Right heart catheterization was notable for normal right ventricular and normal pulmonary artery pressures. Mixed venous oxygen saturation measured from inferior and superior vena cava was 73%, and pulmonary artery oxygen saturation was 76%, resulting in a Qp/Qs ratio of 1.15, suggesting absence of any significant left-to-right shunt.

3. Discussion

Pectus excavatum, a posterior depression of the sternum and costal cartilages, is the most common congenital chest wall

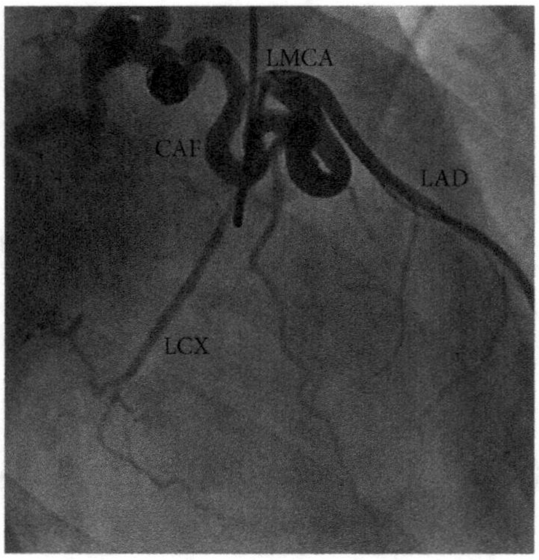

FIGURE 1: Coronary angiogram of the left main coronary artery (LMCA) showing filling of coronary arteriovenous fistula (CAF) originating near the LMCA bifurcation and connecting to the right atrium. LAD: left anterior descending artery; LCX: left circumflex artery.

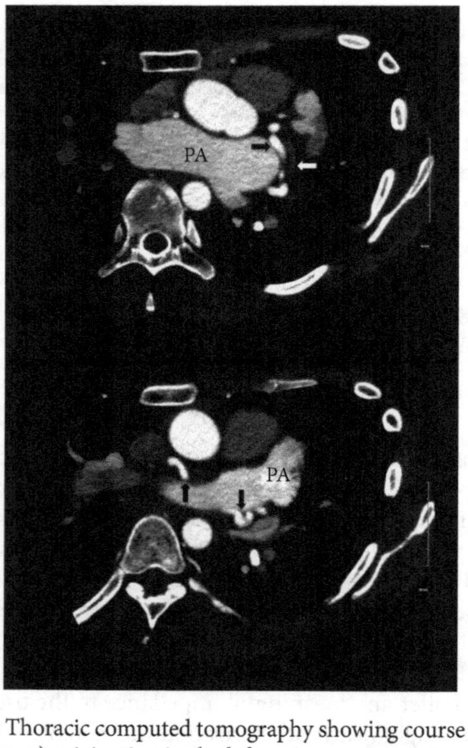

FIGURE 2: Thoracic computed tomography showing course of fistula (black arrows) originating in the left main coronary artery, initially running parallel to left circumflex artery (white arrow), posterior, and above the pulmonary artery (PA) before draining into the right atrium (right atrium not visualized in these sections).

deformity, accounting for over 90% of such cases [1]. Although the exact etiology is not known, there appears to be a genetic contribution due to familial clustering of the disease [2]. In severe cases, right atrial and right ventricular compression from the deformity, as well as reduced lung volumes, result in decreased cardiac output and reduced exercise capacity [3]. Severity of pectus deformity is often measured using pectus index defined as the ratio of maximal transverse

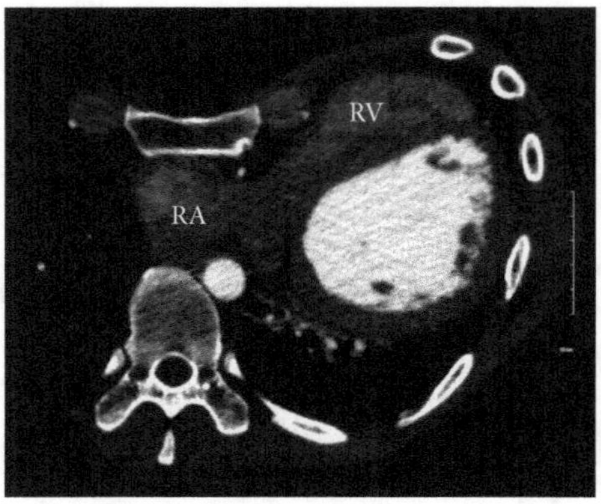

FIGURE 3: Computed tomogram showing pectus excavatum with severe compression and elongation of right atrium (RA) and right ventricle (RV).

diameter to narrowest anterior posterior length of chest (distance between the vertebrae and sternum). A pectus index of greater than 3.0 is considered severe and often used to identify candidates for surgical correction in early years of life before cardiopulmonary complications develop [4]. Colombani showed that besides chest computed tomography and magnetic resonance imaging used for calculating pectus index and assessing the degree of cardiac compression, echocardiography provides additional information on diastolic chamber filling and cardiac function [5]. The author also proposed a criterion for selection of patients for surgical repair of pectus.

Coronary artery to right system fistulae of large size pose a risk of myocardial ischemia via steal phenomenon, as well as congestive heart failure and pulmonary hypertension by causing left-to-right shunt in most patients [6, 7]. Symptoms become apparent in a majority of young adults, frequently developing before the age of 20 [8]. While surgical or interventional treatment is usually reserved for symptoms of myocardial ischemia or congestive heart failure, American College of Cardiology and American Heart Association guidelines recommend that fistulae of large size should be treated regardless of symptoms or clinical manifestations (a class I indication) [9]. In addition, elective closure is also recommended for fistulae detected in early life and fistulae originating from proximal segments of coronary arteries, regardless of their size [7].

In the case mentioned above, the patient was initially deemed a surgical candidate for pectus deformity as well as the coronary fistulae. Further workup including right heart catheterization and transthoracic echocardiogram revealed normal right-sided pressures and normal hemodynamics. A subsequent myocardial perfusion study excluded ischemia. Additionally, patient had maintained a normal functional and exercise capacity for over three decades of his life. This suggested that the coexistence of these two conditions likely resulted in a paradoxical balance, maintaining normal right-sided hemodynamics. Besides being an unusual case of a sizeable coronary fistula in a patient with severe pectus excavatum, the most remarkable aspect of this patient's pathophysiology is the likely neutralizing effect offered by his pectus deformity against development of right-sided overload and possibly vice versa (Figures 2 and 3). These findings led to a very carefully considered decision to allow both congenital deformities be left untreated in this case with no further intervention and conservative management was pursued. The patient remained asymptomatic on follow-up visit and continued to have normal exercise capacity.

Acknowledgments

We thank Dr. Nabeel Porbandarwala from the Department of Radiology, University of Cincinnati College of Medicine, for providing radiographic images and useful insight into the details of the patient's pectus excavatum and coronary fistula. We thank Dr. Saagar Sanghvi and Dr. Muhammad Athar for their help in preparing the manuscript.

References

[1] D. Jaroszewski, D. Notrica, L. McMahon, D. E. Steidley, and C. Deschamps, "Current management of pectus excavatum: a review and update of therapy and treatment recommendations," *Journal of American Board of Family Medicine*, vol. 23, no. 2, pp. 230–239, 2010.

[2] J. Sabiston Jr. and J. Heinle, *Congenital Deformities of the Chest Wall. Textbook of Surgery Philadelphia*, WB Sauders Co, 1997.

[3] H. Gattiker and A. Bühlmann, "Cardiopulmonary function and exercise tolerance in supine and sitting position in patients with pectus excavatum," *Helvetica Medica Acta*, vol. 33, no. 2, pp. 122–138, 1966.

[4] J. A. Haller Jr. and G. M. Loughlin, "Cardiorespiratory function is significantly improved following corrective surgery for severe pectus excavatum. Proposed treatment guidelines," *The Journal of Cardiovascular Surgery*, vol. 41, no. 1, pp. 125–130, 2000.

[5] P. M. Colombani, "Preoperative assessment of chest wall deformities," *Seminars in Thoracic and Cardiovascular Surgery*, vol. 21, no. 1, pp. 58–63, 2009.

[6] G. Dimitrakakis, U. Von Oppell, H. Luckraz, and P. Groves, "Surgical repair of triple coronary-pulmonary artery fistulae with associated atrial septal defect and aortic valve regurgitation," *Interactive Cardiovascular and Thoracic Surgery*, vol. 7, no. 5, pp. 933-934, 2008.

[7] L. A. Latson, "Coronary artery fistulas: how to manage them," *Catheterization and Cardiovascular Interventions*, vol. 70, no. 1, pp. 110–116, 2007.

[8] A. Dursun, R. Demirbag, A. Yildiz, Y. Sezen, I. H. Altiparmak, and R. Yilmaz, "Diagnosis of the left circumflex coronary artery fistula drainage into the left ventricle by echocardiographic color Doppler flow imaging," *International Journal of Cardiology*, vol. 134, no. 3, pp. e85–e86, 2009.

[9] C. A. Warnes, R. G. Williams, T. M. Bashore et al., "ACC/AHA 2008 guidelines for the management of adults with congenital heart disease: executive summary: a report of the American College of Cardiology/American Heart Association Task Force on Practice Guidelines (writing committee to develop guidelines for the management of adults with congenital heart disease)," *Circulation*, vol. 118, no. 23, pp. 2395–2451, 2008.

8

A Large Intrathoracic Hiatal Hernia as a Cause of Complete Heart Block

Ali Abbood, Hareer Al Salihi, Jorge Parellada, Mario Madruga, and S. J. Carlan

Department of Internal Medicine, Division of Academic Affairs and Research, Orlando Regional Healthcare, Orlando, Florida, USA

Correspondence should be addressed to S. J. Carlan; stevecarlan@gmail.com

Academic Editor: Luigi Sciarra

Hiatal hernia is a not uncommon anatomic disorder resulting in portions of the bowel occupying space in the thoracic cavity. There are a number of antecedent risk factors including obesity but not hiatal hernias resulting in symptoms. When symptoms do occur, they can include chest pain, nausea, abdominal pain, and gastroesophageal reflux. Cardiac arrhythmias have also been reported as associated conditions resulting from a hiatal hernia. To date, however, a complete heart block secondary to a hiatal hernia has not been reported. An 88-year-old female with a history of GERD (gastroesophageal reflux disease) was found to have a large hiatal hernia at endoscopy after she presented to the emergency department with nausea and abdominal pain. Prior to her scheduled surgical repair, she developed symptomatic third degree heart block which resolved with nasogastric tube deflation of the gastric contents. After surgical repair of the hiatal hernia, she developed episodes of atrial fibrillation with rapid ventricular response and was started on diltiazem. She eventually converted back to normal sinus rhythm and remained dysrhythmia free. In addition to other known arrhythmias associated with hiatal hernia, a complete heart block can also be seen. Acute management requires deflation of the chest occupying hernia. This appears to be the one of the first reported cases of complete heart block caused by hiatal hernia.

1. Introduction

Hiatal hernia is a common pathology which increases in incidence with age. It is associated with (GERD) gastroesophageal reflux disease, a widespread condition that may present as atypical chest pain. Cases of patients with large hiatal hernia causing electrocardiographic changes have been well documented, manifesting as atrial fibrillation [1], atrial flutter [2], ST segment elevation [3], and others, but to date, there have been no reports of complete heart block caused directly by hiatal hernia. Here, we discuss one of the first reported documented cases of a hiatal hernia causing complete heart block.

2. Case Presentation

An 88-year-old female with a past medical history of gastroesophageal reflux disease, hypertension, and anxiety presented to the emergency department with nausea and abdominal pain after chest X-ray and CT (computed tomography) scan of the abdomen performed at an outside facility showed a large hiatal hernia with possible volvulus or gastric obstruction (Figures 1–3) at an outside facility. She had no past history of known treated cardiac dysrhythmia. Her vital signs were normal, and physical exam was only remarkable for epigastric abdominal pain. The patient was admitted and evaluated with GI series barium study, which showed a thoracic stomach with gastric obstruction. An EGD (esophagogastroduodenoscopy) was performed which confirmed the presence of a large hiatal hernia. Surgical intervention was planned to correct the anatomical defect, but the day prior to her planned surgery, she ate a large meal and became hypotensive, with her 12-lead ECG showing complete heart block (Figure 4). The patient was promptly sent to the intensive care unit (ICU) for monitoring. She had a nasogastric tube inserted for decompression, which converted the complete heart block back to normal sinus rhythm (Figure 5). Three days later, she underwent successful laparoscopic robotic-assisted hiatal hernia repair and gastrostomy tube placement. Postoperatively, the patient had no recurrence of complete heart block, and she was transferred from the

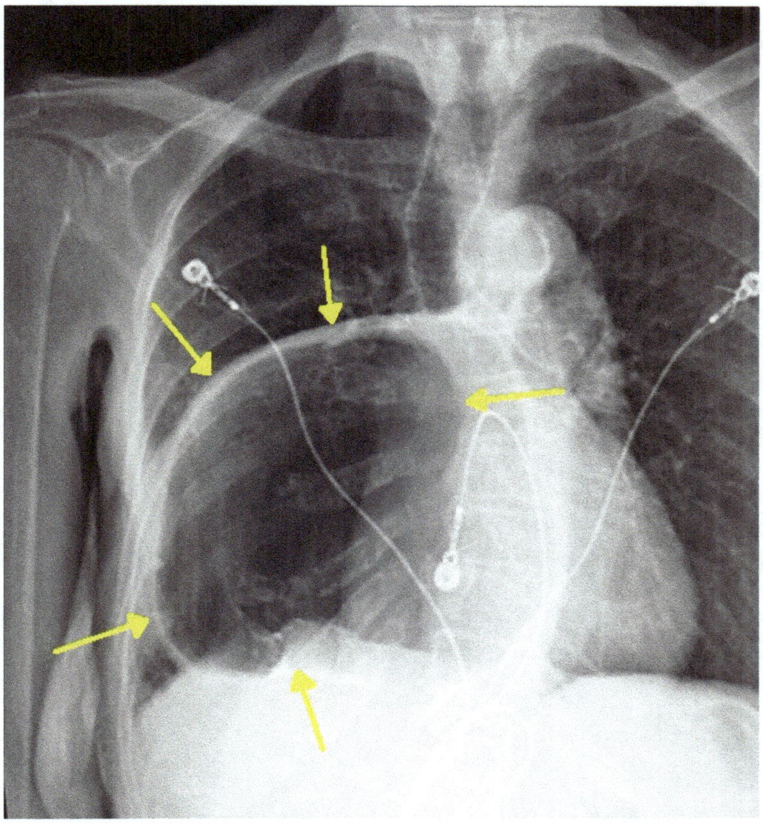

FIGURE 1: Upright chest X-ray showing large intrathoracic hiatal hernia between the yellow arrows.

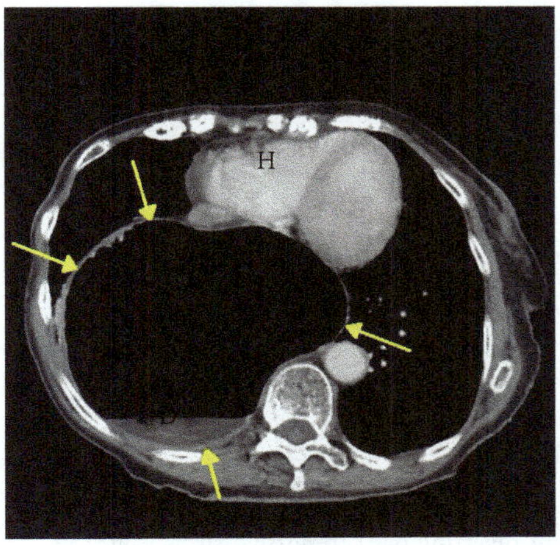

FIGURE 2: Transverse chest CT of the abdomen showing large hiatal hernia with concern for gastric volvulus or gastric outlet obstruction. The large hernia is between the yellow arrows. The heart is "H," and the debris in the bowel is "D."

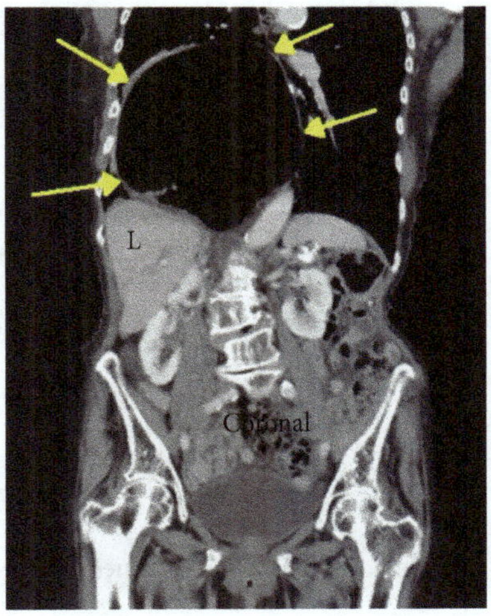

FIGURE 3: Coronal CT of chest and abdomen showing the large hiatal hernia located above the diaphragm with the liver "L" apparent.

ICU to the cardiac unit. There, she proceeded to experience episodes of atrial fibrillation with rapid ventricular response. Echocardiography was performed and was significant for an ejection fraction of 65-69%, moderate aortic stenosis, and pulmonary hypertension. The patient was placed on diltiazem and eventually converted back to normal sinus rhythm. She was discharged to a skilled nursing facility with diltiazem and apixaban and was instructed to follow up with cardiology and thoracic surgery as an outpatient.

3. Discussion

Hiatal hernia is defined as an abnormal protrusion of the stomach above the diaphragm from the esophageal hiatus. While hiatal hernias most often only involve protrusion of the stomach as the protruding organ, it may also contain the transverse colon, small bowel, spleen, or some combination of these. Risk factors for hiatal hernias include obesity, age-related changes in the diaphragm, and increased intra-

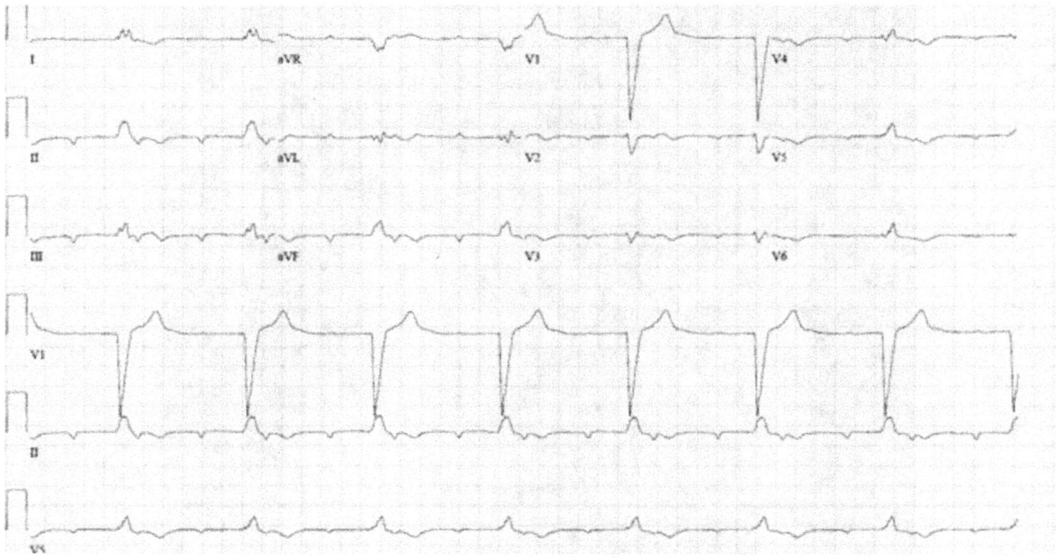

FIGURE 4: 12-lead EKG showing complete heart block.

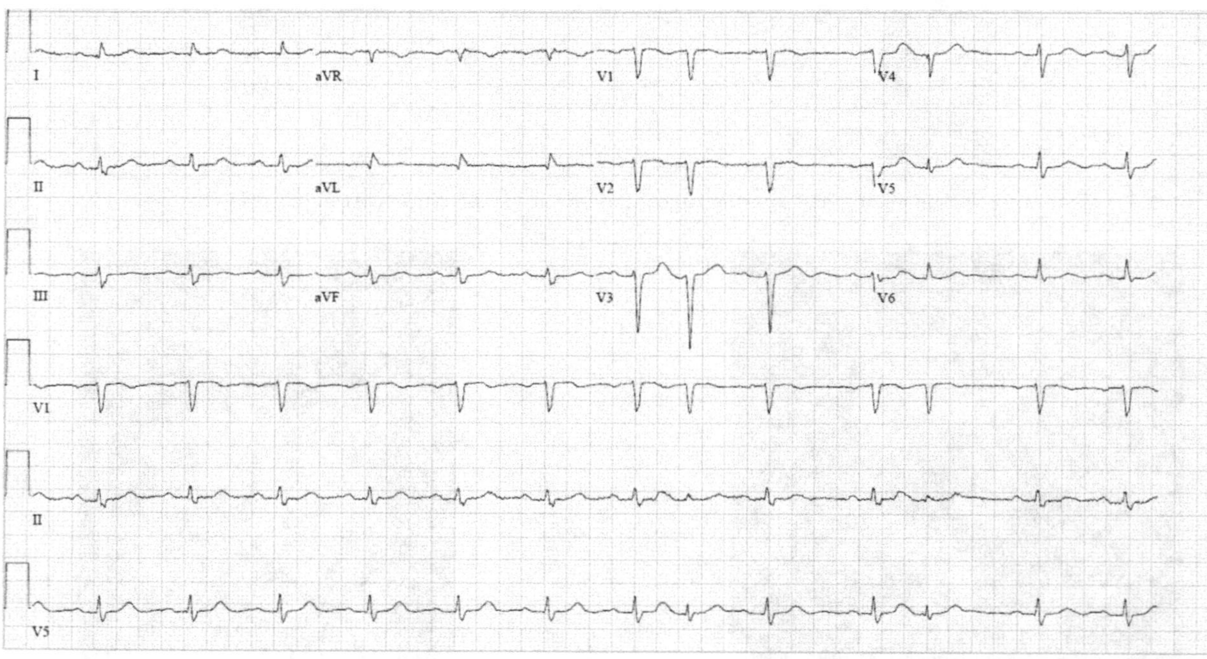

FIGURE 5: 12-lead EKG obtained after NG tube placement and patient reverting back to normal sinus rhythm.

abdominal pressure due to conditions like chronic coughing, constipation, exercising, and lifting heavy objects. Hiatal hernias may be asymptomatic or may present with gastroesophageal reflux disease, dysphagia, odynophagia, hoarseness, or asthma. Extreme cases may cause compression of the heart and pulmonary veins, leading to a presentation of pulmonary edema and cardiac failure [4]. Atrioventricular (AV) block is a cardiac electrical disorder defined as impaired (delayed or absent) conduction from the atria to the ventricles. The severity of the conduction abnormality is described in degrees: first-degree, second-degree, type I (Wenckebach or Mobitz I) or type II (Mobitz II), and third-degree (complete) AV block [5].

Large hiatal hernias can induce electrocardiographic changes, and atrial tachycardia, atrial fibrillation, supraventricular tachycardia, atrial flutter, and T wave changes have all been previously reported, but the exact mechanism of such arrhythmias is not well understood. One current hypothesis suggests that it is the increase in the direct or indirect pressure on the global surface of the heart by the hernia which causes these electrical changes seen on EKG [6]. Another suggests that it is actually due to the compression on the heart by the thoracic stomach causing anatomic conduction block or disruption in the vagal nerve [7]. Intense vagal stimulation has been described before to causing syncope and bradycardia in "swallow syncope syndrome." The pathophysiologic explanation is due to the common innervation of the esophagus and heart by the vagus nerve. The mechanoreceptors in the esophagus sense the distension and send signals along the esophageal plexus vagus nerve to the brainstem and then efferent impulses from the brainstem reach the sinoatrial (SA) node and the AV node, that leads to developing various bradyarrhythmias and temporary reduction of the cardiac output, which in result leads to cerebral hypoperfusion and syncope [8].

The presented patient had a huge hiatal hernia, and the food intake was the trigger for her hypotension and telemetry at that time it showed complete heart block. After the patient had a successful laparoscopic surgery and hiatal hernia repair, she did not develop any recurrent AV blocks. She did have a brief atrial fibrillation episode that converted back to normal sinus rhythm, which can be a postoperative episode as the patient has no history of AFib or palpitations before. Our patient was monitored on telemetry for days prior to discharge, and no recurrent events were recorded. She followed with cardiology outpatient and was on Holter monitor for 2 weeks which showed no significant events and leads to the conclusion that the surgical repair to the hernia resulted in complete resolution of the AV block.

We hypothesize that the hernia has caused a mechanical conduction block on the AV node or an increase in the firing of the vagal nerve by the mechanism mentioned above.

4. Conclusion

We present a rare case of a large hiatal hernia causing complete heart block and symptomatic hypotension resolving with nasogastric tube placement. To our knowledge, this appears to be one of the first cases to report these findings. We performed a MEDLINE search of the English language literature via PubMed from January 1, 1946 to the present, using the MeSH terms and keywords "hiatal hernia," "heart block," and "atrioventricular block." We could find, however, no cases of complete heart block associated with hiatal hernia. We concluded that the symptomatology of the patient was related to compressive effects caused by the hernia.

References

[1] L. Armaganijan, D. Patel, R. D. Lopes et al., "Gastroesophageal reflux and atrial fibrillation: Is there any correlation?," *Expert Review of Cardiovascular Therapy*, vol. 10, no. 3, pp. 317–322, 2012.

[2] D. A. Cristian, A. S. Constantin, M. Barbu, D. Spătaru, T. Burcoş, and F. A. Grama, "Paroxysmal postprandial atrial fibrilation suppressed by laparoscopic repair of a giant paraesophageal hernia compressing the left atrium," *Journal of Gastrointestinal and Liver Diseases*, vol. 24, no. 1, pp. 113–116, 2020.

[3] B. Basir, B. Safadi, R. J. Kovacs, and B. Tahir, "A rare case of transient inferior ST segment elevation," *Heart Views*, vol. 14, no. 3, pp. 117–120, 2013.

[4] C.-W. Siu, M.-H. Jim, H.-H. Ho et al., "Recurrent acute heart failure caused by sliding hiatus hernia," *Postgraduate Medical Journal*, vol. 81, no. 954, pp. 268-269, 2005.

[5] M. E. Josephson, *Clinical cardiac electrophysiology: techniques and interpretations*, Lippincott Williams & Wilkins, Philadelphia, PA, 4th ed. edition, 2008.

[6] N. G. Kounis, G. M. Zavras, P. J. Papadaki et al., "Diaphragmatic herniation of the large bowel associated with unusual clinical and electrocardiographic presentation," *The British Journal of Clinical Practice*, vol. 50, no. 1, pp. 54-55, 1996.

[7] A. Patel, R. Shah, S. Nadavaram, and A. Aggarwal, "Hiatal hernia squeezing the heart to flutter," *The American Journal of Emergency Medicine*, vol. 32, no. 4, pp. 392.e1–392.e2, 2014.

[8] K. S. W. Siew, M. P. Tan, I. N. Hilmi, and A. Loch, "Swallow syncope: a case report and review of literature," *BMC Cardiovascular Disorders*, vol. 19, no. 1, p. 191, 2019.

9

Cardiac Arrest during Transesophageal Echocardiogram (TEE) due to Acute Right Ventricular Failure

Cooper B. Kersey,[1] Fitsumberhan Medhane,[2] Andrew M. Pattock,[1] Linda Liu,[1] Gary Huang,[2] Abhijit V. Lele,[3] and Younghoon Kwon[2]

[1]*University of Washington, Department of Medicine, USA*
[2]*University of Washington, Division of Cardiology, USA*
[3]*University of Washington, Department of Anesthesiology and Pain Medicine, USA*

Correspondence should be addressed to Cooper B. Kersey; kerseycb@uw.edu

Academic Editor: Christopher S. Snyder

The case of a patient who suffered cardiac arrest while undergoing transesophageal echocardiography (TEE) is presented here. A 75-year-old man with moderate right ventricular (RV) dysfunction and pulmonary hypertension became bradycardic and hypotensive after receiving propofol for procedural sedation. His profound hypotension ultimately led to a pulseless electrical activity (PEA) cardiac arrest. TEE images captured immediately prior to cardiac arrest show a severely dilated and hypokinetic RV, consistent with acute right ventricular failure. This case highlights the potentially fatal consequences of procedural sedation in patients with RV dysfunction and pulmonary hypertension.

1. Introduction

The sedation administered during transesophageal echocardiography (TEE) can have profound effects on intraprocedural hemodynamics, particularly in patients with underlying right ventricular (RV) dysfunction or pulmonary hypertension. Current echocardiographic practice guidelines offer no specific recommendations on whether the performing cardiologist or an anesthesiologist should provide sedation for TEE, which can lead to variable types and levels of sedation during procedures [1]. This report demonstrates a case of cardiac arrest during TEE in the setting of RV dysfunction and pulmonary hypertension and briefly reviews TEE-related complications and fatality rates reported in the literature.

2. Case Description

The patient was a 75-year-old man with a body mass index of 23.4 kg/m^2 and an American Society of Anesthesiologists (ASA) class of three. He had a history of end-stage renal disease on hemodialysis and was initially transferred to our hospital from an outside facility for subacute functional decline and encephalopathy. His admission work-up was notable for a leukocytosis of 12,800 cells/μL, *Enterococcus faecalis* bacteremia, and bilateral pleural effusions. His 12-lead electrocardiogram showed sinus rhythm with first-degree atrioventricular block and a right bundle branch block. The patient was started on broad spectrum antibiotics for bacteremia and later narrowed to ampicillin. Repeat blood cultures were negative. On hospital day one, the patient underwent a transthoracic echocardiogram which demonstrated a left ventricular ejection fraction of 45-50% with global systolic dysfunction, moderate RV dysfunction, mild pulmonary hypertension with a pulmonary artery systolic pressure (PASP) of 41 mmHg, and no visible valvular vegetations.

The patient underwent thoracentesis of the right sided pleural effusion, and bacterial cultures of the pleural fluid grew *Enterococcus Faecalis*. Given this multifocal enterococcus infection, TEE was pursued.

On hospital day nine, the patient underwent TEE under monitored anesthesia care. The anesthesia service was

Table 1: The rates of common complications of TEE documented in the literature from a multicenter retrospective review of over 10,000 patients undergoing TEE (Daniel et al.) and a meta-analysis (Côté et al.).

Complication	Frequency	Source of data
Nonsustained ventricular tachycardia	0.03%	Daniel et al. [3]
Transient atrial fibrillation	0.03%	Daniel et al. [3]
Third degree heart block	0.01%	Daniel et al. [3]
Angina	0.01%	Daniel et al. [3]
Cardiac arrest	0.01%	Daniel et al. [3]
Hypoxemia ($SpO_2 < 90\%$)	18%	Côté et al. [2]
Bronchospasm	0.5%	Daniel et al. [3]
Mortality	0.1%	Daniel et al. [3]
Retching	39%	Côté et al. [2]
Esophageal perforation	0.1%	Côté et al. [2]

consulted due to pulmonary hypertension as per the institutional guideline. The patient was connected to standard monitoring as recommended by the ASA. Supplemental oxygen was provided by a face mask, with end-tidal carbon dioxide monitoring. The patient received a total of 70 mg of propofol administered over the first ten minutes of the procedure in boluses of 10 mg-20 mg. Hemodynamically, the patient's blood pressure at the beginning of the procedure was 140/50 mmHg with a pulse in the low 60 s. His blood pressure dropped precipitously after receiving propofol down to 60/40 mmHg fifteen minutes into the procedure. At that point, the patient became bradycardic and went into a PEA cardiac arrest. The TEE probe was withdrawn, and chest compressions were initiated under the advanced cardiac life support algorithm. The patient was intubated, and return of spontaneous circulation (ROSC) was achieved after four rounds of chest compressions and epinephrine administration. The patient's cardiac rhythm then deteriorated into ventricular fibrillation requiring defibrillation and further chest compressions. ROSC was achieved once again, and the patient was transferred to the intensive care unit. Upon review of the images captured by TEE at the onset of PEA arrest, it was noted that the RV was severely dilated with minimal contractile function, and a small pericardial effusion was found (Video 1). Due to the patient's critical condition, his family decided to transition him to comfort measures only.

3. Discussion

Cardiovascular complications from TEE have been documented to occur in 0.08% of cases and cardiac arrest in 1 : 10,000 cases [2, 3] (Table 1). The sedation administered during TEE poses risks particularly to patients with poor cardiac reserve who are sensitive to minor changes in hemodynamics. Determining the appropriate depth of sedation is made difficult by the trade-off between the level of sedation and the patient's tolerance of the TEE probe. If a patient is not sufficiently sedated, they are more likely to have a gag reflex and vagal response to intubation of the TEE probe. An excessive vagal response to the TEE probes can lead to profound vasodilation, systemic hypotension, and a decreased systemic venous return to the right ventricle [4, 5]. On the other hand, patients who are more deeply sedated tend to be more tolerant of the TEE probe but are at higher risk of the adverse hemodynamic and respiratory suppressant effects of the anesthetic agents [2, 4]. One meta-analysis of TEE complications found that hypoxemia (defined as oxygen saturation less than 90%) occurred in 18% of cases [2]. Transient hypoxemia induces pulmonary vasoconstriction, which increases RV afterload and diminishes RV stroke volume [6].

In this case, we suspect that the vasodilatory effects of the propofol led to a profound decrease in RV preload and hypotension. These hemodynamic changes were likely compounded by vagal stimulation of the TEE probe which further contributed to vasodilation and the reduction of RV preload. In a patient with moderate RV dysfunction and pulmonary hypertension, this likely triggered acute RV failure resulting in a PEA arrest (Figure 1). The ideal sedative for a short, minimally invasive procedure like TEE has a quick time to onset, minimal hemodynamic side effects, and a rapid recovery period [7]. Midazolam, fentanyl, ketamine, and propofol are common agents chosen for TEE. However, none of these agents possess all of the characteristics of an ideal sedative agent.

The advantages of using ketamine over propofol include preservation of airway reflexes, maintenance of spontaneous respirations, and sympathetic stimulation, which in turn may allow maintenance of cardiovascular stability. Disadvantages include increased oropharyngeal secretions and neurological side effects such as hallucinations [8]. Propofol, on the other hand, may significantly reduce sympathetic nerve activity and norepinephrine levels at different depths of sedation. These effects result in significant decreases in mean blood pressure of 9% and 18% at moderate and deep sedation, respectively, even in healthy volunteers. Additionally, propofol also reduces reflexive increases in sympathetic nerve activity [9]. Midazolam or fentanyl alone may be insufficient to provide adequate depth of anesthesia. The prevalence of dexmedetomidine use for TEE is unknown, but dexmedetomidine may cause a reduction in pharyngeal muscular tone and respiratory depression similar to propofol, in addition to bradycardia. Dexmedetomidine has been

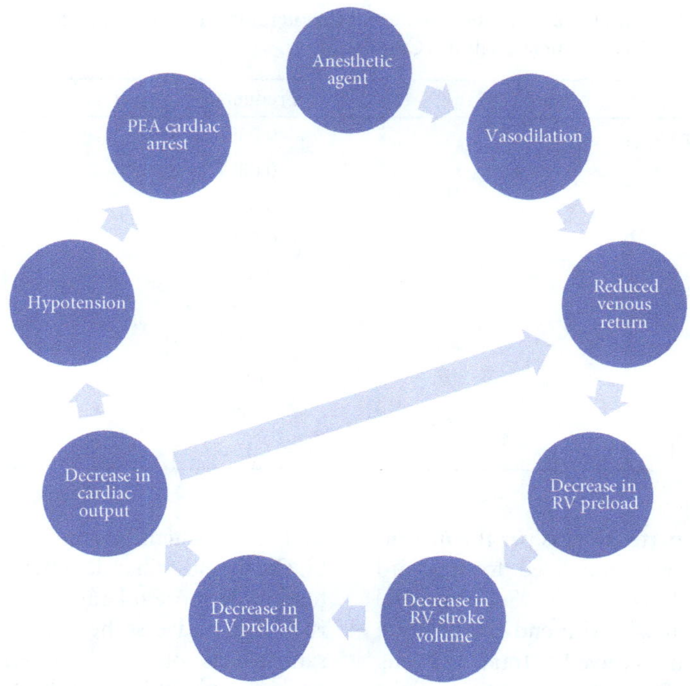

FIGURE 1: A visual representation of the vicious cycle of right ventricular failure that the vasodilatory effects of anesthetic agents can precipitate [15].

shown to provide satisfactory sedation levels, hemodynamic stability, short recovery time, and acceptable patient and practitioner satisfaction during TEE [10, 11].

In addition to understanding the cardiovascular side effects of sedatives, the proceduralist should also be aware of the risks of hypoxia and hypercarbia in precipitating RV dysfunction. Transient hypoxemia may be sufficient to initiate a vicious cycle of RV dysfunction. Similarly, in patients with a native airway undergoing sedation, hypercarbia is also likely not accurately measured despite the use of end-tidal carbon dioxide monitoring.

We present this case to raise awareness of the risks associated with deep sedation during TEE and illustrate the lack of society and institutional guidelines regarding the choice of sedative agents. The ASA score is a validated measure of patients' intraprocedural risk and could be used to predict which patients undergoing TEE are more susceptible to the hemodynamic consequences of general anesthesia [12]. More research into what patient and procedural factors lead to patient morbidity and mortality during TEE is required to inform practice guidelines and ensure patient safety. Additionally, this case would have been an opportunity to implement TEE-guided CPR, which has been shown to be an efficacious way of monitoring resuscitation efforts in the emergency room setting [13].

Based on this case and available literature, we propose that preprocedural evaluation of patients undergoing TEE includes a detailed review of any contemporaneous TTE data. Data suggestive of pulmonary hypertension with or without RV dysfunction should significantly raise the concern for adverse procedural events. The risk of hypotension, hypoxemia, and hypercarbia need to be balanced with the expectation of TEE tolerance and safety, and this should be discussed between the anesthesiologist and cardiologist as well as during the informed consent process. Monitored anesthesia care or general anesthesia with an endotracheally intubated patient may carry unique risks and benefits and thus should be individualized to the patient and the procedure. In patients identified to be at high risk of adverse events from the hemodynamic effects of propofol, topical anesthetics, ketamine, or midazolam may be useful adjuncts. Alternatively, non-propofol-based anesthesia, such as with dexmedetomidine, may be suitable for certain patients. Lastly, the proceduralist must be familiar with the terminology related to monitored anesthesia care, conscious sedation, and general anesthesia. In any given patient, the depth of anesthesia may vary significantly from light sedation to general anesthesia [14].

This case demonstrates the potentially fatal consequences of procedural sedation in patients with RV dysfunction and pulmonary hypertension. Clinicians should be cognizant of the hemodynamic effects of sedative agents, and institutions should work to create evidence-based criteria to decide if patients undergoing TEE will receive moderate sedation, monitored anesthesia care, or general anesthesia.

References

[1] M. D. Cheitlin, W. F. Armstrong, G. P. Aurigemma et al., "ACC/AHA/ASE 2003 guideline update for the clinical application of echocardiography: summary article: a report of the American College of Cardiology/American Heart Association Task Force on Practice Guidelines (ACC/AHA/ASE Committee to Update the 1997 Guidelines for the Clinical Application of Echocardiography)," *Circulation*, vol. 108, no. 9, pp. 1146–1162, 2003.

[2] G. Côté and A. Denault, "Transesophageal echocardiography-related complications," *Canadian Journal of Anaesthesia*, vol. 55, no. 9, pp. 622–647, 2008.

[3] W. G. Daniel, R. Erbel, W. Kasper et al., "Safety of transesophageal echocardiography. A multicenter survey of 10,419 examinations," *Circulation*, vol. 83, no. 3, pp. 817–821, 1991.

[4] S. K. Mathur and P. Singh, "Transoesophageal echocardiography related complications," *Indian Journal of Anaesthesia*, vol. 53, no. 5, pp. 567–574, 2009.

[5] B. K. Khandheria, J. B. Seward, and A. J. Tajik, "Transesophageal echocardiography," *Mayo Clinic Proceedings*, vol. 69, no. 9, pp. 856–863, 1994.

[6] K. J. Dunham-Snary, D. Wu, E. A. Sykes et al., "Hypoxic pulmonary vasoconstriction: from molecular mechanisms to medicine," *Chest*, vol. 151, no. 1, pp. 181–192, 2017.

[7] C. R. M. Barends, A. R. Absalom, and M. Struys, "Drug selection for ambulatory procedural sedation," *Current Opinion in Anaesthesiology*, vol. 31, no. 6, pp. 673–678, 2018.

[8] R. J. Strayer and L. S. Nelson, "Adverse events associated with ketamine for procedural sedation in adults," *The American Journal of Emergency Medicine*, vol. 26, no. 9, pp. 985–1028, 2008.

[9] T. J. Ebert, "Sympathetic and hemodynamic effects of moderate and deep sedation with propofol in humans," *Anesthesiology*, vol. 103, no. 1, pp. 20–24, 2005.

[10] A. Alizadehasl, A. Sadeghpour, Z. Totonchi, R. Azarfarin, S. Rahimi, and A. Hendiani, "Comparison of sedation between dexmedetomidine and propofol during transesophageal echocardiography: a randomized controlled trial," *Annals Of Cardiac Anaesthesia*, vol. 22, no. 3, pp. 285–290, 2019.

[11] J. W. Jung, G. C. Go, S. Y. Jeon et al., "Dexmedetomidine sedation for transesophageal echocardiography during percutaneous atrial septal defect closure in adult," *Journal of Medical Sciences*, vol. 29, no. 6, pp. 1456–1458, 2013.

[12] A. Sankar, S. R. Johnson, W. S. Beattie, G. Tait, and D. N. Wijeysundera, "Reliability of the American Society of Anesthesiologists physical status scale in clinical practice," *British Journal of Anaesthesia*, vol. 113, no. 3, pp. 424–432, 2014.

[13] J. Fair 3rd, M. P. Mallin, A. Adler et al., "Transesophageal echocardiography during cardiopulmonary resuscitation is associated with shorter compression pauses compared with transthoracic echocardiography," *Annals of Emergency Medicine*, vol. 73, no. 6, pp. 610–616, 2019.

[14] J. Apfelbaum, J. Gross, R. Connis et al., "Practice guidelines for moderate procedural sedation and analgesia 2018: a report by the American Society of Anesthesiologists Task Force on moderate procedural sedation and analgesia, the American Association of Oral and Maxillofacial Surgeons, American College of Radiology, American dental association, American Society of Dentist Anesthesiologists, and Society of Interventional Radiology," *Anesthesiology*, vol. 128, no. 3, pp. 437–479, 2018.

[15] F. de Wit, A. L. van Vliet, R. B. de Wilde et al., "The effect of propofol on haemodynamics: cardiac output, venous return, mean systemic filling pressure, and vascular resistances," *British Journal of Anaesthesia*, vol. 116, no. 6, pp. 784–789, 2016.

10

Surgical Strategy for Huge Right Coronary Artery Aneurysm Combined with Left Ventricular Fistula

Takafumi Terada, Yoshimori Araki, Akihiro Kobayashi, and Osamu Kawaguchi

Department of Cardiac Surgery, JA Aichi Koseiren Toyota Kosei Hospital, Aichi, Japan

Correspondence should be addressed to Takafumi Terada; takafumi_terada0828@yahoo.co.jp

Academic Editor: Antonio de Padua Mansur

Coronary artery aneurysms combined with left ventricular fistulas are rare; coronary revascularization strategy after coronary artery aneurysm resection is complex in such cases. We report the surgical repair of a giant right coronary artery aneurysm with a fistula in the left ventricle in a 79-year-old woman diagnosed with an aneurysm 50 mm in diameter. Surgical repair included resection of the coronary artery aneurysm, coronary artery bypass grafting to the posterior descending artery, and isolation of reconstructed right coronary circulation from the fistula. The postoperative course was uneventful; postoperative coronary angiography revealed a patent bypass graft unconnected to the left ventricle.

1. Introduction

Coronary artery aneurysm (CAA), defined as local dilatation of the coronary artery more than 150% of the referred coronary artery, is a rare condition detected in 0.3% to 4.9% of patients who undergo coronary angiography [1, 2].

Coronary artery fistula (CAF), defined as an abnormal direct connection between the coronary artery and cardiac chamber or other great vessels, is also a rare anomaly, with an estimated incidence of 0.002% in the normal population [3, 4].

The coexistence of CAA and CAF to the left ventricle (LV) is extremely rare. In this case, we considered CAA as an indicator of operative repair since its diameter was >50 mm. However, the surgical strategy of coronary reconstruction after aneurysm resection is complicated if closure of the fistula to the LV is impossible.

2. Case Report

A 79-year-old woman, who had been diagnosed with right coronary artery- (RCA-) LV fistula by coronary angiography 20 years ago, was transferred to our hospital for evaluation of an RCA aneurysm revealed by ultrasound cardiography (Figure 1(a)). The fistula flowed into the LV underneath the posterior leaflet of the mitral valve (Figure 1(b)). Although she did not have any symptom, she also had chronic atrial fibrillation. Multidetector computed tomography (MDCT) revealed a giant RCA aneurysm and an abnormal connection between the terminal RCA and LV (Figures 1(c) and 1(d)). Although she was asymptomatic, surgical treatment was recommended because the aneurysm was large; its diameter was 50.8 mm.

3. Operative Procedure

The operation was performed via a median sternotomy. A large RCA aneurysm in the right atrium was observed after pericardiotomy (Figure 2). At the beginning of the surgery, the RCA juts distal to the CAA and encircled with vascular tape. By monitoring transesophageal echocardiography, the inferior wall motion decreased after occlusion of the RCA. Once a graftable terminal branch of the posterior descending artery (PDA) was detected, we decided to create a coronary bypass.

Surgical repair was performed under cardiac arrest with cardiopulmonary bypass. Cardiac arrest was achieved by routine antegrade cardioplegia infusion and additional antegrade infusion with RCA occlusion.

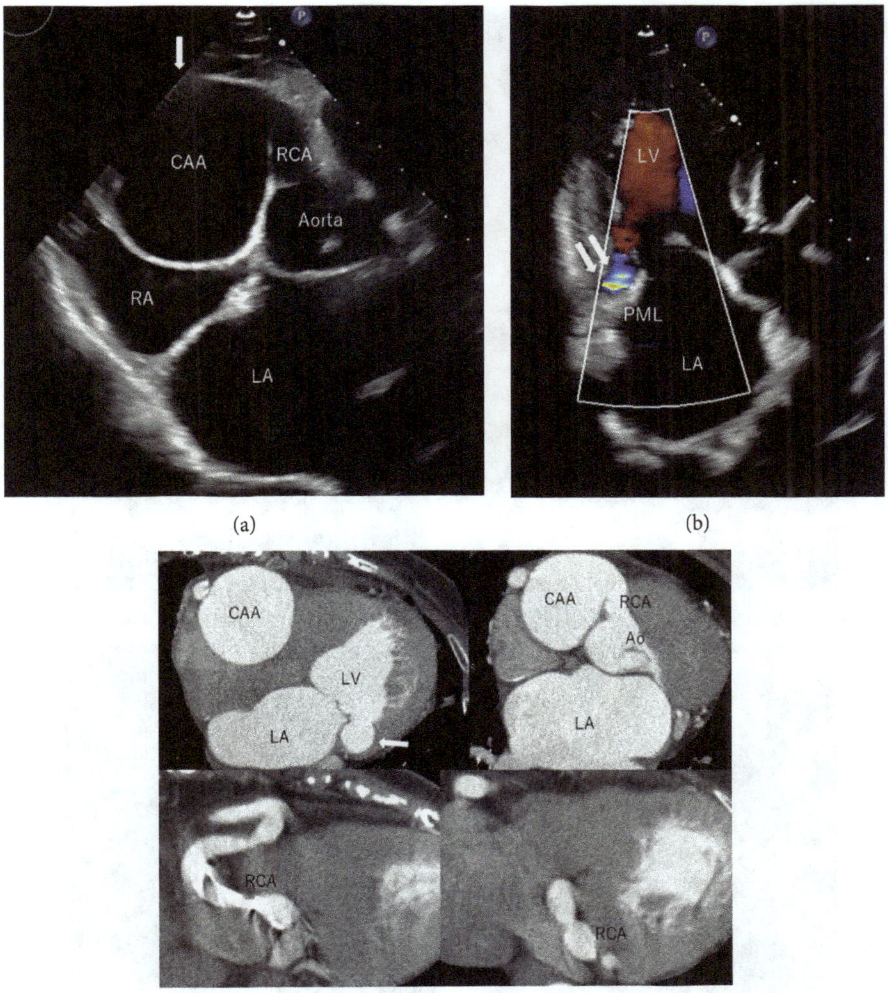

FIGURE 1: (a, b) Preoperative ultrasound echocardiography. CAA (↓) CAF (↓↓). (c) MDCT of coronary artery. CAF (↓). CAA: coronary artery aneurysm; RCA: right coronary artery; RA: right atrium; LA: left atrium; LV: left ventricle; PML: posterior mitral reflet; Ao: ascending aorta.

The Cryo-Maze procedure was performed via a left and right atriotomy. Although an ostium of the RCA-LV fistula was detected behind the posterior mitral leaflet, closure of the fistula seemed impossible or would be incomplete because of infraventricular structures such as the chordae tendineae.

The CAA was incised, and the proximal ostium was closed directly. A coronary artery bypass to the PDA was created using the saphenous vein. (Figures 3(a)–3(d)) The proximal end of the grafted PDA was ligated to avoid stealing to the left ventricle.

The distal end of the RCA aneurysm was ligated from the outside, and direct closure was added from the inside.

Cardiopulmonary bypass support was easily weaned, and the postoperative course was uneventful except for atrial fibrillation was sustained. Postoperative coronary angiography revealed a patent bypass graft without flow into the LV (Figure 4(a)). Postoperative coronary MDCT revealed a partially thrombosed residual RCA connected to the fistula (Figure 4(b)).

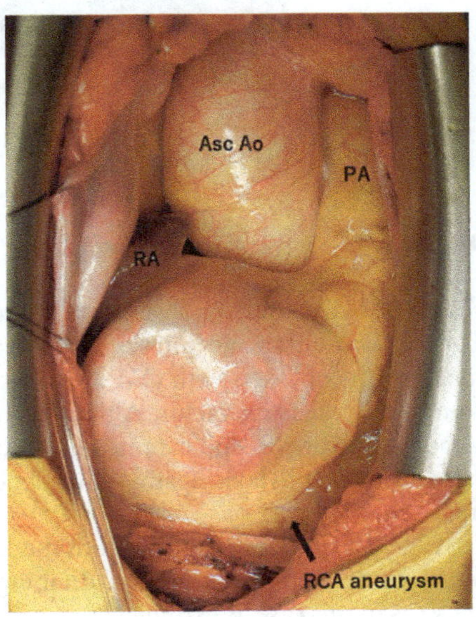

FIGURE 2: Intraoperative view. asc Ao: ascending aorta; PA: pulmonary artery.

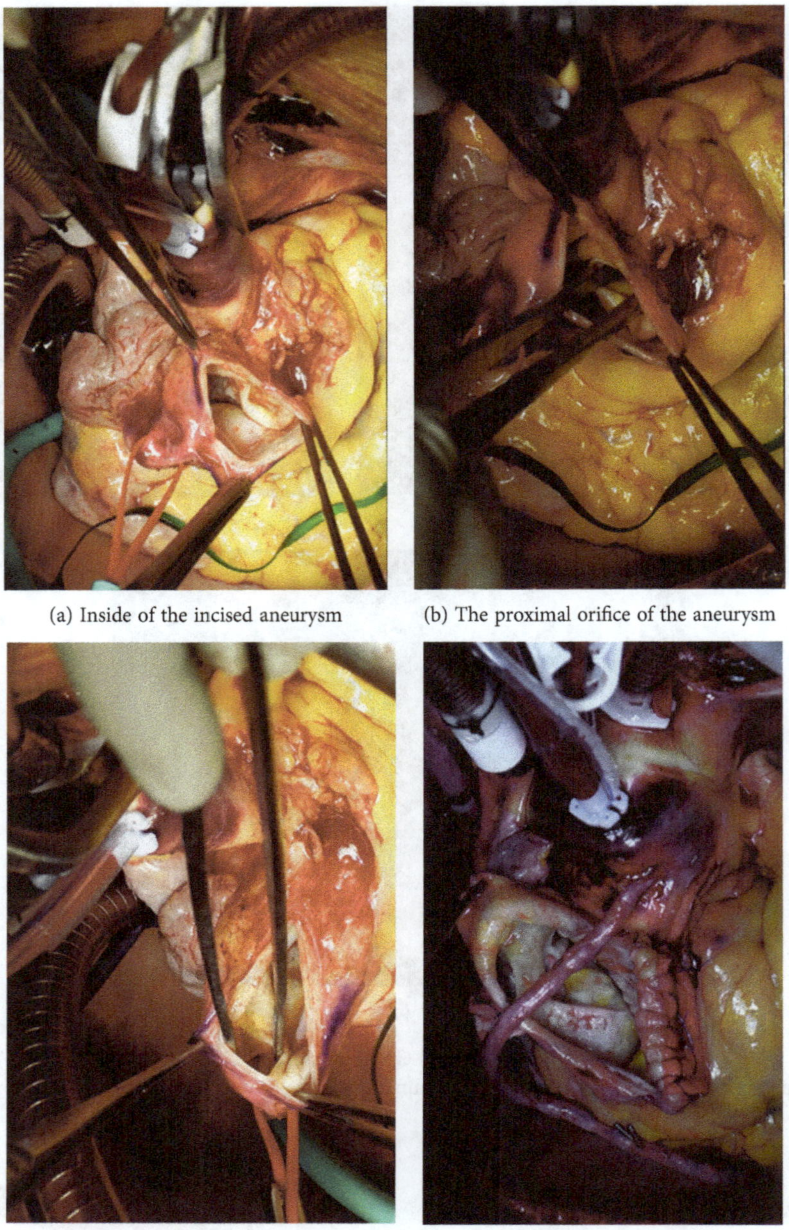

(a) Inside of the incised aneurysm

(b) The proximal orifice of the aneurysm

(c) The distal orifice of the aneurysm

(d) Closed orifices and bypass graft

Figure 3: (a–d) Intraoperative images during the procedure.

4. Comment

The main cause of CAA is atherosclerosis, followed by congenital inflammation, iatrogenic injury, and infection [5]. Most previous reports of CAAs with CAFs report congenital malformation as the causative factor. Although there is no consensus about the surgical indication for CAA, the aim of this treatment is prophylaxis against thromboembolism and rupture.

As for CAFs, 52% of them originate from the RCA, with the right heart being the most common draining site [6]. CAF to the LV, as in this case, is extremely rare and accounts for 4% of CAFs [7]. Volume overloading due to shunt flow, aneurysmal dilatation of the coronary artery, ischemic symptoms due to coronary steal, and so on are considered indications for treatment [4].

Moreover, the cause of our patient's CAA did not seem to be congenital as no aneurysm was detected during previous examinations. The RCA was exposed to antegrade hyperblood flow and direct retrograde systolic blood pressure via CAF, which might induce aneurysmal dilatation of the RCA and diffuse RCA ectasia. The influence of atherosclerotic degeneration could not be ruled out given her age; however, it was not detected in the histopathological examination of the resected aneurysm.

As for her atrial fibrillation, its cause might be CAA compression of the atrium. However, it might be the result of left atrial dilatation caused by similar hemodynamics to

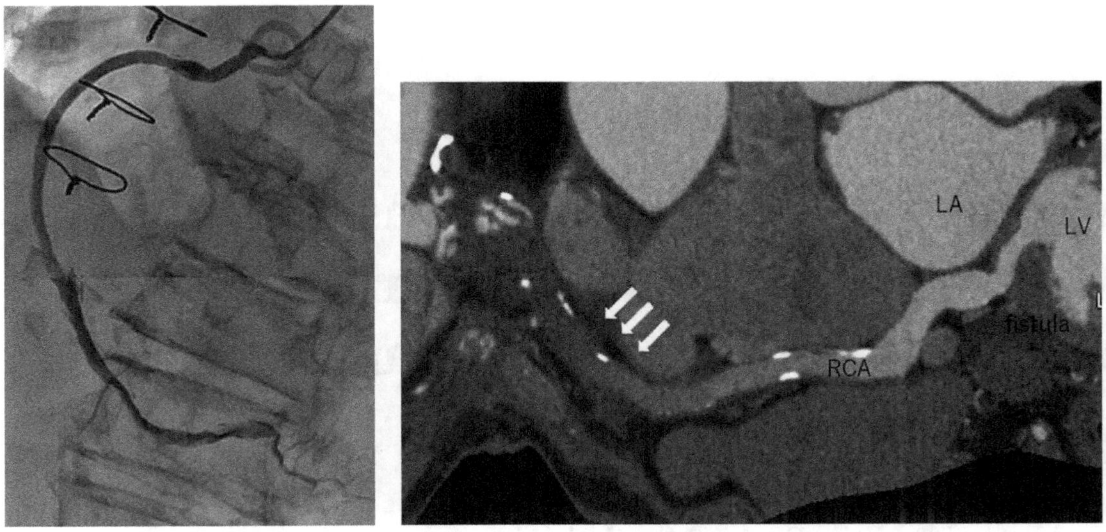

(a) (b)

FIGURE 4: (a, b) Postoperative coronary angiography (a) and MDCT (b).

aortic regurgitation. The latter more likely to be the cause of her atrial fibrillation because her left atrium diameter was 63.0 mm in diameter preoperatively and her atrial fibrillation persisted after resection of the CAA.

Ideally, surgical correction of this anomaly should include resection of the aneurysm, reconstruction of the coronary circulation, and closure of the fistula [8]. As the contraction of the inferior wall decreased after RCA obstruction and a reasonably sized PDA was detected, a coronary artery bypass was created. If no graft vessel can be detected, systolic retrograde blood flow via the fistula may be the only remaining blood supply to the RCA. Furthermore, antegrade cardioplegia infusion with RCA obstruction was added in order to induce cardiac arrest for fear of inadequate distribution due to steal to emptying the LV via the fistula.

Since it was difficult to approach the fistula and the blood supply to the atrioventricular node artery might depend on direct blood flow from the LV in our case, closure of the fistula was finally abandoned. We investigated the prognosis of residual RCA with fistula; however, postoperative coronary MDCT revealed partially thrombosed residual RCA with a fistula. As the residual RCA close to the fistula is exposed to systemic pressure from the LV, careful long-term follow-up is essential for detection of residual fistula and RCA ectasia.

Consent

The patient gave a written informed consent.

Acknowledgments

We would like to thank Editage (http://www.editage.com) for English language editing.

References

[1] P. S. Swaye, L. D. Fisher, P. Litwin et al., "Aneurysmal coronary artery disease," *Circulation*, vol. 67, no. 1, pp. 134–138, 1983.

[2] B. Lima, S. K. Varma, and J. E. Lowe, "Nonsurgical management of left main coronary artery aneurysms: report of 2 cases and review of the literature," *Texas Heart Institute Journal*, vol. 33, no. 3, pp. 376–379, 2006.

[3] P. Angelini, "Coronary artery anomalies—current clinical issues: definitions, classification, incidence, clinical relevance, and treatment guidelines," *Texas Heart Institute Journal*, vol. 29, no. 4, pp. 271–278, 2002.

[4] L. Luo, S. Kebede, S. Wu, and G. A. Stouffer, "Coronary artery fistulae," *The American Journal of the Medical Sciences*, vol. 332, no. 2, pp. 79–84, 2006.

[5] M. Syed and M. Lesch, "Coronary artery aneurysm: a review," *Progress in Cardiovascular Diseases*, vol. 40, no. 1, pp. 77–84, 1997.

[6] J. E. Lowe, H. M. Oldham Jr., and D. C. Sabiston Jr., "Surgical management of congenital coronary artery fistulas," *Annals of Surgery*, vol. 194, no. 4, pp. 373–380, 1981.

[7] S. A. Said, "Current characteristics of congenital coronary artery fistulas in adults: a decade of global experience," *World Journal of Cardiology*, vol. 3, no. 8, pp. 267–277, 2011.

[8] C. V. Mangukia, "Coronary artery fistula," *The Annals of Thoracic Surgery*, vol. 93, no. 6, pp. 2084–2092, 2012.

11

Incidental Finding and Endovascular Repair of a Left Internal Mammary Artery Aneurysm following a Multivessel Coronary Artery Bypass Graft

Osayi Lawani,[1] Jiries Ganim,[2] and Rick Ganim[3]

[1]*HCA Houston Healthcare-Kingwood, USA*
[2]*University of Southern California, USA*
[3]*Vital Heart & Vein, USA*

Correspondence should be addressed to Osayi Lawani; osayi.lawani@hcahealthcare.com

Academic Editor: Filippo M. Sarullo

True aneurysms discovered within the internal mammary artery are extremely rare and typically have an asymptomatic occurrence. Their presentation and management have also been variable due to their low incidence, decreased detection, or lack of documentation. They have a high risk for morbidity or mortality as they can possibly rupture with increasing size and thus become life-threatening. Coronary CT angiography is the most definitive test for confirming and finding complications related to the aneurysm. With an increase in the aging population and advancement in the techniques used in coronary artery bypass grafting, it is likely that the rate of recorded occurrence of aneurysms and pseudoaneurysms will increase. Endovascular repair is currently the most favored treatment modality. In this report, we describe a case of a 74-year-old male who was incidentally found to have a left internal mammary artery aneurysm following complaints of chest pain related to another nearly occluded grafted vessel. To the best of our knowledge, and following an extensive literature review, this is likely the first documented case of a true aneurysm found within a left internal mammary artery bypass graft. The patient recovered well following placement of a covered stent; however, upon follow-up one year later, he was found to have stenosis of the same vessel, which was subsequently treated without further complication.

1. Introduction

Aneurysms manifesting from the internal mammary artery (IMA) are a very rare occurrence. Although they are usually small, these aneurysms will have an increased risk of rupture which can be life-threatening [1]. Other possible complications include hemothorax, thromboembolism, compression of adjacent structures, myocardial infarction, and possible death. Aneurysms in the IMA are typically found incidentally on cardiac angiography. Characteristically, these aneurysms grow slowly and silently, making this a highly underdiagnosed disease process [2].

The left IMA (LIMA) is the vessel used most to bypass a significant stenosis of the left anterior descending (LAD) artery [3]. Advantages of using the LIMA over a saphenous vein graph are long-term patency and survival rates greater than 90% beyond 10 years and decreased postoperative mortality [4]. The exact cause of an IMA aneurysm is unknown, however, it can be traumatic or iatrogenic in origin, caused by progressive atherosclerosis, or due to connective tissue disorders such as Marfan, Loeys-Dietz, and Ehlers-Danlos syndromes [5]. In this report, we present a case of an elderly male who was found to have a large aneurysm located in a LIMA to LAD artery graft following a coronary bypass procedure 6 months prior.

2. Case History

A 74-year-old male with a past medical history of coronary artery disease with cardiac stenting, peripheral artery disease with femoral popliteal bypass, hypertension, hyperlipidemia, diabetes mellitus, chronic kidney disease, deep vein thrombosis, and distant history of heavy tobacco use, presented to a local emergency department with complaints of symptoms that were suggestive of unstable angina. Cardiology was consulted and a left heart catheterization was performed.

The left main had mild diffuse plaquing. The LAD was of large caliber, and in the midsection at the takeoff of a large diagonal branch, there were stents in the artery and in the ostium of the diagonal branch, which had about 60% and 90% in-stent restenosis, respectively. The left circumflex artery was small in caliber, and in the proximal section there was 85% stenosis. The ostium of the first obtuse marginal branch had 70% stenosis. The right coronary artery was occluded in its midsegment, and the distal coronary system was able to perfuse left-to-right collateral circulation. Finally, the left internal mammary artery was widely patent. Given the multivessel coronary artery disease and small caliber of the left circumflex artery, it was recommended that the patient be evaluated by cardiothoracic surgery for a coronary artery bypass graft (CABG).

Six months later, the patient presented to his cardiologist with complaints of intermittent episodes of nitroglycerin-responsive, substernal chest pain that radiated down both arms with strenuous activity. The patient had undergone a six-vessel CABG five months earlier without any residual complications to date. Home medications included dual antiplatelet therapy, antihypertensives, antianginal agents, and a lipid-lowering agent. An electrocardiogram showed normal sinus rhythm, occasional premature atrial contractions, and no ischemic changes. Laboratory results showed elevated troponin I. He was subsequently admitted to the hosptial for cardiac catheterization.

The distal left main had 40-50% stenosis just proximal to the bifurcation of the LAD and left circumflex arteries. The proximal-to-mid portion of the LAD continued to have 60% in-stent restenosis. The ostium of the diagonal branch also continued to have 90% in-stent restenosis. The proximal portion of the left circumflex had increased stenosis from 85% to 99%, and the midsegment was now occluded. The right coronary artery remained occluded in its midsegment with collateral circulation. A saphenous vein graft to the right coronary artery had 50% stenosis. A saphenous vein graft to the obtuse marginal branch in the mid-to-distal segment had 95% stenosis. A LIMA graph to the LAD was patent; however, there was a large aneurysm within the LIMA with TIMI-3 blood flow (Figure 1). The culprit vessel causing the intermittent episodes of chest pain was felt to be the saphenous vein graph to the obtuse marginal branch, and a drug-eluting stent was placed.

As for the large aneurysm found in the LIMA, it was decided that it would either be treated by surgical repair or by percutaneous intervention at a later date. The patient was discharged home to continue dual antiplatelet therapy and start aggressive blood pressure and lipid control. Three weeks later, the patient returned to the hospital to undergo repair of the large aneurysm found in the LIMA to LAD bypass graft. Following multiple discussions with and evaluation by cardiothoracic surgery, it was concluded that the patient would best benefit from placing a covered stent to

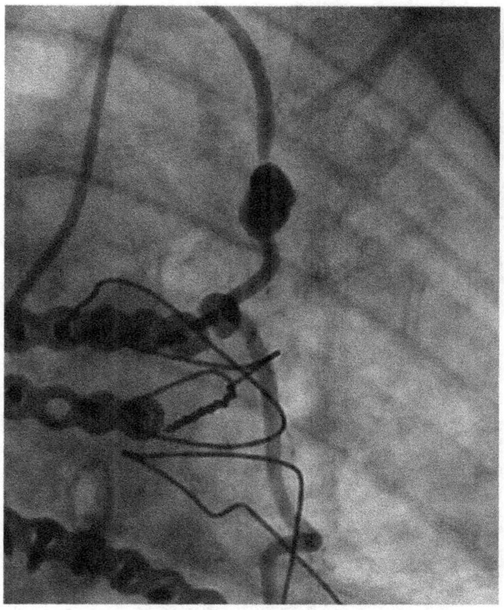

FIGURE 1: Large aneurysm in the left internal mammary artery to the left anterior descending artery bypass graft.

repair the aneurysm. Intravascular ultrasound was used to determine the size and length of the lesion. A 2.8×19 mm covered stent was placed in the midsegment of the aneurysm (Figure 2). Postintervention angiography showed TIMI-3 blood flow with no residual aneurysm or stenosis (Figures 3 and 4). The patient was discharged the following day and instructed to continue dual antiplatelet therapy and aggressive blood pressure and lipid control.

One year later, the patient presented to the hospital with complaints of chest pain and was diagnosed with non-ST elevation myocardial infarction. During cardiac catheterization, he was found to have approximately 75% in-stent restenosis of the LIMA covered stent that was located in the midsegment of the graft. There continued to be complete resolution of the prior aneurysm. Repair within the stenosed section was performed with a 3.0×20 mm drug-eluting stent. Postintervention showed no residual stenosis and TIMI-3 blood flow. Ultimately, the patient was discharged home to continue lifelong dual antiplatelet therapy with aggressive blood pressure and lipid control.

3. Discussion

Arterial aneurysms usually occur in elderly men, as well as in individuals that have uncontrolled high blood pressure [6]. They are also typically asymptomatic, small, and do not pose a significant health risk [6]. The most common clinical presentation of a symptomatic graft aneurysm is chest pain and hemoptysis [7].

3.1. Epidemiology. A modest number of reported cases of these aneurysms have been documented since 1978, with 51.9 years noted as a mean age of occurrence (Table 1) [8]. Aneurysms and pseudoaneurysms found in the IMA are seldomly seen outside of ailments involving hereditary diseases, infections, iatrogenic causes, vasculitis, persistent atherosclerosis, or physical trauma [9]. It is an increased likelihood that

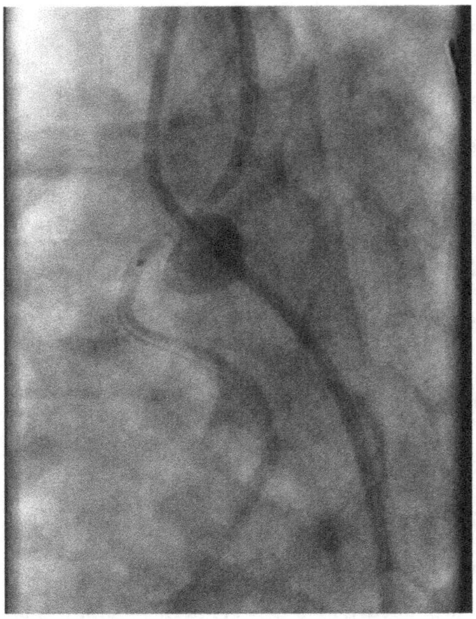

FIGURE 2: Covered stent placement in the midsegment of a large left internal mammary artery bypass graft aneurysm.

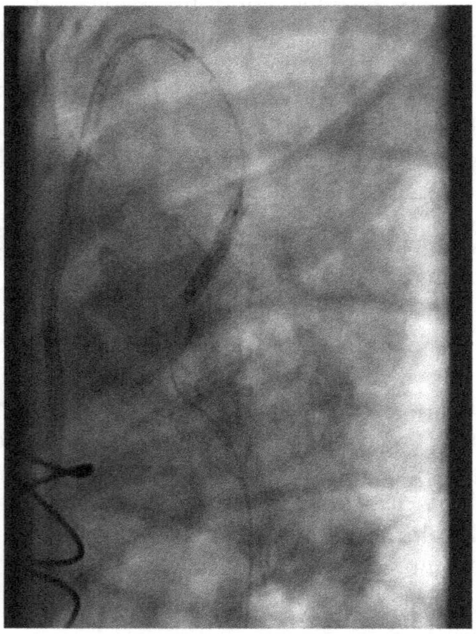

FIGURE 3: Stent placement within the left internal mammary artery bypass graft.

graft endothelial dysfunction, atherosclerotic changes, and changes in the orientation of the medial smooth muscle have some role in late aneurysm development [9].

IMAs are fundamentally ideal for use during bypass grafting due to a decreased tendency for spasms and reduced development of atherosclerosis [4]. Procedurally, the LIMA is removed from the chest wall and the proximal end remains attached to the subclavian artery, with the distal end newly connected to the LAD distal to the site of occlusion (Figure 5) [4]. One theory suggests that skeletonization of the IMA to preserve sternal blood perfusion in fact deprives the grafted artery of possible long-term sustainability because it adversely affects its resistance to atherosclerosis by affecting its original nerve supply, vasa vasorum, and lymphatic drainage [10]. With this theory, it may be a disadvantage to perform grafting with this method in comparison to using pedicled grafting or covered stents in a person with a known history of severe atherosclerosis [10].

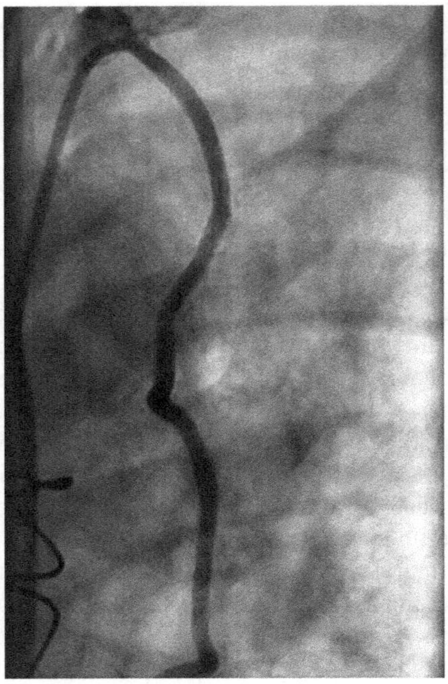

FIGURE 4: Postintervention angiography showing no residual aneurysm or stenosis in the left internal mammary artery bypass graft.

3.2. Causes. The IMA's pregrafting location adjacent to the sternum provides increased susceptibility to penetrating injury, blunt chest trauma, and iatrogenic injury [6]. A few case reports have described the existence of these aneurysms following pacemaker lead placement or a complicated central venous catheter placement [11]. An idiopathic IMA aneurysm without a recent medical history to explain its occurrence is extremely rare [11]. IMA aneurysms can be classified into various groups such as early versus late presentation [12].

Early IMA graft aneurysms may be due to tension at the site of anastomosis or may be related to an implanted graft infection. Other causes include technical errors during anastomosis, intimal hyperplasia, direct trauma from a median sternotomy, or from atheroma formation [11]. It is likely that the patient in this case developed a LIMA aneurysm in a short time following his CABG due to iatrogenic trauma related to grafting. Late graft aneurysms are likely secondary to progressive or accelerated atherosclerotic degeneration that is due to patient medication noncompliance or resistance to treatment. IMA grafts, however, are usually resistant to the formation of atherosclerosis, which contributes to longer patency rates when compared to subclavian vein grafts [4].

3.3. Diagnosis. Aneurysms that are symptomatic pose a challenge diagnostically because they may present as congestive heart failure or acute coronary syndrome [12]. Having an

TABLE 1: Previously reported artery aneurysms [8].

Study (year)	Location	Etiology	Management	Discovery
Otter and Stam [5] (1978)	Left internal mammary artery	Unknown	Left lateral thoracotomy and ligation	"Coin lesion" on chest X-ray
Chan and Fermanis [1] (1995)	Left internal mammary artery	Unknown	Angiographic embolization	Spontaneous hemothorax
Kugai and Chibana [8] (1999)	Left internal thoracic artery	Atherosclerosis	Internal thoracic artery aneurysmectomy and reconstruction	"Angina"
Lindblom et al. [14] (2013)	Left internal thoracic artery	Unknown	Endovascular coiling	Left-sided shoulder pain radiating to chest
Heyn et al. [15] (2014)	Left internal mammary artery	Thrombotic obliterated aneurysm	Open surgical resection	Preoperative chest X-ray
Present case (2018)	Left internal mammary artery	Iatrogenic trauma during bypass grafting	Covered stent	Incidental finding during cardiac catheterization

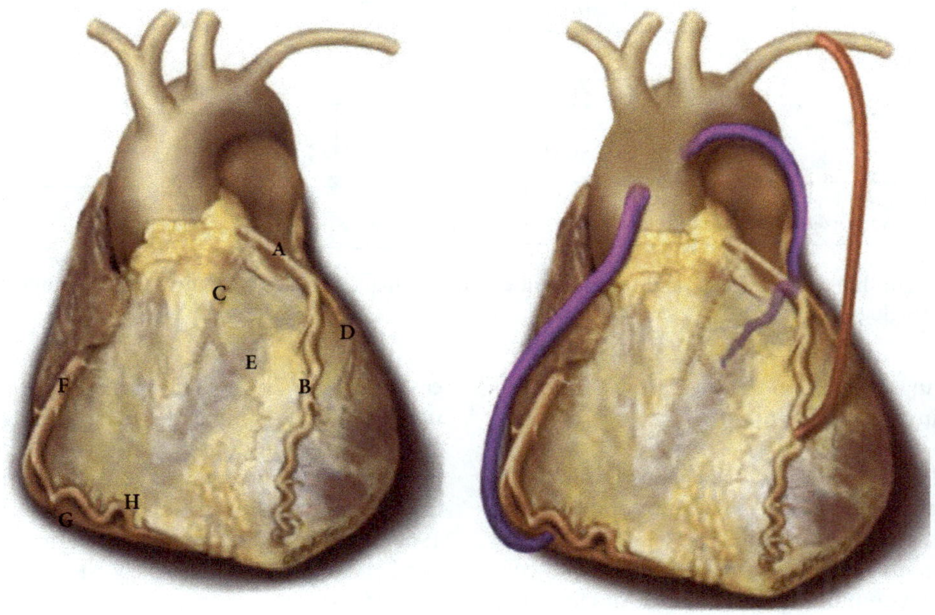

(a) (b)

FIGURE 5: (a) Normal anatomy of the coronary arteries: (A) left coronary artery, (B) left anterior descending artery, (C) left circumflex artery, (D) diagonal artery, (E) obtuse marginal branch of the left circumflex artery, (F) right coronary artery, (G) posterior descending artery, and (H) acute marginal branch of the right coronary artery. (b) Left internal mammary artery graft from its origin at the subclavian artery proximally and grafted to the left anterior descending artery distally (in red) [4]. This figure is reproduced from Frazier, A., Qureshi, F., Read, K. M., Gilkeson, R. C., Poston, R. S., & White, C. S. (2005). Coronary Artery Bypass Grafts: Assessment with Multidetector CT in the Early and Late Postoperative Settings. Radiographics, 25(4), 881-896 (under the Creative Commons Attribution License/public domain).

asymptomatic clinical course, no current guidelines for screening, initial presentation of sudden death from rupture, and incidental finding on diagnostic imaging are some reasons that may contribute to the underdiagnosing of this phenomena [2]. Late presentation is also another reason that these aneurysms are likely to be missed. About 90% of saphenous vein graph aneurysms manifest greater than five years following bypass surgery, with a mean time of about 13 years before final diagnosis [2].

Reportedly, about 50% of aneurysm cases can be observed incidentally on chest X-ray and will show a hilar or mediastinal mass [4]. In one report, a pulmonologist documented that a patient that was referred to him for an evaluation of a coin lesion noted on imaging in fact was discovered to have an IMA aneurysm [5]. Other diagnostic modalities include echocardiogram, contrast-enhanced thoracic CT scan, CT angiography, and MRI angiography. The definitive imaging test for confirming an aneurysm is coronary artery CT angiography, as it will show the extent of the aneurysm, local mass effect, and will note a change in the vasculature [7]. Findings may be obscured if there is a mural thrombus involved [13]. In coming years, increased early identification of bypass aneurysms will likely be reported due to continuous improvement of long-term outcomes following coronary

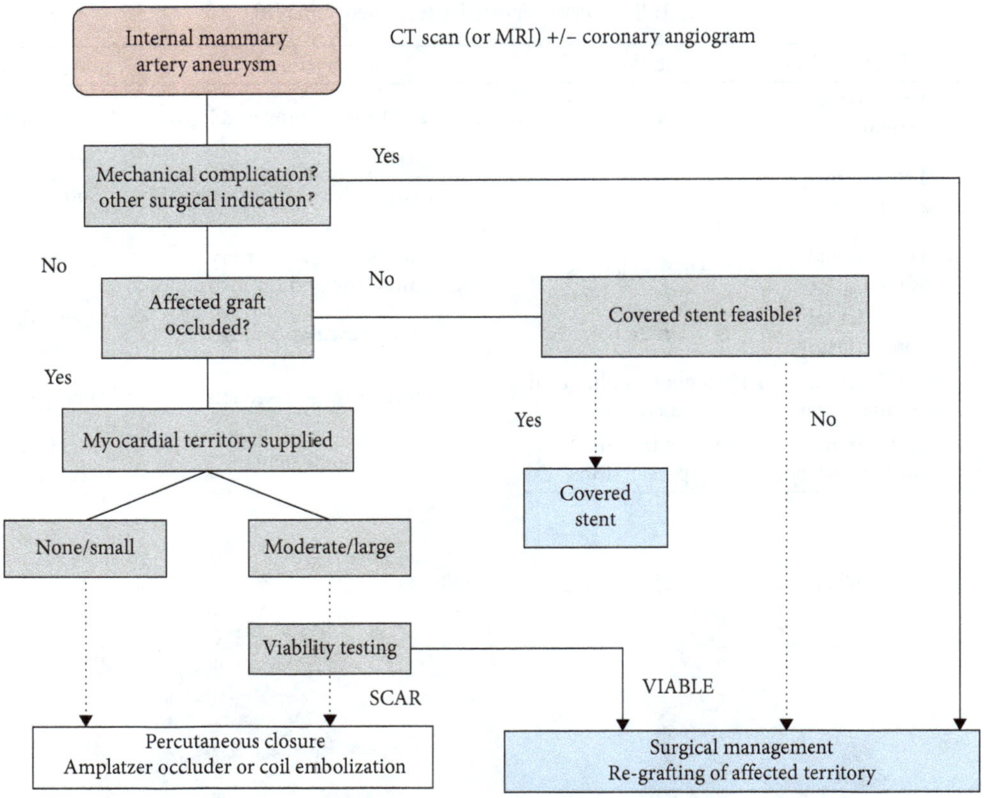

Figure 6: Suggested algorithm for assessment and treatment of an internal mammary artery aneurysm. CT: computed tomography; MRI: magnetic resonance imaging [7].

artery bypass grafting and due to the increasing sophistication of diagnostic investigations [6].

3.4. Treatment. When a patient is diagnosed with an IMA aneurysm, it is highly recommended to begin prompt therapy to prevent life-threatening complications [11]. About 20% of patients with saphenous vein aneurysms are treated with conservative management comprising of risk factor modification, secondary prevention, and surveillance [2]. Reducing the risk of mass effect, thromboembolism, rupture, and myocardial ischemia are the main goals of treatment [2]. Options for invasive treatment are surgical repair or percutaneous approaches, which include vascular coil embolization, covered stenting, and vascular occlusion (Figure 6) [7]. Covered stenting has a major advantage in that it protects distal flow patency, unlike other percutaneous options. Surgery should be immediately considered if the patient has a high risk of rupture or if the aneurysm is causing compressive complications [2]. Surgical techniques include ligation of the aneurysm or resection of the aneurysm with or without bypass revascularization [2]. At a minimum, patients should receive a complete cardiac evaluation by an interventional cardiologist and a cardiac surgeon [7].

4. Conclusion

IMA aneurysms represent a very rare complication following a CABG. It has a high potential for morbidity and mortality, and the risk of complications will likely rise with the size of the aneurysm [2]. Increased attention to and awareness of this disease process will hopefully facilitate earlier diagnosis. Coronary CT angiography is the most definitive test for not only confirming but also discovering possible complications stemming from the aneurysm [13]. With continued improvement in long-term outcomes following bypass grafting since the 1960s, and with an increase in the aging population undergoing bypass surgery, it is likely that the incidence of documented IMA aneurysms or pseudoaneurysms will grow [7, 12]. Endovascular treatment is especially effective for the severely ill and elderly population, with the number of successful aneurysm cases treated with this method continuing to rise [6]. Following an extensive literature review, and to the best of our knowledge, this is the first documented case of a true aneurysm found within a LIMA bypass graft. It is our hope that this review will further assist clinicians in increasing accurate evaluation and management of this rare disease process.

Authors' Contributions

Osayi Lawani's contributions consisted of conceptualization, data curation, investigation, creation of the original draft, review and editing, and visualization. Rick Ganim's contributions consisted of supervision, conceptualization, methodology, validation, and review and editing of the original draft. Jiries Ganim contributed in data curation, investigation, and review and editing of the original draft.

Acknowledgments

The authors would like to especially thank John Washington IV, Laura Tinnell, Misty Jennings, and Richard Shannon.

References

[1] L. W. Chan and G. G. Fermanis, "Spontaneous hemothorax caused by an internal mammary artery aneurysm," *The Australian and New Zealand Journal of Surgery*, vol. 66, no. 5, pp. 332-333, 1996.

[2] J. T. Connell, "Saphenovenous graft aneurysm: a rare complication of CABG," *Case Reports in Cardiology*, E. Ercan, Ed., vol. 2017, Article ID 8101489, 2017.

[3] S. J. Head, T. M. Kieser, V. Falk, H. A. Huysmans, and A. P. Kappetein, "Coronary artery bypass grafting: part 1—the evolution over the first 50 years," *European Heart Journal*, vol. 34, no. 37, pp. 2862–2872, 2013.

[4] A. Frazier, F. Qureshi, K. M. Read, R. C. Gilkeson, R. S. Poston, and C. S. White, "Coronary artery bypass grafts: assessment with multidetector CT in the early and late postoperative settings," *Radiographics*, vol. 25, no. 4, pp. 881–896, 2005.

[5] G. D. Otter and J. Stam, "Aneurysm of internal mammary artery," *Thorax*, vol. 33, no. 4, pp. 526-527, 1978.

[6] M. Miyazaki, H. Nagamine, H. Hara, H. Sugita, and Y. Kawase, "Successful treatment of a right internal mammary artery aneurysm with thoracoscopic surgery," *Journal of Vascular Surgery Cases and Innovative Techniques*, vol. 5, no. 3, pp. 269–272, 2019.

[7] D. Ramirez, B. Hibbert, T. Simard et al., "Natural history and management of aortocoronary saphenous vein graft aneurysms," *Circulation*, vol. 126, no. 18, pp. 2248–2256, 2012.

[8] T. Kugai and M. Chibana, "Non-trauma-induced aneurysm of the left internal thoracic artery with ischemic heart disease-a case report and review of the literature," *Japan Journal of Cardiovascular Surgery*, vol. 28, no. 4, pp. 260–263, 1999.

[9] I. K. Klair and J. Palomino, "Giant saphenous vein coronary artery bypass graft aneurysm," *American Journal of Respiratory and Critical Care Medicine*, vol. 189, no. 5, pp. 8-9, 2014.

[10] J. Francis, "Skeletonized internal mammary graft vs pedicled graft," in Cardiac Surgery, Kozhikode, Kerala, India, 2018, July 2020, https://johnsonfrancis.org/professional/skeletonized-internal-mammary-graft-vs-pedicled-graft/.

[11] T. Almerey, R. Paz-Fumagalli, H. Farres, W. A. Oldenburg, and A. G. Hakaim, "Idiopathic internal mammary artery aneurysm in the setting of aberrant right subclavian artery," *Journal of Vascular Cases and Innovative Techniques*, vol. 3, no. 4, pp. 251–253, 2017.

[12] M. Doyle, D. L. Spizarny, and D. E. Baker, "Saphenous vein graft aneurysm after coronary artery bypass surgery," *American Journal of Roentgenology*, vol. 168, pp. 747–749, 1996.

[13] C. Burke, S. Shalhub, and B. W. Starnes, "Endovascular repair of an internal mammary artery aneurysm in a patient with SMAD-3 mutation," *Journal of Vascular Surgery*, vol. 62, no. 2, pp. 486–488, 2015.

[14] R. Lindblom, V. Zemgulis, A. Lilieqvist, and R. Nyman, "Even small aneurysms can bleed: a ruptured small idiopathic aneurysm of the internal thoracic artery," *Interactive Cardiovascular and Thoracic Surgery*, vol. 17, no. 3, pp. 583–585, 2013.

[15] J. Heyn, H. Zimmermann, A. Klose, B. Luchting, C. Hinske, and M. S. Azandaryani, "Idiopathic internal mammary artery aneurysm," *Journal of Surgical Case Reports*, vol. 12, pp. 1–3, 2014.

A Case of a 50-Year-Old Woman with Typical Fabry Disease who Showed Serial Electrocardiographic and Echocardiographic Changes over a 17-Year Period

Su Nam Lee, Gee-Hee Kim, and Ki-Dong Yoo

Division of Cardiology, Department of Internal Medicine, St. Vincent's Hospital, The Catholic University of Korea, Seoul, Republic of Korea

Correspondence should be addressed to Gee-Hee Kim; jiheekim@catholic.ac.kr

Academic Editor: Man-Hong Jim

Fabry disease (FD) is a progressive, X-linked lysosomal storage disorder caused by a deficiency of α-galactosidase A activity. Affected individuals accumulate globotriaosylceramide and glycosphingolipids in the lysosomes and cytoplasm of cells throughout the body, leading to major organ failure and premature death. Cardiac involvement includes left ventricular hypertrophy, arrhythmia, endothelial dysfunction at vascular wall, and cardiomyopathy. The diagnosis of FD can be difficult and there is often a long lag time between symptoms and diagnosis. Here, we present a case of a 50-year-old woman with typical Fabry disease who showed serial electrocardiographic and echocardiographic changes over 17 years prior to diagnosis with Fabry disease.

1. Introduction

Fabry disease (FD) is a progressive inherited metabolic disorder. Deficient activity of lysosomal α-galactosidase A (α-GLA) results in progressive accumulation of globotriaosylceramide (Gb3) and related glycosphingolipids within lysosomes and, ultimately, leads to multiorgan dysfunction of the cardiac, renal, and cerebrovascular systems [1, 2]. Life- threatening cardiovascular or cerebrovascular complications limit life expectancy [3]. Therefore, early diagnosis of FD before cardiocerebrovascular irreversible organ damage occurs is important. However, the diagnosis of FD is difficult and is made at approximately 13.7 and 16.3 years in males and females, respectively, after the onset of symptoms [4]. Cardiac involvement includes left ventricular hypertrophy (LVH), arrhythmia, angina, and dyspnea. Electrocardiographic (ECG) changes in patients with FD are frequent and include LVH, ST segment depression, T wave inversion, short PR interval, prolonged QTc intervals, intermittent supraventricular tachycardia, ventricular tachycardia, atrioventricular (AV) node blocks, and bundle branch blocks [5, 6].

Here, we report a case of a 50-year-old woman who showed serial electrocardiographic and echocardiographic changes over 17 years prior to diagnosis with typical FD.

2. Case Presentation

In 2000, a 34-year-old woman without disease was referred due to epigastric discomfort. A physical examination revealed no abnormal findings. Endoscopic examination showed normal findings. An electrocardiogram (ECG) showed regular sinus rhythm with a normal PR interval (160 ms) and no LVH by the Sokolow-Lyon index (28 mm) (Figure 1(a)). The Sokolow-Lyon index for LVH defined as *S* in V1+R in V5 or V6 (whichever is larger) ≥ 35 mm [7].

The patient was repeatedly admitted to our hospital from 2003 to 2010 (Table 1).

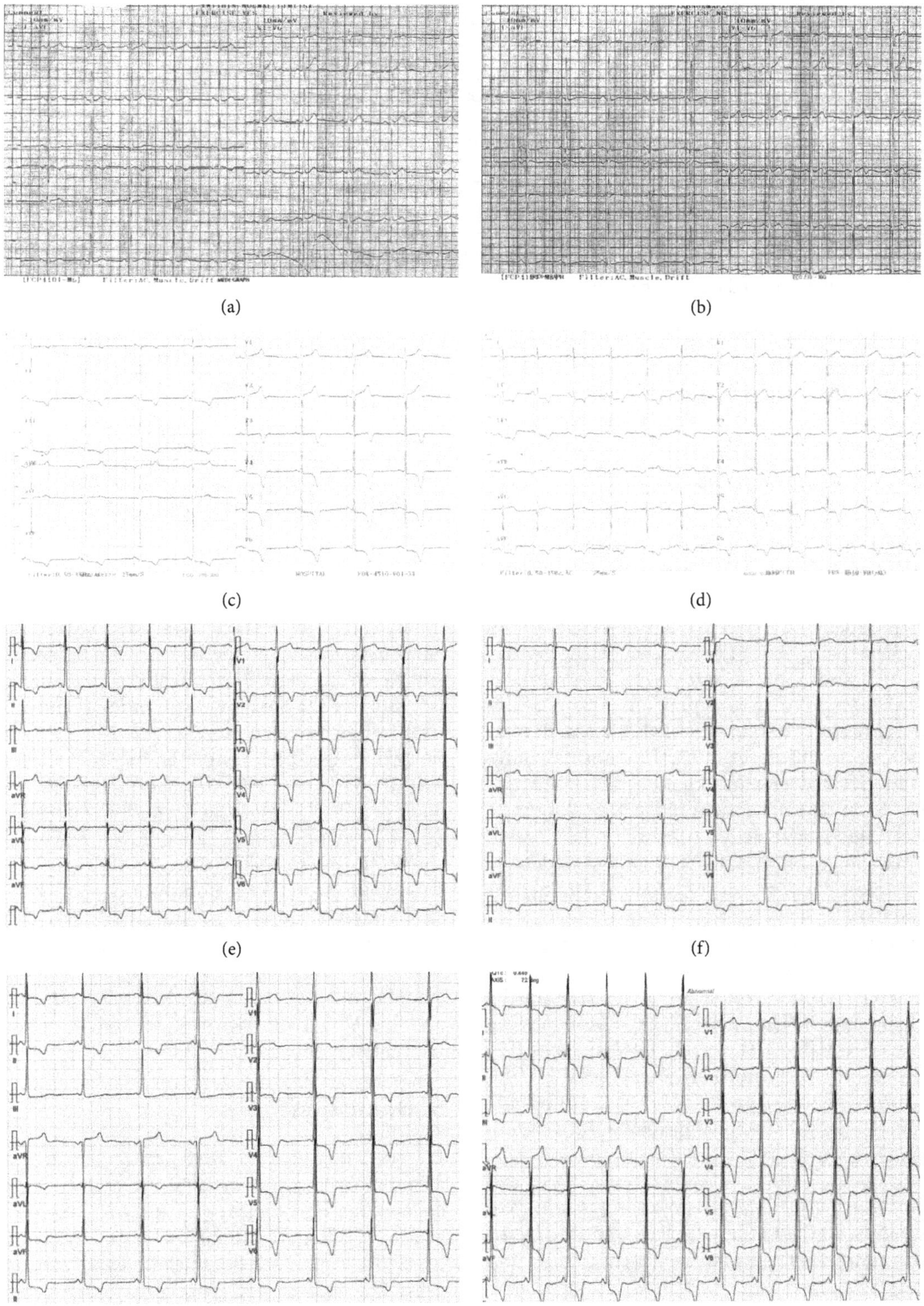

FIGURE 1: Serial electrocardiographic changes. (a) In 2000: PR interval 160 ms, LVH criteria (Sokolow-Lyon index) 28 mm. (b) In 2003: PR interval 160 ms, LVH criteria (Sokolow-Lyon index) 36 mm. (c) In 2007: PR interval 160 ms, LVH criteria (Sokolow-Lyon index) 38 mm. (d) In 2008: PR interval 120 ms, LVH criteria (Sokolow-Lyon index) 47 mm. (e) In 2010: PR interval 120 ms, LVH criteria (Sokolow-Lyon index) 46 mm. (f) In 2014: PR interval 100 ms, LVH criteria (Sokolow-Lyon index) 50 mm. (g) In 2016: PR interval 100 ms, LVH criteria (Sokolow-Lyon index) 63 mm. (h) In 2017: PR interval 100 ms, LVH criteria (Sokolow-Lyon index) 67 mm.

Table 1: Hospitalization history between 2003 and 2010.

Year	Age	Symptoms	Evaluation
2003	37	Palpitation and chest discomfort	ECG: a normal PR interval (160 ms) and LVH (36 mm) by the Sokolow criteria with T wave inversion on V4-6 (Figure 1(b)) Thyroid function test: normal Transthoracic echocardiography (TTE): concentric LVH Treadmill test: normal 24-hour Holter monitoring: normal
2007	41	Palpitation and chest discomfort	ECG: LVH (38 mm) by the Sokolow-Lyon index but a normal PR interval (160 ms) (Figure 1(c)) 24-hour Holter monitoring: normal Myocardial stress single-photon emission computed tomography: normal
2008	42	Palpitation and chest discomfort	ECG: a short PR interval (120 ms) and marked LVH (47 mm) by the Sokolow-Lyon index (Figure 1(d)) Coronary angiography: myocardial bridging in the mid portion of the left anterior descending artery
2010	44	Palpitation and chest discomfort	ECG: a short PR interval (120 ms) and marked LVH (46 ms) by the Sokolow-Lyon index (Figure 1(e)) TTE: concentric LVH (Figures 2(a) and 2(b))

*ECG: electrocardiography; LVH: left ventricular hypertrophy.

In 2014, the patient was referred to our hospital with dyspnea and chest pain. An ECG showed a shorter PR interval (100 ms) and more severe LVH (50 mm) by the Sokolow-Lyon index than the previous examinations (Figure 1(f)). Laboratory testing revealed a normal creatine phosphokinase (CPK) level (132 U/L; normal range 60-190 U/L), an elevated creatine kinase- (CK-) MB isoenzyme level of 15.44 ng/mL (normal range 0.1-6.7 ng/mL), and a slightly elevated lactate dehydrogenase (LDH) level of 302 U/L (normal range 140-271 U/L). TTE revealed LVH and partially decreased LV global longitudinal strain rates (Figures 2(c) and 2(d)).

In 2016, the patient was again hospitalized with chest discomfort. The blood pressure was normal. An ECG showed a short PR interval (100 ms) and severe LVH (63 mm) by the Sokolow-Lyon index (Figure 1(g)). Laboratory testing revealed elevated CK-MB (15.21 ng/mL; normal range 0.1-6.7 ng/mL), LDH (494 U/L; normal range 140-271 U/L), and brain natriuretic peptide (pro-BNP) levels (2223 pg/mL; normal range < 115 pg/mL) with a normal CPK level of 151 U/L (normal range 60-190 U/L). Creatinine was normal and the 24-hour creatinine clearance ratio (Ccr) was 101.1 mL/min/1.73m^2. TTE showed a thicker LV wall than the previous results. In addition, TTE revealed marked decreased LV longitudinal strain rates (Figures 2(e) and 2(f)). Magnetic resonance imaging findings showed a delayed enhancement at the basal segment of LV lateral wall and LVH, and thus, FD was suspected (Figures 3(a) and 3(b)). Ophthalmic examination showed cornea verticillata (Figure 4). We measured α-GLA in patient's blood plasma using a fluorometric enzyme assay. Leukocyte α-GLA was significantly reduced to 10.6 nmol/h/mg protein (normal range > 35 nmol/h/mg protein). We identified one hemizygous mutation in exon 6 of GLA, c.969delC (p.Leu324 Trpfs*24). Therefore, this patient was diagnosed with classic FD.

In 2017, the patient was admitted to cardiology for enzyme replacement therapy (ERT). Before ERT, an ECG still showed a short PR interval (100 ms) and extreme LVH (67 mm) by the Sokolow-Lyon index (Figure 1(h)). Laboratory testing revealed elevated CK-MB/CPK (38.91 ng/mL; normal range 0.1-6.7 ng/mL/272 U/L; normal range 60-190 U/L), LDH (289 U/L; normal range 140-271 U/L), and pro-BNP level (2853 pg/mL; normal range < 115 pg/mL). Eight months after ERT, ECG still showed a short PR interval and extreme LVH. TTE still showed LVH but a marked improvement of LV longitudinal strain rates (Figures 2(g) and 2(h)). The patient's family members also underwent genetic testing, and the patient's two sons were diagnosed with classic FD (Figure 5). We summarized the organ involvement and changes of Gb3 and lysoGb3 biomarkers of the affected family member in Tables 2 and 3.

3. Discussion

FD was identified in 1898 by Anderson and Fabry [8]. This inborn error of metabolism is characterized by either an absence or deficiency of α-GLA activity. The enzyme substrate, Gb-3, accumulates in a variety of cell types, including capillary endothelial, renal, cardiac, and nerve cells. The first clinical symptoms occur during childhood or adolescence and include a burning pain originating in the extremities, fever of unknown origin, hypohidrosis, and gastrointestinal symptoms, such as abdominal cramps and diarrhea [9]. More specific manifestations, such as angiokeratoma and asymptomatic corneal opacities, usually present in late adolescence. Neurological, cardiac, and renal complications develop in the third or fourth decade [2].

Early signs of cardiac involvement may be present during adolescence. These signs include a shortened PR interval,

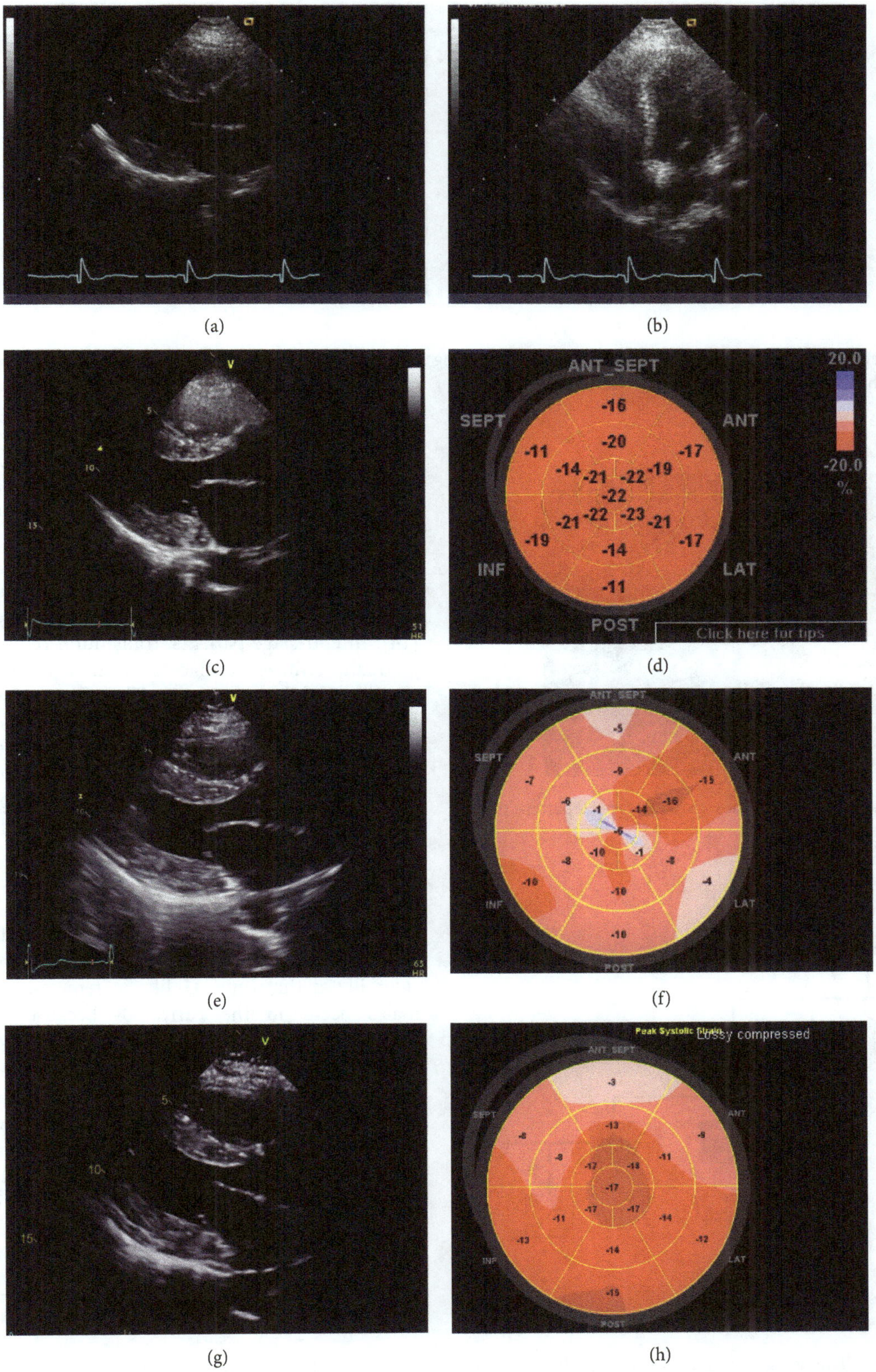

FIGURE 2: Transthoracic echocardiogram. Echocardiography showed concentric LVH in 2010 (a, b). In 2014, transthoracic echocardiography (TTE) revealed LVH (c) and partially decreased left ventricular (LV) global longitudinal strain rates (d). In 2016, TTE showed LVH (e) and marked decreased LV longitudinal strain rates (f). Eight months after ERT, TTE still showed LVH (g) but a marked improvement of LV longitudinal strain rates (h).

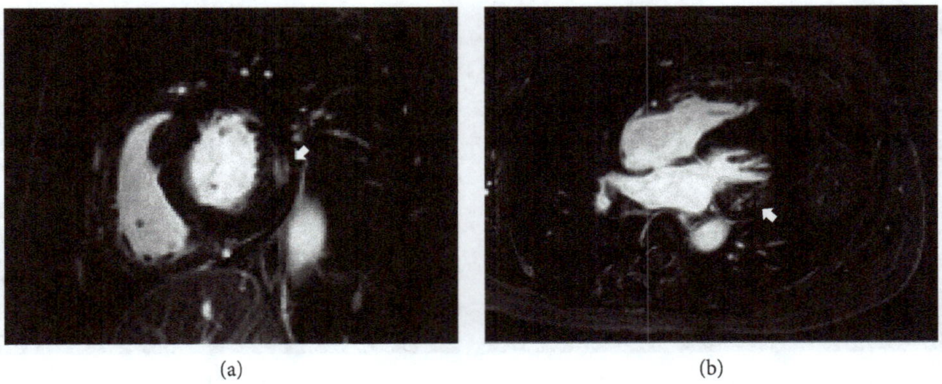

Figure 3: Magnetic resonance imaging. Magnetic resonance imaging showed delayed enhancement (arrows) at the basal segment of LV lateral wall. (a) Short axis view. (b) 4-chamber view.

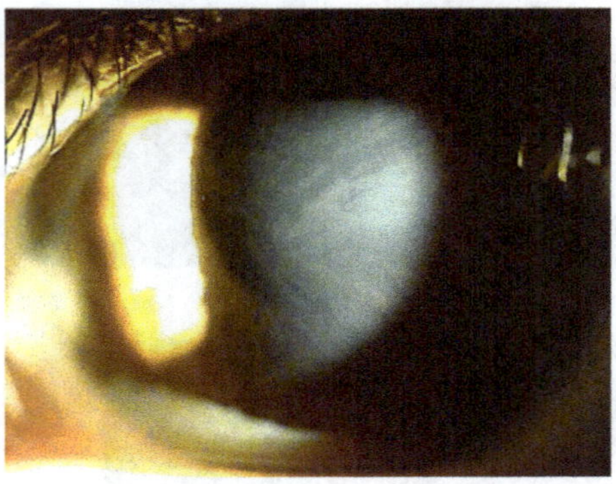

Figure 4: Cornea. Subepithelial lines show the typical pattern of the so-called "cornea verticillata".

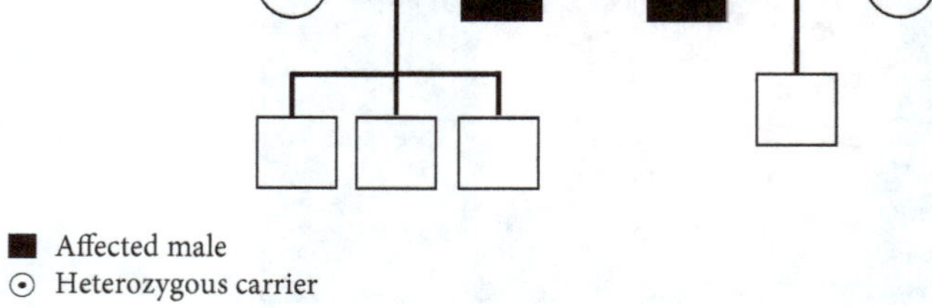

Figure 5: The pedigree of the patient's family.

arrhythmias, impaired heart rate variability, and mild valvular insufficiency [10]. Cardiac symptoms including LVH, arrhythmia, angina, and dyspnea are reported in approximately 40-60% of patients with FD [5, 6]. With an ECG, these early-stage patients had shorter PQ intervals due to a shortening of the P-wave duration as compared to age- and heart rate-matched healthy controls [11, 12]. LVH most commonly manifests at an average age of 32 years in men and 40 years in women [13].

Progressive myocardial fibrosis develops with both interstitial and replacement fibrosis as the patient ages [14]. In end-stage patients, transmural replacement fibrosis gradually reduces cardiac function to the stage of congestive heart failure [13, 15]. Therefore, early diagnosis of FD is important, although the diagnosis of FD is difficult and there is often a long lag time between symptoms and diagnosis. Males are diagnosed at a median age of 24 years old and females at a median age of 31 years old. Diagnoses are made after 15 years for males and 18 years for females after the onset of symptoms [16].

In this case, changes in ECG had been observed in the patient's late 30s, specifically a shortened PR interval and severe LVH. We should have tested for FD in this patient with unexplained LVH. However, we did not consider FD at that time. Unlike in females, ECG changes in males occur in the early 30s because the activity of enzyme is lower than that in female. Gender differences are one of the reasons why it is difficult to diagnose FD. In female patients, the progression toward hypertrophy is prolonged, whereas the development of fibrosis and regional functional abnormalities progresses simultaneously. However, in males, LVH and concomitant reduction in longitudinal function appear in adolescence and both two processes lead to replacement fibrosis [17, 18].

4. Conclusion

This case has not been reported previously, showing a series of long-term electrocardiographic changes prior to FD diagnosis. We reported here that serial ECG and TTE changes over 17 years were observed before the patient was diagnosed with FD. Physicians should be aware of the importance of electrocardiographic and echocardiographic changes, especially PR interval and LVH, in the diagnosis of FD.

TABLE 2: Organ involvements of the affected family member.

Variables	Patient	First son	Second son
Age at diagnosis	50	32	31
Sex	Female	Male	Male
Mutation	Exon 6 p.Leu324Trpfs*24	Exon 6 p.Leu324Trpfs*24	Exon 6 p.Leu324Trpfs*24
Leukocyte α-galactosidase (nmol/h/mg protein)	10.6	2.2	4.4
PR interval on ECG	0.127	0.141	0.157
LVH on ECG	(+)	(+)	(+)
TTE	LVH	LVH	LVH
Delayed enhancement on heart MRI	(+), basal segment	(-)	(-)
Proteinuria (mg/24 h)	60	473	416
Cornea verticillata	(+)	(+)	(+)
Angiokeratoma	(+)	(+)	(+)
Anhidrosis	(-)	(-)	(+)
Chronic neurotic pain	(+)	(+)	(+)
Brain involvement	(-)	(-)	(-)

*ECG: electrocardiography; TTE: transthoracic echocardiography; LVH: left ventricular hypertrophy; MRI: magnetic resonance imaging.

TABLE 3: The changes of Gb3 and lysoGb3 biomarkers of the affected family member.

	Base	3 months	6 months	9 months	12 months
Gb3 (μg/mL, normal range 3.9-9.9 μg/mL)					
Patient	7.4	5.3	6.5	7	7.3
First son	14.1	8.8	6.3	7.1	7.7
Second son	8.5	7.7	6.4	7.6	5.8
LysoGb3 (ng/mL, normal range $\leq$ 1.74 ng/mL)					
Patient	Not checked	7.82	8.13	7.14	8.05
First son	Not checked	30.4	20.8	24.3	30.8
Second son	Not checked	36	25.7	32.5	28

*Gb3: globotriaosylceramide.

Disclosure

This case was presented at the poster session of the Lysosomal Disease Symposium 2018 (14th Annual WORLD Symposium) held in San Diego, United States, February 2018.

Acknowledgments

We acknowledge the helpful support of all authors.

References

[1] C. C. Sweeley and B. Klionsky, "Fabry's disease: classification as a sphingolipidosis and partial characterization of a novel glycolipid," *Journal of Biological Chemistry*, vol. 238, pp. 3148–3150, 1963.

[2] D. P. Germain, "Fabry disease," *Orphanet Journal of Rare Diseases*, vol. 5, no. 1, p. 30, 2010.

[3] R. Schiffmann, D. G. Warnock, M. Banikazemi et al., "Fabry disease: progression of nephropathy, and prevalence of cardiac and cerebrovascular events before enzyme replacement therapy," *Nephrology Dialysis Transplantation*, vol. 24, no. 7, pp. 2102–2111, 2009.

[4] A. Mehta, R. Ricci, U. Widmer et al., "Fabry disease defined: baseline clinical manifestations of 366 patients in the Fabry Outcome Survey," *European Journal of Clinical Investigation*, vol. 34, no. 3, pp. 236–242, 2004.

[5] C. Kampmann, F. Baehner, C. Whybra et al., "Cardiac manifestations of Anderson-Fabry disease in heterozygous females," *Journal of the American College of Cardiology*, vol. 40, no. 9, pp. 1668–1674, 2002.

[6] A. Linhart, T. Paleček, J. Bultas et al., "New insights in cardiac structural changes in patients with Fabry's disease," *American Heart Journal*, vol. 139, no. 6, pp. 1101–1108, 2000.

[7] M. Sokolow and T. P. Lyon, "The ventricular complex in left ventricular hypertrophy as obtained by unipolar precordial and limb leads," *American Heart Journal*, vol. 37, no. 2, pp. 161–186, 1949.

[8] H. Fabry, "Angiokeratoma corporis diffusum–Fabry disease: historical review from the original description to the introduction of enzyme replacement therapy," *Acta Paediatrica*, vol. 91, no. 439, pp. 3–5, 2002.

[9] R. J. Hopkin, J. Bissler, M. Banikazemi et al., "Characterization of Fabry disease in 352 pediatric patients in the Fabry Registry," *Pediatric Research*, vol. 64, no. 5, pp. 550–555, 2008.

[10] C. Kampmann, C. M. Wiethoff, C. Whybra, F. A. Baehner, E. Mengel, and M. Beck, "Cardiac manifestations of Anderson-Fabry disease in children and adolescents," *Acta Paediatrica*, vol. 97, no. 4, pp. 463–469, 2008.

[11] M. Namdar, C. Kampmann, J. Steffel et al., "PQ interval in patients with Fabry disease," *The American Journal of Cardiology*, vol. 105, no. 5, pp. 753–756, 2010.

[12] M. Namdar, J. Steffel, M. Vidovic et al., "Electrocardiographic changes in early recognition of Fabry disease," *Heart*, vol. 97, no. 6, pp. 485–490, 2011.

[13] A. Linhart, C. Kampmann, J. L. Zamorano et al., "Cardiac manifestations of Anderson-Fabry disease: results from the international Fabry outcome survey," *European Heart Journal*, vol. 28, no. 10, pp. 1228–1235, 2007.

[14] H. Hasegawa, H. Takano, S. Shindo et al., "Images in cardiovascular medicine. Transition from left ventricular hypertrophy to massive fibrosis in the cardiac variant of Fabry disease," *Circulation*, vol. 113, no. 16, pp. e720–e721, 2006.

[15] C. Kampmann, A. Linhart, F. Baehner et al., "Onset and progression of the Anderson-Fabry disease related cardiomyopathy," *International Journal of Cardiology*, vol. 130, no. 3, pp. 367–373, 2008.

[16] W. R. Wilcox, J. P. Oliveira, R. J. Hopkin et al., "Females with Fabry disease frequently have major organ involvement: lessons from the Fabry Registry," *Molecular Genetics and Metabolism*, vol. 93, no. 2, pp. 112–128, 2008.

[17] M. Niemann, S. Herrmann, K. Hu et al., "Differences in Fabry cardiomyopathy between female and male patients: consequences for diagnostic assessment," *JACC: Cardiovascular Imaging*, vol. 4, no. 6, pp. 592–601, 2011.

[18] K. Selthofer-Relatic, "Time of Anderson-Fabry disease detection and cardiovascular presentation," *Case Reports in Cardiology*, vol. 2018, Article ID 6131083, 5 pages, 2018.

13

Debate of Percutaneous Coronary Intervention versus Coronary Artery Bypass Grafting in a Multimorbidity Patient with Complex Coronary Lesions

Sotirios Mitsiadis, Nikolaos Miaris, Antonios Dimopoulos, Anastasios Theodosis-Georgilas, Spyridon Tsiamis, Nikolaos Patsourakos, Nikolaos Papakonstantinou, and Evangelos Pisimisis

Department of Cardiology, "Tzaneio" General Hospital of Piraeus, Piraeus, Greece

Correspondence should be addressed to Nikolaos Miaris; nmiaris@gmail.com

Academic Editor: Ertugrul Ercan

Background. While complete revascularization in coronary artery disease is of high priority, the method of implementation in patients with complex coronary lesions and multiple comorbidities is not directed by published guidelines. *Case Presentation.* A 53-year-old female with a chronic total occlusion of the right coronary artery and a bifurcation lesion of the left anterior descending artery and the first diagonal branch, presented with non-ST elevation myocardial infarction. Her past medical history concerned thymectomy and prior chest radiation for thymoma, myasthenia gravis, peripheral artery disease, and cervical cancer treated with surgery and radiation. Although SYNTAX score II favored surgical revascularization, the interventional pathway was finally successfully followed. However, it was complicated with vessel perforation and tamponade managed with pericardiocentesis. *Conclusion.* Comorbidities are not all involved in common risk models and require individualization until more evidence comes to light.

1. Introduction

Complete revascularization (CR) in patients with multivessel coronary artery disease (CAD) is a crucial prognostic factor that should be taken into consideration in the decision between percutaneous coronary intervention (PCI) and coronary artery bypass grafting (CABG), as it is associated with reduced cardiovascular mortality regardless of the method of implementation [1, 2]. Frequently, the best reperfusion strategy has to be considered with prudence, as CABG in patients with comorbidities may be accompanied by an increased risk for adverse outcomes, which is also high when performing PCI in very complex lesions along with a lower success rate in those cases [3, 4]. The aim of this paper is to present the case of a female patient with two-vessel CAD and such lesion complexity that created skepticism over interventional management, while on the other hand, her simultaneous comorbidities were actually discouraging the surgical option.

2. Case Presentation

A 53-year-old woman presented to our emergency department with non-ST elevation myocardial infarction (NSTEMI). She was a 30-pack-year smoker and dyslipidemic on ezetimibe. Her past medical history involved peripheral artery disease (PAD), cervical cancer treated with surgery and radiotherapy 9 years before admission, myasthenia gravis (MG) currently on steroids and pyridostigmine, and thymoma managed with thymectomy (complicated with a myasthenic crisis) and radiotherapy one year before admission.

Four months preceding her current admission, the patient had been hospitalized with non-ST elevation acute coronary syndrome (NSTEACS) and diagnosed with two-vessel CAD that involved a bifurcation lesion extending from the left anterior descending (LAD) artery to the first diagonal branch (D1) and a proximal total occlusion of the right

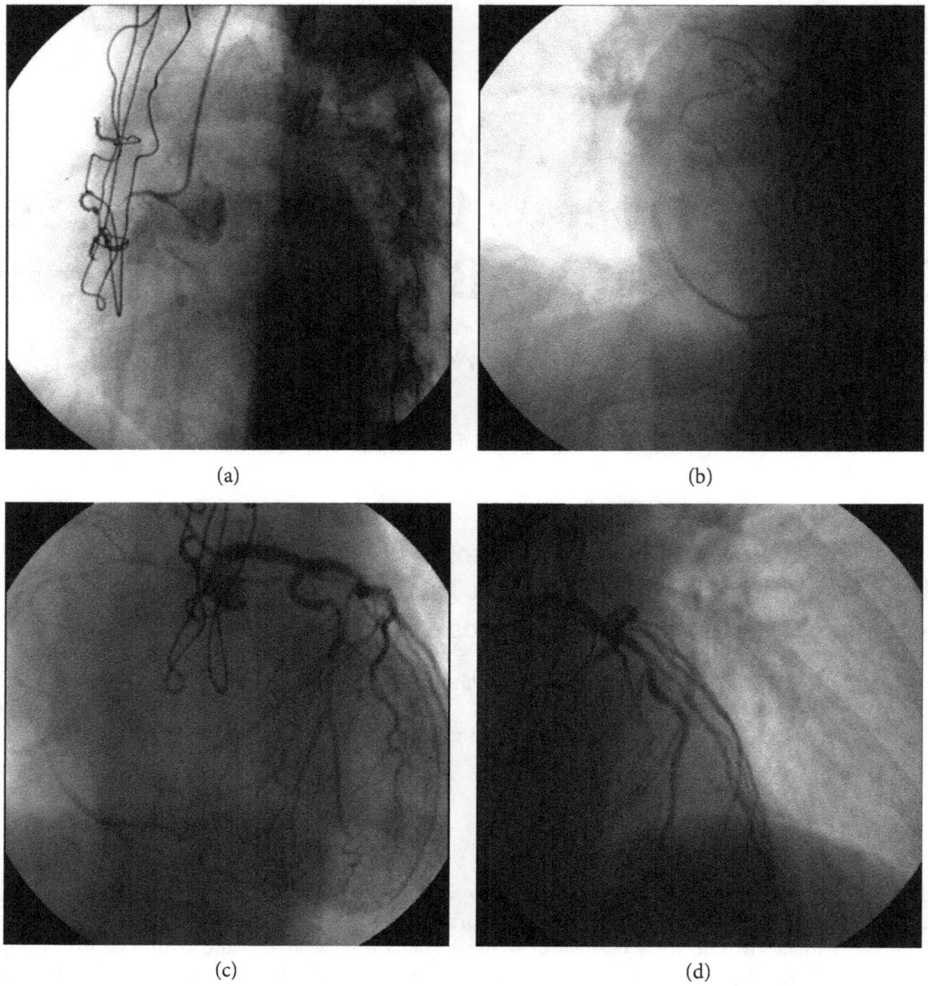

FIGURE 1: Coronary angiography of the patient. (a) CTO of RCA. (b, c) Collaterals from LAD to RCA territory. Retrograde filling of RCA. (d) LAD/D1 bifurcation lesion.

coronary artery (RCA). Lesion complexity indicated reperfusion with CABG, which was then rejected by the patient, and optimal medical treatment was finally adopted.

On admission, the patient presented with chest pain, dynamic electrocardiography changes in multiple precordial leads, and elevated serum cardiac troponin I levels (maximum level of 250 ng/L, cutoff level of 15 ng/L), while mild left ventricular dysfunction (ejection fraction of 45-50%) and inferior wall hypokinesis were revealed by echocardiography. A new invasive coronary angiography (ICA) showed no significant changes in comparison with previous findings (Figure 1).

At this stage, the most beneficial reperfusion strategy should be followed. Although the common risk stratification models indicated an intermediate surgical risk (EuroSCORE II 1.2%, STS score 8.4%) and the SYNTAX scores favored CABG (SYNTAX score I was 23, SYNTAX score II was 39.4 for PCI with 4-year mortality of 14.4% and 21 for CABG with 4-year mortality of 3.3%), our patient's comorbidities made the actual surgical risk higher than that typically calculated. On the other hand, the implementation of a successful PCI was challenging with a high periprocedural risk, as coronary lesions were complex; they concerned, firstly, a chronic total occlusion (CTO) of the RCA and secondly, an acute-angled bifurcation lesion involving the LAD and a major diagonal branch (D1) with diffuse disease extending more than 15 mm from its ostium. Those bifurcation characteristics made the use of a complex 2-stent technique unavoidable.

The final joint decision of the Heart Team and the patient was the interventional approach, while the surgical option was kept as a minor alternative. Although computed tomography angiography could provide some more information, this was not feasible. Based on the ICA, the Japanese CTO score of the RCA lesion was calculated to be 0, as it would be the first attempt of PCI in a short-length CTO lesion with tapered entry and without calcification or bending within the segment. Our strategy involved beginning with the CTO PCI of the RCA due to its favorable anatomical features and in order to avoid any complications of the donor artery and afterwards, continuing with the PCI of the LAD/D1 bifurcation lesion.

At the same time, another issue was the lack of a second arterial access, as there was a patent left radial artery, whereas the right radial artery was occluded following the previous ICA and the common femoral arteries were severely diseased

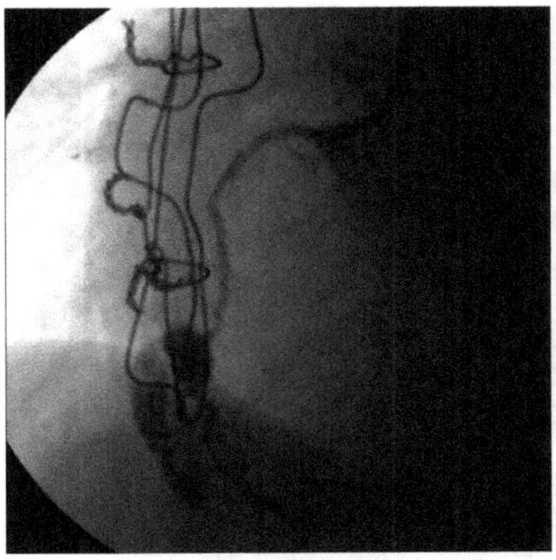

FIGURE 2: Ellis type III RCA perforation.

(radiation-induced PAD). Patient's frailty and the fact that we wanted to avoid any complications of the brachial arteries made us proceed with a single left radial artery access using the antegrade wire escalation technique. The proximal lesion of the RCA was crossed, and a stiff guidewire was advanced to the distal vessel with a free wire movement. After having confirmed the position of the guidewire with two consecutive vertical views, a predilatation with a 1.5/15 mm semicompliant balloon was performed. Unfortunately, an Ellis type III perforation of the vessel was caused (Figure 2), as the balloon predilatation was found to have been implemented in an acute marginal branch that ran parallel to the main vessel [5]. Inflating a balloon proximally to the perforation was intended to stop further blood extravasation. Nevertheless, the patient soon became severely symptomatic with hemodynamic compromise because of rapid fluid accumulation into the pericardial cavity. Urgent pericardiocentesis under fluoroscopic guidance (Figure 3) fortunately stabilized the patient. Restoration of blood flow was finally achieved with the deployment of three drug-eluting stents after wiring the lumen of the RCA. The final angiographic result of the CTO PCI of the RCA was very good (TIMI flow grade 3) (Figure 4), and the patient was transferred to the coronary care unit being hemodynamically stable and asymptomatic.

A week later, the patient reentered the catheterization laboratory. The severity of the LAD lesion was assessed with fractional flow reserve (FFR) measurement that turned out to be 0.8. Double kissing crush technique using two stents was adopted due to the anatomical features of the bifurcation lesion that involved a large lumen diagonal branch with rich blood distribution arising at a steep angle from LAD (steep angle between D1 and LAD distal to the bifurcation).

An excellent angiographic result was finally succeeded (Figure 4), and 3 days later, the patient was discharged being asymptomatic. Eighteen months later, she still remains in the same good asymptomatic condition.

3. Discussion

The therapeutic strategy in patients with CAD and comorbidities is challenging and should be individualized based on the anatomical and functional characteristics of coronary arterial lesions, technical feasibility, and perioperative risk. Besides, after having been fully informed regarding revascularization alternatives, patient's will play the major role.

As mentioned above, our patient had plenty of comorbidities and even though the usual perioperative risk scores seemed to be intermediate and the SYNTAX score II indicated CABG for myocardial revascularization, there actually exist many features that are not taken into account by these risk models. MG and the history of myasthenic crisis experienced when operated with thymectomy, the prior sternotomy and thoracic radiation therapy creating uncertainty about the patency of the left internal mammary artery, and the long-term treatment with steroids discouraged essentially the option of CABG in our case.

MG is a rare disease caused by autoantibody-mediated blockade of the neuromuscular junction resulting in muscle disability [6]. Such patients are unpredictably resistant or sensitive to various anesthetic medications and may develop either a myasthenic crisis, which is an exacerbation of the disease, or a cholinergic crisis caused by cholinesterase inhibitor overdose [6]. Both conditions may need endotracheal intubation, while surgery may be by itself a triggering factor of myasthenic crisis frequently requiring immediate immunomodulating treatment [6].

There is an ongoing discussion regarding whether prior chest radiation exposure increases adverse outcomes of patients undergoing cardiac surgery. According to Wu et al., increased long-term mortality was observed in patients with prior thoracic radiation exposure treated with cardiac surgery [7]. In particular, the authors concluded with considering other treatment options as more appropriate in such cases. In contrast, Fender et al. demonstrated in their study that surgical revascularization in such patients could be performed as safely as in the control group [8]. Nevertheless, multiple studies conclude with the adverse effect of radiotherapy on internal mammary artery integrity and on its potential usage in CABG, which is a major factor of long-term survival [8, 9]. So, preoperative angiographic evaluation of the integrity of the graft may be considered.

Another field of discrepancy is whether repeat sternotomy portends a poorer prognosis. While some studies report that intraoperative injury can occur in as many as 9-9.1% of redo sternotomies, other authors report much lower risk [10–12]. Although redo sternotomies have been traditionally thought to carry higher mortality rate than first-time operations, this cannot be supported by all ongoing research and neither can its association with intraoperative injuries [10–13]. In either case, detailed preoperative planning including computed tomography scans may be very beneficial, along with a proper surgery technique such as hemisternotomy [12].

CR with complex PCI is a common practice nowadays and is associated with favorable outcomes concerning both morbidity and mortality. Farooq et al. showed that residual CAD with SYNTAX score greater than 8 following PCI was a determinant of 5-year mortality [14]. According to the 2018 guidelines of the European Society of Cardiology and the European Association for Cardio-Thoracic Surgery on myocardial revascularization, the choice of CABG instead

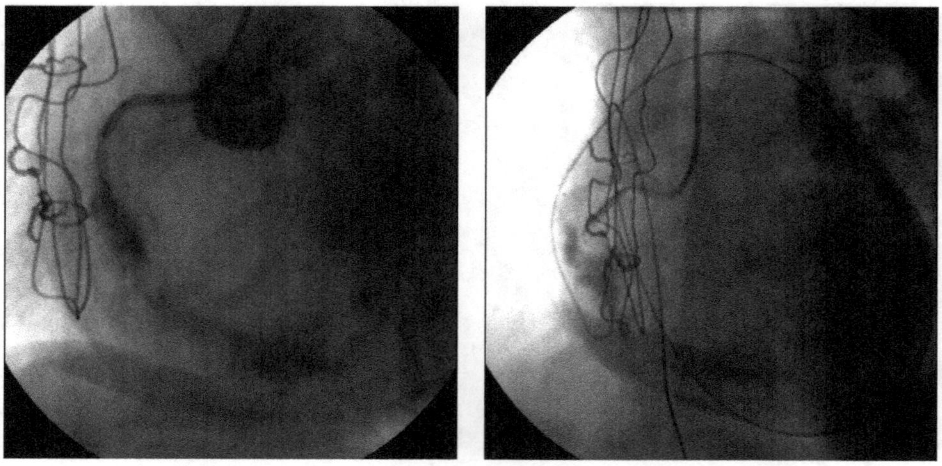

(a) (b)

FIGURE 3: (a) Extravasation causing cardiac tamponade. (b) Urgent pericardiocentesis under fluoroscopic guidance.

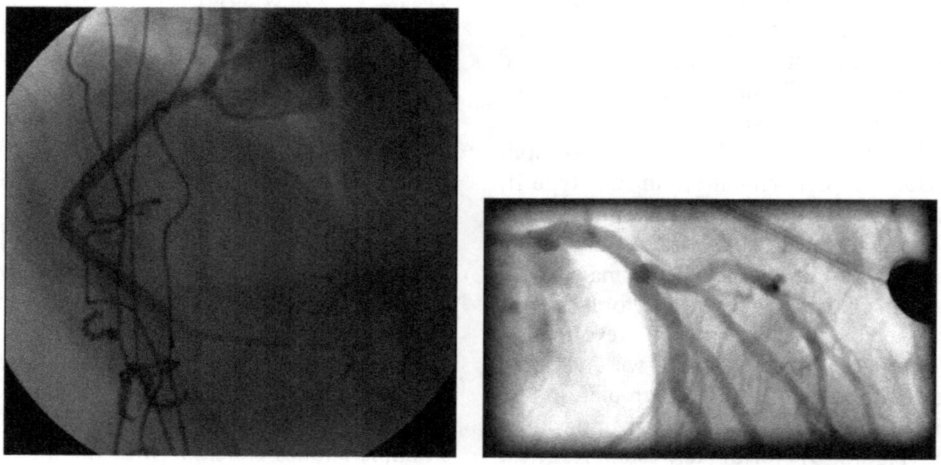

(a) (b)

FIGURE 4: Final angiographic results. (a) CTO PCI of RCA; (b) PCI of LAD/D1 bifurcation lesion.

of PCI should be guided by the potential for achieving CR [15]. Moreover, FAME and FAME 2 studies showed that the goal of CR via PCI should be preferably directed by functional characteristics and not by anatomical ones [15–17]. However, complex PCI procedures are associated with higher rates of complications; therefore, operators must be well prepared regarding not only the preprocedural planning but also the intervention itself in order to achieve a high quality result and deal with possible complications [4].

CTO PCI is a rapidly growing field of interventional cardiology that needs particular attention in safety issues. After obtaining dual contrast injection, several factors such as the position and the morphological features of the proximal and distal cap, the lesion length, the presence of branches, and retrograde techniques adequacy have to be assessed prior to the intervention [18]. However, PAD and the frailty of our patient made it hard to obtain a second arterial access that proved an unwise decision after all. Then, the similar course of RCA and acute marginal branches may mislead even an experienced operator. Imaging devices such as intravascular ultrasound may have beneficial contribution in proper wire crossing and balloon dilation. As regards complications, Patel et al. showed in their study that vessel perforation seemed to be the most common concern among cardiologists, whereas death and tamponade were their second and third most frequent single responses accordingly [19]. Consequently, urgent pericardiocentesis is a life-saving skill that all interventional cardiologists should be familiar with, while readily available pericardiocentesis kits in combination with either fluoroscopic or echocardiographic guidance may facilitate the procedure.

Last but not least, there comes the reliability of FFR in evaluating the severity of LAD lesions prior to and following the CTO PCI of RCA. Even though FFR in the culprit vessel is not reliable in the acute phase of ST-elevation myocardial infarction [20, 21], transient microvascular dysfunction is likely to be more limited in NSTEACS, so lesions in both the culprit and the nonculprit arteries may be reliably evaluated with FFR in those cases [20–22]. Then, as shown in Figure 1, the RCA territory is supplied by collaterals from the LAD. This results in larger total blood supply from the LAD compared to this vessel's supply in case of patent RCA. Regarding CTOs, the supply of the occluded-vessel territory depends on the patency and flow of the donor artery. When the last is affected by intermediate stenosis, FFR in the donor artery may normalize after successful PCI of the vessel with the CTO [23, 24]. Therefore, CTO recanalization followed by reassessment of the donor artery stenosis seems to be the proposed treatment plan in these cases [24].

In conclusion, although the common risk score models guiding the decision between PCI and CABG are helpful, in fact, they do not take into account various patient comorbidities. Individualization, case-by-case analysis, and patient's wishes are the key points of the therapeutic strategy. The evolution of PCI techniques, particularly in the field of CTO, makes interventional treatment possible in cases that were formerly managed exclusively with CABG. Nevertheless, this nonsurgical approach does not lack complications that every catheterization laboratory should be adequately trained to deal with.

Abbreviations

CABG: Coronary artery bypass grafting
CAD: Coronary artery disease
CR: Complete revascularization
CTO: Chronic total occlusion
D1: First diagonal branch
FFR: Fractional flow reserve
ICA: Invasive coronary angiography
LAD: Left anterior descending
MG: Myasthenia gravis
NSTEACS: Non-ST elevation acute coronary syndrome
NSTEMI: Non-ST elevation myocardial infarction
PAD: Peripheral artery disease
PCI: Percutaneous coronary intervention
RCA: Right coronary artery.

References

[1] C. De Innocentiis, M. Zimarino, and R. De Caterina, "Is complete revascularisation mandated for all patients with multivessel coronary artery disease?," *Interventional Cardiology Review*, vol. 13, no. 1, pp. 45–50, 2017.

[2] R. D. Vieira, W. Hueb, B. J. Gersh et al., "Effect of complete revascularization on 10-year survival of patients with stable multivessel coronary artery disease: MASS II trial," *Circulation*, vol. 126, no. 11, Supplement_1, pp. S158–S163, 2012.

[3] D. Scrutinio and P. Giannuzzi, "Comorbidity in patients undergoing coronary artery bypass graft surgery: impact on outcome and implications for cardiac rehabilitation," *European Journal of Preventive Cardiology*, vol. 15, no. 4, pp. 379–385, 2009.

[4] J. R. Estrada, J. D. Paul, A. P. Shah, and S. Nathan, "Overview of technical and cost considerations in complex percutaneous coronary intervention," *Interventional Cardiology Review*, vol. 9, no. 1, pp. 17–22, 2011.

[5] S. G. Ellis, S. Ajluni, A. Z. Arnold et al., "Increased coronary perforation in the new device era: incidence, classification, management, and outcome," *Circulation*, vol. 90, no. 6, pp. 2725–2730, 1994.

[6] L. Blichfeldt-Lauridsen and B. D. Hansen, "Anesthesia and myasthenia gravis," *Acta Anaesthesiologica Scandinavica*, vol. 56, no. 1, pp. 17–22, 2012.

[7] W. Wu, A. Masri, Z. B. Popovic et al., "Long-term survival of patients with radiation heart disease undergoing cardiac surgery: a cohort study," *Circulation*, vol. 127, no. 14, pp. 1476–1485, 2013.

[8] E. A. Fender, P. Chandrashekar, J. J. Liang et al., "Coronary artery bypass grafting in patients treated with thoracic radiation: a case–control study," *Open Heart*, vol. 5, no. 1, article e000766, 2018.

[9] F. D. Loop, B. W. Lytle, D. M. Cosgrove et al., "Influence of the internal-mammary-artery graft on 10-year survival and other cardiac events," *The New England Journal of Medicine*, vol. 314, no. 1, pp. 1–6, 1986.

[10] C. B. Park, R. M. Suri, H. M. Burkhart et al., "Identifying patients at particular risk of injury during repeat sternotomy: analysis of 2555 cardiac reoperations," *The Journal of Thoracic and Cardiovascular Surgery*, vol. 140, no. 5, pp. 1028–1035, 2010.

[11] P. I. Ellman, R. L. Smith, M. E. Girotti et al., "Cardiac injury during resternotomy does not affect perioperative mortality," *Journal of the American College of Surgeons*, vol. 206, no. 5, pp. 993–997, 2008.

[12] A. Lemaire, G. Batsides, S. Saadat et al., "Effect of repeat sternotomy on cardiac surgery outcomes," *Annals of Surgery and Perioperative Care*, vol. 1, no. 1, p. 1001, 2016, https://austinpublishinggroup.com/annals-surgery/fulltext/aspc-v1-id1001.php.

[13] S. Launcelott, M. Ouzounian, K. J. Buth, and J.-F. Légaré, "Predicting in-hospital mortality after redo cardiac operations: development of a preoperative scorecard," *The Annals of Thoracic Surgery*, vol. 94, no. 3, pp. 778–784, 2012.

[14] V. Farooq, P. W. Serruys, C. V. Bourantas et al., "Quantification of incomplete revascularization and its association with five-year mortality in the synergy between percutaneous coronary intervention with taxus and cardiac surgery (SYNTAX) trial validation of the residual SYNTAX score," *Circulation*, vol. 128, no. 2, pp. 141–151, 2013.

[15] ESC Scientific Document Group, "2018 ESC/EACTS guidelines on myocardial revascularization," *European Heart Journal*, vol. 40, no. 2, pp. 87–165, 2019.

[16] P. A. L. Tonino, B. De Bruyne, N. H. J. Pijls et al., "Fractional flow reserve versus angiography for guiding percutaneous coronary intervention," *The New England Journal of Medicine*, vol. 360, no. 3, pp. 213–224, 2009.

[17] P. Xaplanteris, S. Fournier, N. H. J. Pijls et al., "Five-year outcomes with PCI guided by fractional flow reserve," *The New England Journal of Medicine*, vol. 379, no. 3, pp. 250–259, 2018.

[18] E. S. Brilakis, J. A. Grantham, S. Rinfret et al., "A percutaneous treatment algorithm for crossing coronary chronic total occlusions," *JACC. Cardiovascular Interventions*, vol. 5, no. 4, pp. 367–379, 2012.

[19] S. M. Patel, R. V. Menon, M. N. Burke et al., "Current perspectives and practices on chronic total occlusion percutaneous coronary interventions," *The Journal of Invasive Cardiology*, vol. 30, no. 2, pp. 43–50, 2018.

[20] W. F. Fearon, "Percutaneous coronary intervention should be guided by fractional flow reserve measurement," *Circulation*, vol. 129, no. 18, pp. 1860–1870, 2014.

[21] W. F. Fearon, B. De Bruyne, and N. H. J. Pijls, "Fractional flow reserve in acute coronary syndromes," *Journal of the American College of Cardiology*, vol. 68, no. 11, pp. 1192–1194, 2016.

[22] J. Layland, D. Carrick, M. McEntegart et al., "Vasodilatory capacity of the coronary microcirculation is preserved in selected patients with non-ST-segment-elevation myocardial infarction," *Circulation. Cardiovascular Interventions*, vol. 6, no. 3, pp. 231–236, 2013.

[23] H. Matsuo and Y. Kawase, "Physiological impact of CTO recanalization assessed by coronary pressure measurement: a case report," *Catheterization and Cardiovascular Interventions*, vol. 82, no. 4, 2013.

[24] R. Sachdeva, M. Agrawal, S. E. Flynn, G. S. Werner, and B. F. Uretsky, "Reversal of ischemia of donor artery myocardium after recanalization of a chronic total occlusion," *Catheterization and Cardiovascular Interventions*, vol. 82, no. 4, 2013.

Acute Coronary Syndrome after 17 Years of Bare Metal Stent Implantation: "Very" Very Late Stent Thrombosis

Raghavendra Rao K,[1] S. Reddy,[1] J. R. Kashyap,[1] K. Vikas,[1] Hithesh Reddy,[1] and Vadivelu Ramalingam[2]

[1]*Department of Cardiology, Government Medical College and Hospital, Sector 32, Chandigarh 160030, India*
[2]*Department of Cardiology, Velammal Medical College Hospital and Research Institute, Madurai 625009, India*

Correspondence should be addressed to Raghavendra Rao K; sarjubmc90@gmail.com

Academic Editor: Alfredo E. Rodriguez

Very late stent thrombosis (VLST) is a catastrophic and life-threatening complication after percutaneous coronary intervention which presents as an acute coronary syndrome with significantly high mortality and morbidity. VLST is a rare entity with drug-eluting stents and even rarer with bare metal stents. The exact pathophysiologic mechanism of VLST after BMS implantation is not known although various mechanisms have been proposed. Recently, in-stent neoatherosclerosis with intimal plaque rupture has been proposed as a potential mechanism of VLST after BMS. We report a rare case of VLST occurring 17 years after BMS implantation with angiographic and intravascular imaging evidence which provides insight into the mechanisms of VLST.

1. Introduction

Coronary stents are the mainstay of percutaneous coronary interventions and have significantly reduced the rates of restenosis and acute vessel closure [1]. Drug-eluting stents (DES) are preferred over bare metal stents (BMS) since DES significantly reduces in-stent restenosis (ISR) by inhibiting neointimal proliferation. However, stent thrombosis (ST) remains an uncommon but catastrophic complication which usually presents as acute coronary syndrome (ACS) with STEMI (ST elevation myocardial infarction) though it can also present as sudden death, arrhythmias, or acute heart failure [2]. Incidence of stent thrombosis has markedly reduced with the use of dual antiplatelet therapy (DAPT) and adequate optimization of stent implantation [1]. According to the Academic Research Consortium criteria and classification, ST is classified according to the time since stent implantation. Acute ST occurs during the stenting procedure or within the subsequent 24 hours, subacute ST occurs between 1 and 30 days after implantation, late ST occurs between 1 month and 1 year, and very late ST occurs more than 1 year after the procedure [3]. A new term "very (or extreme) very late stent thrombosis (VVLST)" was suggested when ST occurred after five years of stent implantation [2, 4]. Very late stent thrombosis (VLST) occurs more frequently with DES than with BMS, and majority of VLST occurs within 1–4 years of stent implantation. VLST occurring after five years of stent implantation is an exceedingly rare phenomenon, and it is still a rarer entity with BMS [2, 5]. We report a case of "very" very late stent thrombosis occurring 17 years after BMS implantation which presented as acute ST segment elevation myocardial infarction.

2. Case Report

A 76-year-old man first reported in the year 2000 with acute-onset retrosternal chest pain of 24-hour duration. Electrocardiogram showed ST segment elevation in the inferior leads with normal sinus rhythm. Apart from diabetes mellitus, other conventional risk factors like obesity, hypertension, smoking, and family history of ischemic heart disease were absent. Routine investigations were within normal limits. Echocardiogram revealed inferior wall hypokinesia with an ejection fraction of 40% with no mitral regurgitation. After

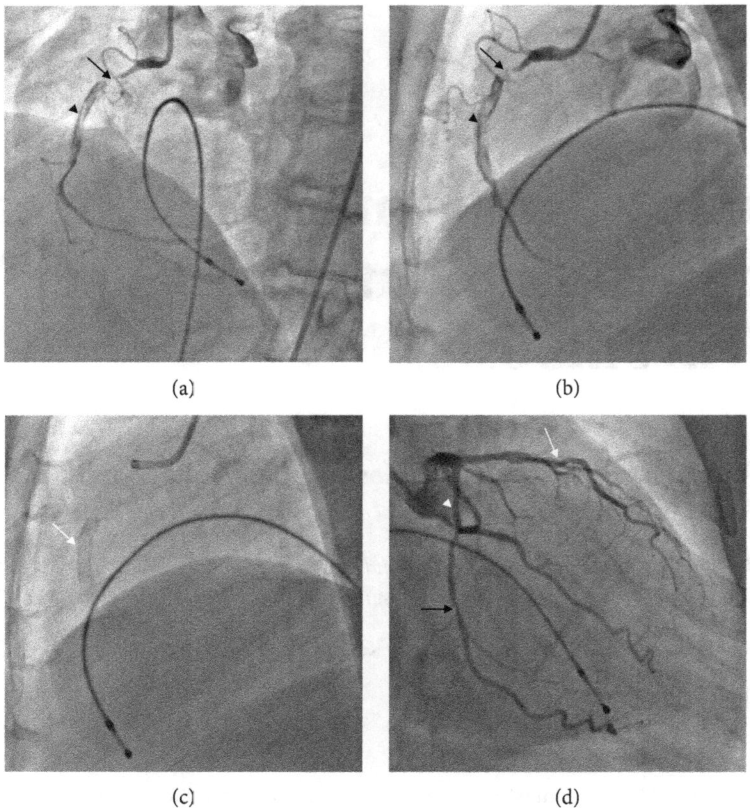

Figure 1: (a) Coronary angiography showing RCA in LAO cranial view with maximum stenosis just proximal to the native bare metal stent (black arrow) and thrombosis within the stent (black arrowhead). (b) RCA in lateral view with 95% stenosis (black arrow) and thrombus inside the stent (black arrowhead). (c) Native bare metal stent (white arrow). (d) RAO caudal view shows plaque in LAD (white arrow) with 30% stenosis in the proximal LCX (white arrowhead) and 50% stenosis in the obtuse marginal artery (black arrow).

receiving a loading dose of aspirin (325 mg), clopidogrel (600 mg), and atorvastatin (80 mg), the patient was taken up for coronary angiography. Coronary angiography revealed a normal left main artery (LM), left circumflex artery (LCX), and left anterior descending artery (LAD). The right coronary artery (RCA) had a significant stenosis in the midsegment, and the patient underwent PCI to RCA with implantation of a bare metal stent (BMS) in the mid-RCA. Drug-eluting stents (DES) were not available at that point of time anywhere in the country. His recovery was uneventful and was discharged on the 4th day on daily aspirin (150 mg), clopidogrel (75 mg), metoprolol (25 mg), atorvastatin (80 mg), and oral hypoglycemic agents. He was on a regular follow-up every 3–6 months since the time of his first coronary intervention. Clopidogrel was stopped after 12 months, and he was advised to continue other medications. The patient remained asymptomatic and was on a regular medical follow-up with no discontinuation of medical therapy at any point of time.

In January 2017, the patient presented to us with sudden-onset chest pain radiating to the left shoulder of one-hour duration and an episode of syncope. His pulse rate was 40/min regular, and his blood pressure is 90/60 mmHg. Electrocardiogram showed sinus bradycardia with ST elevations in leads II, III, and aVF. The cardiac enzyme troponin T was positive, and echocardiography showed hypokinesia of the inferior wall with no mitral regurgitation and a left-ventricular ejection fraction of 45%. Blood sugars were well controlled with normal renal function tests and a hemogram. The patient underwent temporary pacemaker insertion in view of the syncopal episode and bradycardia. Coronary angiography revealed proximal LAD plaque, proximal LCX 30% stenosis, and obtuse marginal 50% stenosis. In proximal RCA 95% stenosis, the mid-RCA stent was thrombus laden extending to the distal RCA. A posterior descending artery (PDA) and posterior left ventricle (PLV) branches were normal (Figures 1(a)–1(d)). He was given loading doses of aspirin (325 mg), clopidogrel (600 mg), and atorvastatin (80 mg) and was taken up for primary PCI to RCA via a right femoral approach. The right coronary artery was engaged with a Judkins right guiding catheter (6 French, 3.5), and the lesion was crossed using a 0.014″ BMW guidewire (Balance Middleweight Universal wire, Abbott Vascular, CA, USA). An IVUS (Eagle Eye® Platinum digital IVUS catheter, Volcano Corporation, CA, USA) pullback was taken from distal RCA which showed thrombus extending from proximal to distal RCA. There was plaque rupture at the proximal stent edge and thrombus. Within the stent, there was neoatherosclerosis in the midregion with intimal plaque rupture, spotty calcification, and thrombosis (Figures 2(a)–2(e)). Significant plaque burden and thrombus were also noted in the distal RCA. Eptifibatide (GP IIbIIIa inhibitor) infusion was started, and manual thrombus aspiration was done using a 6 French

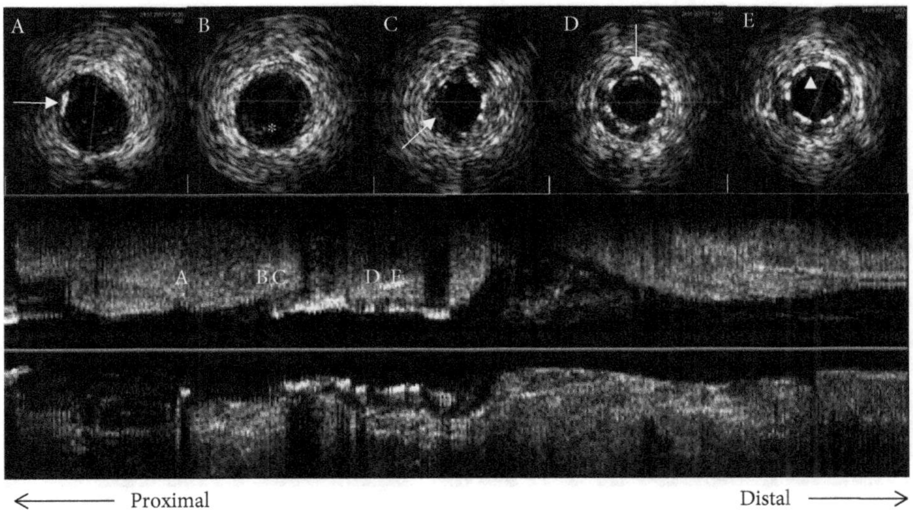

FIGURE 2: Cross-sectional and longitudinal views: baseline IVUS pullback images from distal to proximal RCA demonstrating (a) an arc of calcium in the proximal RCA (white arrow), (b) a site of plaque rupture at the proximal stent edge (white asterisk), (c) thrombus inside the stent (white arrow), (d) spotty calcification within the stent (white arrow), stent struts (black arrow), and (e) a site of plaque rupture within the stent (white arrowhead).

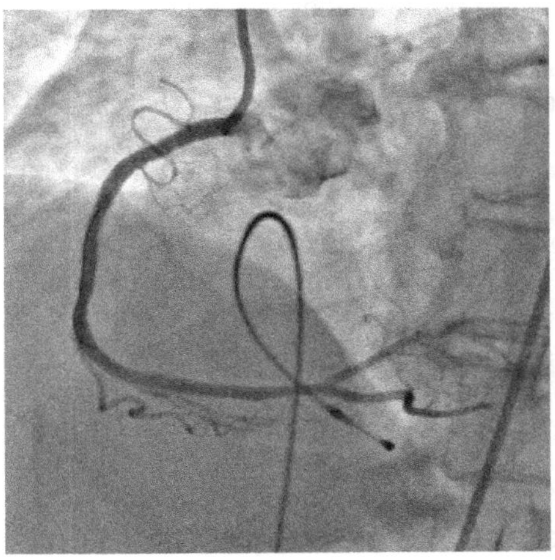

FIGURE 3: Final angiographic view post-PCI showing adequate stent expansion with good distal opacification.

Thrombuster II® (Kaneka Corporation, Osaka, Japan). The lesion was predilated with a SPRINTER® semicompliant 2.5 × 15 mm balloon (Medtronic, Minneapolis, USA) from distal to proximal RCA at 10-12 atm. The stent Xience Prime (2.75 × 38 mm) (2nd-generation everolimus-eluting stent, Abbott Vascular, CA, USA) was deployed in mid-RCA to distal RCA at 10 atm, the second stent Xience Prime (3 × 38 mm) was deployed in proximal RCA to mid-RCA at 12 atm overlapping with the previous stent, and the third stent Xience Prime (3.5 × 28 mm) was deployed from ostial to proximal RCA at 12 atm overlapping with the previous stent. Postdilatation of the distal to ostial RCA stents was done using SPRINTER® noncompliant balloons (Medtronic, Minneapolis, USA) (2.75 × 9 mm, 3 × 12 mm, and 3.5 × 12 mm) successively at 12-18 atm. Postprocedure angiography showed TIMI III flow (Figure 3), and an IVUS pullback was taken which showed good stent strut apposition (Figures 4(a)–4(e)). The patient was discharged in a stable condition on dual antiplatelets and statins.

3. Discussion

VLST is an exceedingly rare complication of PCI with recent studies showing an incidence of approximately 0.5% per year with BMS that reaches up to 2% per year with DES. Most cases present as an ST segment elevation myocardial infarction carrying high morbidity and mortality with an annual mortality rates of 10% to 20% [6, 7]. We present a case of "very" very late stent thrombosis occurring 17 years after implantation of a bare metal stent. Our case highlights the importance that the underlying pathophysiologic mechanisms are multifactorial. To the best of our knowledge, this is the first case to report with the longest duration after bare metal stent implantation to thrombosis with an intravascular imaging guidance. Earlier, Acibuca and colleagues reported a case of BMS thrombosis occurring after two decades; however, in their report, intravascular ultrasound (IVUS) was not done and the exact duration was not clear [8]. Our case is unique as IVUS was performed and we demonstrated that multiple factors are responsible for plaque rupture leading to VLST such as (a) persistent peristent strut chronic inflammation leading to plaque rupture at the proximal stent edge, (b) neoatherosclerosis inside the stent which led to plaque rupture, and (c) the presence of calcium suggesting longer duration of the atherosclerotic plaque and subsequent plaque rupture due to a calcified nodule.

Earlier, Sarkees et al. had reported VLST occurring 13 years after BMS implantation which occurred upon termination of antiplatelet therapy [9]. History of discontinuation of antiplatelet therapy was not there in our case. Randomized trials have shown that the incidence of stent thrombosis within the first year of implantation is identical in patients

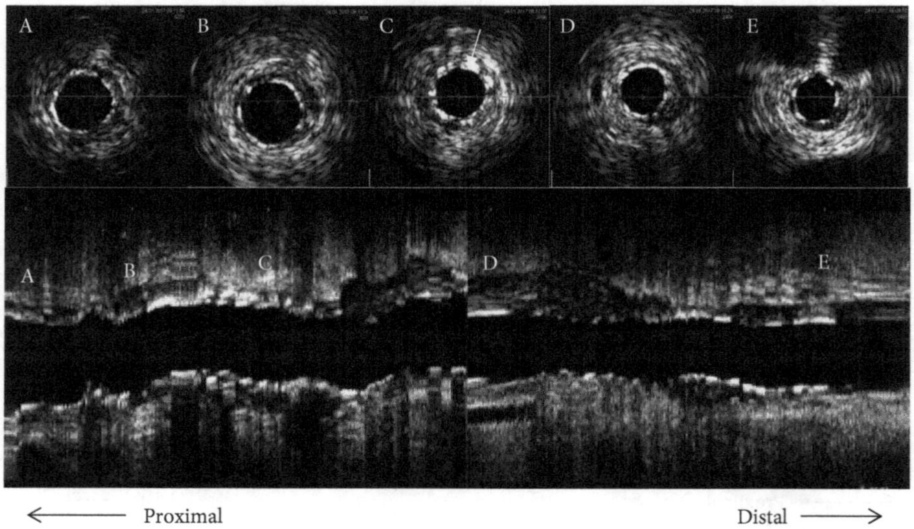

FIGURE 4: Poststenting IVUS pullback showing adequate stent expansion with an MLD/CSA (minimum lumen diameter/cross-sectional area) of (a) 3.13 mm/8.43 mm^2 at the proximal RCA, (b) 3.23 mm/8.92 mm^2 at the previous stent proximal edge, (c) 2.85 mm/6.46 mm^2 at the stent overlapping region (white arrow), (d) 2.54 mm/5.49 mm^2 at the distal RCA, and (e) 2.39 mm/4.78 mm^2 at the very distal RCA.

with DES and those with BMS. However, after 1 year, a modest increase is observed in VLST after DES implantation compared to that after BMS implantation [10]. The exact pathophysiologic mechanism for VLST after BMS implantation is not known, but various mechanisms have been proposed. BMS have a rapid endothelialization after implantation which is usually completed by 3 to 6 months unlike DES which takes a longer period; hence, the inflammatory response does not seem to be the triggering cause of VLST with BMS [5, 11, 12].

Of the various hypotheses proposed for VLST after BMS implantation, the most important and plausible mechanism being in-stent neoatherosclerosis and subsequent plaque rupture which presents as an ACS and the histological features are indistinguishable between patients with VLST and patients with ACS unrelated to stent thrombosis [6]. Yumoto et al. showed that VLST after BMS might be caused by a thrombus formation subsequent to a calcified atherosclerotic plaque rupture [11]. Stent strut malapposition and positive arterial remodeling and late acquired stent malapposition have also been suggested as probable etiologies for VLST after BMS [13]. Late stent malapposition occurs with both DES and BMS though it is more common after DES implantation and increases the risk of VLST [12]. In the present case, there was no clear IVUS evidence of stent malapposition. Metallic stent struts being a foreign body can induce persistent peristrut chronic inflammation which can accelerate atherosclerotic changes and subsequent plaque rupture [14]. Long-term follow-up studies using intravascular imaging guidance after BMS implantation have shown that the neointima transforms into lipid-laden tissue with narrowing of the lumen, expansion of the neovascularization into the intima, calcification, and advanced atherosclerotic changes like intimal disruption with thrombus formation leading to ACS [15]. Our case showed the presence of calcium in both the native vessel and the stented segment along with evidence of neointimal rupture, plaque rupture at the proximal stent edge possibly due to peristent strut inflammation, and superimposed thrombus formation.

4. Conclusion

Based on our case study and IVUS analysis, we conclude that multiple mechanisms contribute to VLST after BMS implantation predominantly due to neoatherosclerotic plaque rupture, peristent strut chronic inflammation leading to plaque rupture, and calcific atherosclerotic plaque rupture. All the above mechanisms either alone or in combination may lead to plaque rupture eventually causing acute coronary syndrome.

References

[1] R. Jaffe and B. H. Strauss, "Late and very late thrombosis of drug-eluting stents: evolving concepts and perspectives," *Journal of the American College of Cardiology*, vol. 50, no. 2, pp. 119–127, 2007.

[2] S. Gupta, "Very very late stent thrombosis: 9.5 years after DES implantation," *Indian Heart Journal*, vol. 68, Supplement 2, pp. S39–S43, 2016.

[3] D. E. Cutlip, S. Windecker, R. Mehran et al., "Clinical end points in coronary stent Trials," *Circulation*, vol. 115, no. 17, pp. 2344–2351, 2007.

[4] A. Kaliyadan, H. Siu, D. L. Fischman et al., ""Very" very late stent thrombosis: acute myocardial infarction from drug-eluting stent thrombosis more than 5 years after implantation," *The Journal of Invasive Cardiology*, vol. 26, no. 9, pp. 413–416, 2014.

[5] S. Windecker and B. Meier, "Late coronary stent thrombosis," *Circulation*, vol. 116, no. 17, pp. 1952–1965, 2007.

[6] M. S. Herrera, J. A. Restrepo, A. F. Buitrago, M. G. Mejía, and J. H. Díaz, "Very late bare metal stent thrombosis," *Case Reports in Critical Care*, vol. 2013, Article ID 856095, 2 pages, 2013.

[7] E. J. Armstrong, D. N. Feldman, T. Y. Wang et al., "Clinical presentation, management, and outcomes of angiographically documented early, late, and very late stent thrombosis," *JACC: Cardiovascular Interventions*, vol. 5, no. 2, pp. 131–140, 2012.

[8] A. Acibuca, D. M. Gerede, and V. K. Vurgun, "Bare-metal stent thrombosis two decades after stenting," *Cardiovascular Journal of Africa*, vol. 26, no. 4, pp. e19–e21, 2015.

[9] M. L. Sarkees, A. A. Bavry, J. M. Galla, and D. L. Bhatt, "Bare metal stent thrombosis 13 years after implantation," *Cardiovascular Revascularization Medicine*, vol. 10, no. 1, pp. 58-59, 2009.

[10] G. W. Stone, J. W. Moses, S. G. Ellis et al., "Safety and efficacy of sirolimus- and paclitaxel-eluting coronary stents," *The New England Journal of Medicine*, vol. 356, no. 10, pp. 998–1008, 2007.

[11] K. Yumoto, T. Anzai, H. Aoki et al., "Calcified plaque rupture and very late stent thrombosis after bare-metal stent implantation," *Cardiovascular Intervention and Therapeutics*, vol. 26, pp. 252–259, 2011.

[12] J. Kotani, M. Awata, S. Nanto et al., "Incomplete neointimal coverage of sirolimus-eluting stents: angioscopic findings," *Journal of the American College of Cardiology*, vol. 47, no. 10, pp. 2108–2111, 2006.

[13] A. Caixeta, V. C. Braga, and G. S. Mintz, "Very late stent thrombosis with bare-metal stent: identifying severe stent malapposition and underexpansion by intravascular ultrasound," *Einstein (São Paulo)*, vol. 11, no. 3, pp. 364–366, 2013.

[14] K. Inoue, K. Abe, K. Ando et al., "Pathological analyses of long-term intracoronary Palmaz-Schatz stenting: is its efficacy permanent?," *Cardiovascular Pathology*, vol. 13, no. 2, pp. 109–115, 2004.

[15] M. Takano, M. Yamamoto, S. Inami et al., "Appearance of lipid-laden intima and neovascularization after implantation of bare-metal stents: extended late-phase observation by intracoronary optical coherence tomography," *Journal of the American College of Cardiology*, vol. 55, no. 1, pp. 26–32, 2009.

15

QT Independent Ventricular Tachycardia Induced by Arsenic Trioxide

Vicken Zeitjian[1] **Carmel Moazez,**[2] **Waqas Arslan,**[3] **and Mehrdad Saririan**[4]

[1]*Department of Cardiovascular Diseases, University of Texas San Antonio Health Science Center, 7703 Floyd Curl Dr. San Antonio, TX 78229, USA*
[2]*Department of Internal Medicine, Creighton University Maricopa Medical Center, 2601 E. Roosevelt St. Phoenix, AZ 85006, USA*
[3]*Department of Hematology and Oncology, Creighton University Maricopa Medical Center, 2601 E. Roosevelt St. Phoenix, AZ 85006, USA*
[4]*Department of Cardiovascular Diseases, Creighton University Maricopa Medical Center, 2601 E. Roosevelt St. Phoenix, AZ 85006, USA*

Correspondence should be addressed to Vicken Zeitjian; zeitjian@uthscsa.edu

Academic Editor: Konstantinos P. Letsas

Arsenic trioxide (ATO) is commonly known to cause QT prolongation with resultant ventricular tachycardia (VT). VT, independent of QT prolongation, can be a complication of ATO. We present a 46-year-old female who received ATO and during her hospital course had intermittent nonsustained VT. All usual causes of VT were considered including reduced EF < 35%, ischemia, electrolyte abnormalities, medications, and genetic polymorphisms; however, no specific cause was found. After stopping therapy, the episodes of nonsustained VT ceased indicating that there is an association between ATO and VT.

1. Introduction

Arsenic trioxide (ATO) is commonly known to cause QT prolongation with resultant ventricular tachycardia (VT); however, it is the preferred treatment in combination with all-trans retinoic acid for acute promyeloctyic leukemia. VT, independent of QT prolongation, is a complication of ATO. Here, we present a case of nonsustained VT without QT prolongation due to ATO. This is the second paper exploring the association of nonsustained VT and ATO due to a mechanism different than prolonged QT.

2. Case

A 46-year-old Hispanic female presented with a chief complaint of generalized fatigue, vaginal bleeding, gingival bleeding, and nasal bleeding for 2 weeks. On exam, she was tachycardic and had conjunctival pallor. She had several areas of ecchymosis over her extremities and abdomen and scattered petechiae across the chest. Labs were significant for a hemoglobin of 7.7 g/dL, white blood cells of 3.3/μL, platelets of 3 K/μL, and blasts of 37%. Peripheral smear showed progranulocytes and auer rods. Fluorescent in situ hybridization was done on bone marrow showing promyelocytic leukemia-retinoic acid receptor alpha (PML-RARA) positivity indicating acute promyelocytic leukemia.

She was started on all-trans retinoic acid (ATRA) and ATO for intermediate risk APL with treatment length until remission or up to 60 days, whichever came first. A combination of ATRA and ATO was chosen based on their efficacy of obtaining remission compared to ATRA combined with standard chemotherapy. Initial electrocardiogram (EKG) showed sinus tachycardia with a heart rate of 110 and corrected QT (QTc) interval of 434 ms. On day 26 of ATO treatment, she complained of palpitations and began having episodes of asymptomatic nonsustained VT on telemetry (Figure 1). EKG was done which was unable to capture the VT. The rhythm was sinus with QTc of 447 ms. Potassium was 4 mg/dL and magnesium was 2.3 mg/dL. She had no family history of sudden cardiac death or related long QT sequelae. Baseline EKG had a normal QTc.

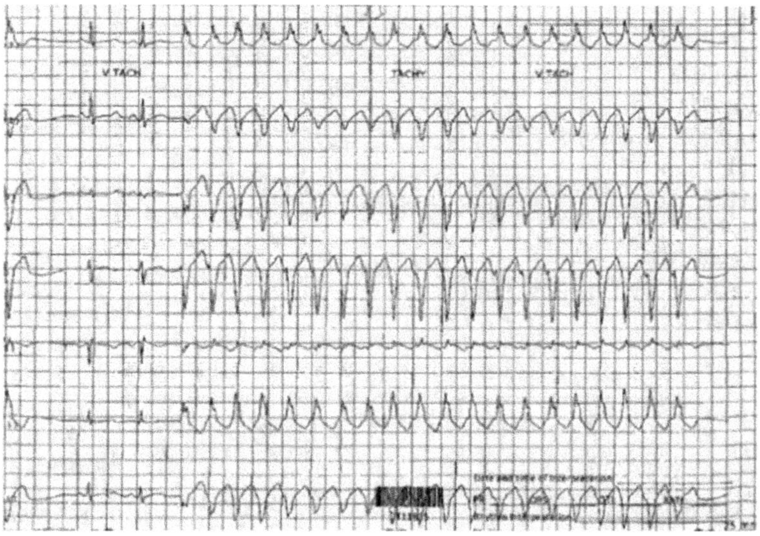

FIGURE 1: Nonsustained monomorphic ventricular tachycardia.

She had a transthoracic echocardiogram, which showed no structural heart disease and a normal ejection fraction. We considered the option of discontinuing ATO; however, our oncology consultants felt strongly about the need to continue combination ATRA and ATO because the patient had at least intermediate risk APL. She was started on nadolol 40 mg daily as off-label treatment given that ATO continuation was necessary for up to 60 days. We chose 40 mg as the starting dose, which is the minimum dose of nadolol with plans of uptitrating if VT was not suppressed. Since there were no further reoccurrences of nonsustained VT, we did not have to increase the dose. Episodes of nonsustained VT were decreased after starting nadolol. Nadolol was chosen as a once daily beta-blocker based on its efficacy of reducing ventricular ectopy and tachycarrhythmias. Fortunately, the patient was able to continue cancer treatment to completion. The patient completed 60 days of ATO treatment with weekly QTc monitoring and was continued on nadolol until completion of treatment.

3. Discussion

ATO has been known to cause VT due to related long QT. However, through this case and literature review, we propose that ATO is also associated with VT independent of prolonged QT. QT prolongation, VT, heart block, and sudden cardiac death have been reported with ATO use. Prolonged QT is the most common and occurs in 26-93% of cases. It commonly occurs after 1-5 weeks of therapy and usually returns to baseline after 8 weeks from the last infusion [1, 2].

In our case, all usual causes of VT were considered including reduced EF < 35%, ischemia, electrolyte abnormalities, medications, idiopathic VT, and genetic polymorphisms; however, no specific cause was found. No invasive studies were performed given that after discontinuation of ATO, the episodes of VT ceased leading us to believe that there is an association.

Ducas et al. presented the first case of VT during ATO treatment independent of QTc. Their investigation for reversible causes of VT was also negative leading the authors to believe ATO as a cause of VT [3]. Arsenic cardiotoxicity is a known pathology well described in the National Comprehensive Cancer Network (NCCN). Per NCCN recommendations, a 12 lead EKG, creatinine, and electrolytes including potassium, magnesium, and calcium are required prior to commencement of therapy. During treatment, weekly EKG and electrolytes should be monitored. Target levels include a QTc of <460 ms (in females), potassium greater than 4 mmol/L, and magnesium greater than 0.74 mmol/L [3, 4].

Current ESC guidelines recommend discontinuing or lowering the dosing of ATO in patients with prolonged QTc > 500 ms to prevent torsade de pointes. Also, providers should perform weekly EKGs and check electrolytes while patients are receiving ATO. Our patient developed VT independent of prolonged QTc, and therefore, we opted to not discontinue or reduce her treatment, as she did not have a prolonged QTc [5].

ATO is known to uncouple cardiac mitochondrial oxidative phosphorylation due to competing with inorganic phosphate for ATP formation. Intracellular ATP will become depleted, and the cardiac $I_{K\text{-}ATP}$ will be activated as a compensatory mechanism. These channels increase potassium conduction and stabilize the resting membrane potential. As a result, there is a shorter action potential with decreased calcium influx and preservation of intracellular energy. ATO is also a potent blocker of I_{Kr} and I_{Ks} which activate delayed rectified potassium channels [6]. Delayed rectified potassium channels are responsible for ventricular repolarization and stabilization of membrane potential. With disruption of the normal function of these channels and multiple potassium currents, electrical instability may result in malignant tachyarrhythmias [7].

We conclude that ATO may induce VT with and without association of QT prolongation. ATO's intrinsic properties affecting potassium ion channels are the likely cause of VT occurrence. After completing ATO, she has been free of ventricular tachycardia for the last 6 months.

4. Conclusion

We conclude that ATO may induce VT independent of QTc prolongation. Previous studies in patients on ATO have shown VT to be dependent on QTc prolongation. Our paper is the 2nd reported case documenting the association between VT and ATO independent of the QTc interval. This clinical observation supports close telemetry monitoring in patients who report palpitations as VT may be the underlying etiology. The mechanism of VT remains unclear, and therefore, further studies at an ionic level may help investigate VT and ATO association.

Authors' Contributions

All authors contributed significantly in writing this manuscript.

References

[1] E. T. H. Yeh and C. L. Bickford, "Cardiovascular complications of cancer therapy: incidence, pathogenesis, diagnosis, and management," *Journal of the American College of Cardiology*, vol. 53, no. 24, pp. 2231–2247, 2009.

[2] J. T. Barbey, "Cardiac toxicity of arsenic trioxide," *Blood*, vol. 98, no. 5, pp. 1632–1634, 2001.

[3] M. R. O'Donnel, F. R. Appelbaum, and S. E. Coutre, *NCCN Clinical Practice Guidelines in Oncology: acute myeloid leukemia*, National Comprehensive Cancer Network, 2010.

[4] R. A. Ducas, M. D. Seftel, J. Ducas, and C. Seifer, "Monomorphic ventricular tachycardia caused by arsenic trioxide therapy for acute promyelocytic leukaemia," *The Journal of the Royal College of Physicians Edinburgh*, vol. 41, no. 2, pp. 117-118, 2011.

[5] J. L. Zamorano, P. Lancellotti, R. D. Muñoz et al., "2016 ESC Position Paper on cancer treatments and cardiovascular toxicity developed under the auspices of the ESC Committee for Practice Guidelines: the task force for cancer treatments and cardiovascular toxicity of the European Society of Cardiology (ESC)," *European Heart Journal*, vol. 37, no. 36, pp. 2768–2801, 2016.

[6] B. Drolet, C. Simard, and D. M. Roden, "Unusual effects of a QT-prolonging drug, arsenic trioxide, on cardiac potassium currents," *Circulation*, vol. 109, no. 1, pp. 26–29, 2004.

[7] L. Chen, K. J. Sampson, and R. S. Kass, "Cardiac delayed rectifier potassium channels in health and disease," *Cardiac Electrophysiology Clinics*, vol. 8, no. 2, pp. 307–322, 2016.

16

Posterior Reversible Encephalopathy Syndrome Associated with Tacrolimus in Cardiac Transplantation

Julián Alejandro Rivillas[1] **Stephania Galindo-Coral**[2,3] **Francisco Arias-Mora**[4] **Juan David Lopez-Ponce de Leon**[2] **Noel Alberto Florez-Alarcón**[2] **Pastor Olaya-Rojas**[2] **and Juan Esteban Gomez-Mesa**[2]

[1]*Resident of Neurology, Universidad Icesi, Cali, Colombia*
[2]*Cardiology Department, Fundación Valle del Lili Hospital Universitario, Cali, Colombia*
[3]*Clinical Research Center, Fundación Valle del Lili Hospital Universitario, Cali, Colombia*
[4]*Neurology Department, Fundación Valle del Lili Hospital Universitario, Cali, Colombia*

Correspondence should be addressed to Juan Esteban Gomez-Mesa; juan.gomez.me@fvl.org.co

Academic Editor: Yigit Canga

Background. Neurological complications occur between 50 and 70% of patients with heart transplantation, including cerebrovascular events, infections, seizures, encephalopathy, and neurotoxicity due to pharmacological immunosuppression. Mortality associated with cerebrovascular complications is 7.5% in the first 30 days and up to 5.3% after the first month and up to the first year after transplantation. *Case Reports.* Three heart-transplanted patients (2 men and 1 woman) treated with tacrolimus were identified. They presented with posterior reversible encephalopathy syndrome on days 5, 6, and 58 posttransplantation, respectively. In these reported cases, no sequelae were observed at 6 months follow-up. *Conclusions.* Posterior reversible encephalopathy syndrome as a neurological complication in patients with HT occurred early after the procedure. Early diagnosis and treatment might reduce the risk of serious complications and mortality.

1. Background

Heart transplantation (HT) is a therapeutic option in patients with advanced and refractory heart failure. In Latin America, this procedure has been performed in more than 8,000 patients, in more than 85 institutions in 13 Latin American countries since 1968 [1, 2]. The current worldwide survival rate is up to 90% for the first year, with a median survival of 14 years. The patient's quality of life improves significantly, and up to 30% of them may reintegrate into working life [3]. After HT, different complications may occur, affecting the survival and functionality of patients, such as graft rejection, infections, neoplasms, high blood pressure, kidney disease, and neurological complications [4, 5].

Neurological complications occur between 50% and 70% of patients with HT when transient and mild effects are included. Most may occur within the first 30 days after the procedure and include cerebrovascular events, infections, seizures, encephalopathy, and neurotoxicity due to immunosuppressive medication. Neurological involvement is of particular concern because of its impact on patients' functional prognosis and survival [6, 7]. The most severe neurological complications are ischemic stroke followed by infection. Mortality associated with cerebrovascular complications is 7.5% in the first 30 days and up to 5.3% after the first month and up to the first year after transplantation. It can be as high as 20% in cases of opportunistic infections and cerebrovascular events [5, 8–10].

The most frequently maintained immunosuppressive agents used in heart transplants are corticosteroids, calcineurin inhibitors, and antimetabolites. Corticosteroids induce commonly acute neuropsychiatric symptoms including delirium, sleep disorders, depression, and cognitive decline. Cyclosporine and tacrolimus are both calcineurin inhibitors

Table 1: Description of patients with PRES after heart transplant.

	Case 1	Case 2	Case 3
Gender	Male	Male	Female
Age (years)	27	67	29
Etiology of HF	Becker muscular dystrophy	Ischemic heart disease	Chagas' heart disease
Onset of PRES symptoms (days)	6	5	58
Symptoms	Decreased visual acuity, generalized tonic-clonic seizures, altered level of consciousness	Blurred vision generalized tonic-clonic seizures, altered level of consciousness	Blurry vision generalized tonic-clonic seizures, altered level of consciousness, severe headache
Previous drugs	Tacrolimus MMF, methylprednisolone, TMP/SMX, acyclovir, vancomycin	Tacrolimus MMF, methylprednisolone, TMP/SMX, acyclovir, vancomycin, ceftriaxone	Tacrolimus MMF, prednisone, TMP/SMX, acyclovir, diltiazem, losartan
Hemoglobin (mg/dl)	9.0	10	8.5
Leukocytes (cel/ml)	6,470	8,540	14,130
Platelets (cel/ml)	130,000	140.000	441,000
Creatinine (mg/dl)	0,9	0,8	0,88
Sodium (mEq/l)	141	139	135
Potassium (mEq/l)	3.9	4.0	5.97
Glycemia (mg/dl)	138	165	145
Tacrolimus (ng/dl)	2.6	8.9	17.4
Brain MR	Bilateral and symmetrical parietal and occipital cortical-subcortical hyperintensities in the FLAIR and T2 sequences (Figure 1)	Asymmetric cortical hyperintensities in the parietal and occipital lobes (Figure 2)	Hyperintense lesions of posterior cortical and subcortical predominance without abnormal enhancements with the contrast agent (Figure 3)
Management	Discontinuing tacrolimus, starting cyclosporine, levetiracetam	Discontinuing tacrolimus, starting cyclosporine, levetiracetam	Discontinuing tacrolimus, starting cyclosporine, levetiracetam
Recurrence of symptoms at 6 months	None	None	None

HF: heart failure; PRES: posterior reversible encephalopathy syndrome; HT: heart transplantation; MMF: mycophenolate mofetil; TMP/SMX: trimethoprim-sulfamethoxazole; NMR: nuclear magnetic resonance.

and can induce encephalopathy, seizures, akinetic mutism, and posterior reversible encephalopathy syndrome. Mycophenolate mofetil and azathioprine are antimetabolites. Mycophenolate mofetil does not have a significant direct neurotoxicity, but it may cause headaches on first doses. Azathioprine is rarely used for heart transplantation [6].

2. Clinical Case Reports

Three cases of HT patients with PRES associated with the use of tacrolimus observed at different times after the procedure are described in a cohort of 223 heart transplant patients in a Colombian hospital. Clinical and radiological information is in Table 1 and Figures 1–3.

3. Discussion

PRES was initially described in 1996 [11] and has ever since been associated with clinical conditions such as high blood pressure, eclampsia, infections, autoimmune diseases, and the use of immunosuppressive drugs. The underlying pathophysiological mechanisms are not clear, but differences have been described in the vascular sympathetic innervation of the anterior and posterior brain circulation with a variable degree in the self-regulation capacity in the presence of external noxae as changes in cerebral perfusion pressure, microangiopathy, and toxic effects (i.e., tacrolimus). These tissue insults favor vasogenic edema in the parietal and occipital lobes occur [12]. In PRES associated with CI, vasoconstricting effects and direct endothelial damage have been described, which cause capillary leakage due to disruption of the blood-brain barrier, which ultimately causes cerebral vasogenic edema [13]. This effect is thought to be related to an intrinsic factor of inhibition of calcineurin widely expressed in the central nervous system. The absence of hypertension crisis and normal serum calcineurin values at diagnosis in reported cases in this article supports that hypothesis. The occurrence of PRES after heart transplantation is typically on the first 30 days after surgery with great variation among studies [14]. In published cases reviewed for this article, we found a median of 14 days after heart transplantation. Two of the cases presented here were below

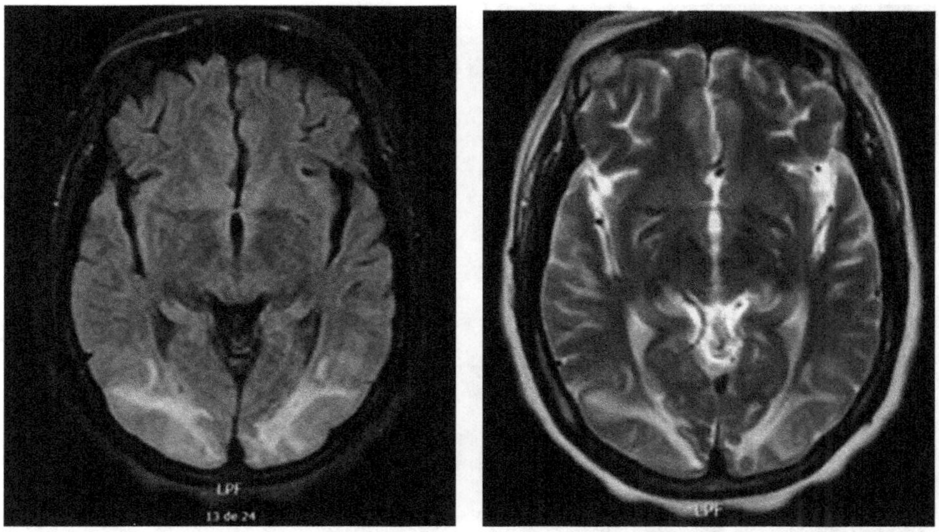

(a) (b)

Figure 1: Brain MR of case 1. (a) Fluid-attenuated inversion recovery sequence showing occipital hyperintensities in occipital gyri. (b) T2-weighted sequence of the same patient showing hyperintensities in the occipital lobe.

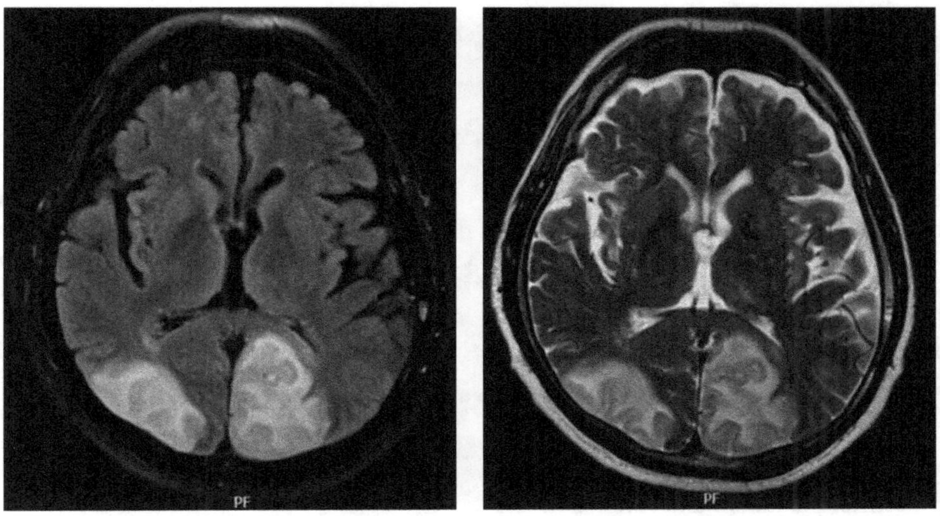

(a) (b)

Figure 2: Brain MR of case 2. (a) Fluid-attenuated inversion recovery sequence showing extensive bilateral asymmetrical occipital hyperintensities in the occipital lobe and (b) its representation on T2-weighted sequence.

this mean time (Table 2). Since most of the reported cases are single-center case series, it is difficult to estimate the true incidence of the problem. Available data indicate that the incidence of PRES syndrome after solid organ transplantation was estimated to be between 1% and 6% [15], but more recent studies estimated it at 0.49% to 1.6% for heart transplants [16] At the end of 2020, our group had performed 223 heart transplants, so we calculate a cumulative incidence of 1.3 cases per 100 transplants since the start of the program in 1994.

3.1. Clinical Features, Imaging, and Histological Findings. PRES is characterized by an alteration of the level of consciousness, seizures, headache, visual disturbances, neurological deficit, and status epilepticus. Fugate and Rabinstein [17] proposed a 7-category list for patients with PRES: encephalopathy, seizure, headache, visual disturbance, focal neurological deficits, status epilepticus, and nausea/vomiting. All of the patients reported by us lacked the three latter. The typical triad of headache, visual disturbances, and seizures was present in all three reported cases. This triad seems to be present in 77% of cases according to previous studies. Other common symptom combination is seizures/encephalopathy (38%), seizures/headache (22.5%), and seizures/visual disturbances (14%) [17].

Brain resonance usually reports bilateral and asymmetric hyperintensities in T2-FLAIR sequences of the occipital and parietal regions, but transient lesions can also be found in the anterior region, cerebellum, centrum semiovale, pons, and hippocampus. Also, coexistent ischemic lesions can be

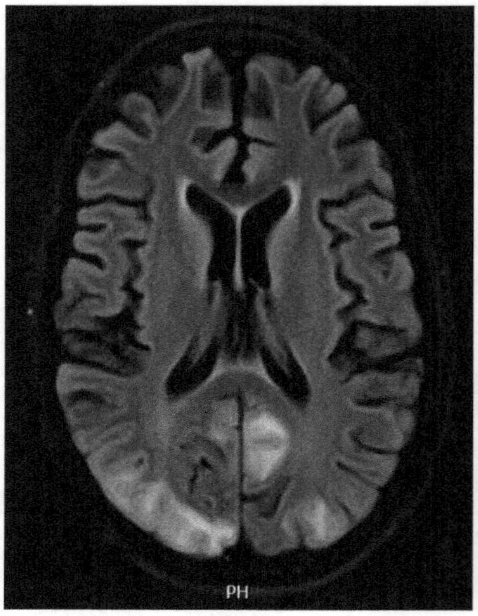

(a)

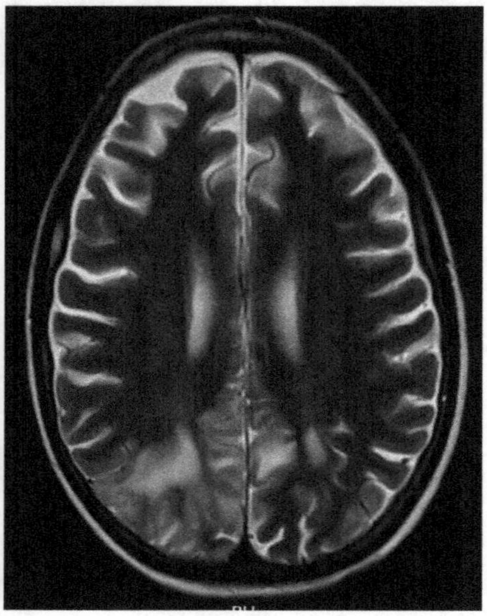

(b)

FIGURE 3: Brain MR of case 3. (a) Fluid-attenuated inversion recovery sequence showing occipitoparietal hyperintensities and (b) its representation in T2-weighted sequence.

present [18]. All reported cases showed typical brain MRI findings, but case 2 presented asymptomatic lesions in the frontal lobe. These findings may support a hypothesis of global alteration of the blood-brain barrier with posterior predominance. No other atypical or hemorrhagic lesions such as those described by McKinney et al. were found [19].

Histopathological findings of cellular edema, disruption of the blood-brain barrier, and, in some cases, necrosis are also observed [20]. These findings help to understand the pathophysiology of the disease but are rarely used in clinical practice. No histopathology information is available for our cases.

3.2. Risk Factors. The onset of symptoms usually occurs during the first month posttransplantation and rarely after the first year despite the chronic use of CI and dose titration during follow-up. The immediate postsurgical period and the following 30 days are critical, since the patient has been suffering from a chronic and debilitating disease with a significant compromise of the functional reserve and subsequently undergoes a major surgery with varying degrees of hemodynamic compromise, tissue hypoperfusion, and administration of immunosuppressive drugs. The reason for the greater incidence of PRES within the first 30 days is not known, but it may be favored by all the factors mentioned above [17]. Two of the reported cases developed PRES during the first 30 days and the other after 58 days, which was associated with a longer hospitalization time and evidence of graft dysfunction in the mediate the postoperative period. Other risk factors frequently reported as hemorrhage and diffusion restriction were not found in our patients [21].

3.3. PRES and Calcineurin Inhibitors. The harmful effects of CI on the endothelium do not seem to be dose-dependent, since many reported cases show normal serum tacrolimus levels at the time of PRES diagnosis (Table 1). That is the case of reported patients. They also lacked a history of hypertensive crises. Similar findings are reported by Song et al. [22]. In contrast, the systematic review performed by this same author reveals a history of hypertension in 69% of patients with PRES after transplantation. The reports of patients with cyclosporine-associated neurotoxicity included headache, seizures, and encephalopathy, and nausea is not necessarily associated with radiological findings of PRES [23, 24]. A trend toward an earlier occurrence and higher likelihood of PRES in the presence of normal drug levels in transplant recipients receiving cyclosporine than those receiving tacrolimus (median time to onset; 12 vs. 26 days and 40%, 8/20 vs. 25.8%, 8/31) [22].

3.4. PRES Treatment and Prognosis. Despite the lack of a general guideline, switching from tacrolimus to cyclosporine is a common measure in the cases published to date. Cyclosporine is effective in preventing organ rejection but has also a risk of causing PRES and other types of neurotoxicity [14]. However, given its high availability in developing countries, it is frequently used in cases of intolerance or adverse effect with other calcineurin inhibitors. Remarkably, in the six-month follow-up, our patients did not present relapse or any other type of neurotoxicity. It is feasible to think that the immunosuppressant is a factor in the early stages after surgery that contributes to the development of PRES but it is not the only cause. Implant rejections were not reported. Consequently, this strategy may seem to be safe and effective for the management of tacrolimus-associated PRES [25–27]. Other approaches include switching to sirolimus, everolimus, mycophenolate mofetil, or hydrocortisone and lowering the dose of immunosuppressive agent. Classically, a low incidence of sequelae, mortality, and recurrence has been described, as evidenced in these three cases. However, some

Table 2: Reported cases compared with reported cases in Literature.

Ref	Sex	Age (years)	Days post-HT	Tacrolimus	Steroids	MMF	Sequelae
Reported cases							
—	M	27	6	Yes	Yes	Yes	No
—	M	67	5	Yes	Yes	Yes	No
—	F	29	58	Yes	Yes	Yes	No
Cases in literature							
1	F	68	14	Yes	No	Yes	No
1	M	19	44	Yes	No	Yes	No
2	F	26	7	Yes	Yes	Yes	No
2	M	33	15	Yes	Yes	Yes	No
3	M	52	8	Yes	Yes	Yes	Yes
4	M	37	16	Yes	Yes	Yes	No
5	F	32	5	Yes	Yes	Yes	No
6	F	30	45	No	Yes	Yes	No
7	F	22	5	Yes	No	Yes	No
8	M	10	10	Yes	Yes	Yes	No
9	F	54	14	Yes	No	Yes	No
10	M	18	150	Yes	Yes	Yes	No
11	F	20	60	Yes	Yes	Yes	No
12	M	10	4	Yes	Yes	Yes	No
13	M	12	4	Yes	Yes	Yes	No

Ref: reference; HT: heart transplantation; MMF: mycophenolate mofetil.

reports report mortality and neurological sequelae as high as 15% especially when it is not identified and treated early and appropriately [28] (Table 2).

4. Conclusions

Neurological complications as PRES in HT patients can occur early after the procedure. Early diagnosis and treatment reduce the risk of more serious outcomes and associated mortality. CI-associated PRES in HT patients is a neurological complication that should be suspected when early "typical manifestations" of an altered level of consciousness, visual disturbances, and seizures appear. The timely diagnosis and treatment of events, change of immunosuppressive therapy to cyclosporine, and multidisciplinary follow-up could reduce the incidence of sequelae.

Abbreviations

CI: Calcineurin inhibitors
HF: Heart failure
HT: Heart transplantation
MMF: Mycophenolate mofetil
NMR: Nuclear magnetic resonance
PRES: Posterior reversible encephalopathy syndrome
TMP/SMX: Trimethoprim-sulfamethoxazol.

References

[1] K. Osorio, *Informe anual Red de Donación y Trasplantes, Colombia*, National Health Institute of Colombia, 2016.

[2] M. Kittleson and J. Kobashigawa, "Cardiac Transplantation: Current Outcomes and Contemporary Controversies," *JACC: Heart Failure*, vol. 5, no. 12, pp. 857–868, 2017.

[3] R. Dhar, "Neurologic complications of transplantation," *Neurocritical Care*, vol. 28, no. 1, pp. 4–11, 2018.

[4] A. A. Pruitt, "Neurologic complications of transplantation," *CONTINUUM: Lifelong Learning in Neurology*, vol. 23, pp. 802–821, 2017.

[5] L. H. Lund, K. K. Khush, W. S. Cherikh et al., "The Registry of the International Society for Heart and Lung Transplantation: Thirty-fourth Adult Heart Transplantation Report—2017; Focus Theme: Allograft ischemic time," *The Journal of Heart and Lung Transplantation*, vol. 36, no. 10, pp. 1037–1046, 2017.

[6] M. Pizzi and L. Ng, "Neurologic complications of solid organ transplantation," *Neurologic Clinics*, vol. 35, no. 4, pp. 809–823, 2017.

[7] M. Acampa, P. E. Lazzerini, F. Guideri, R. Tassi, and G. Martini, "Ischemic stroke after heart transplantation," *Journal of Stroke*, vol. 18, no. 2, pp. 157–168, 2016.

[8] A. Heroux and S. V. Pamboukian, "Neurologic aspects of heart transplantation," *Handbook of Clinical Neurology*, vol. 121, pp. 1229–1236, 2014.

[9] D. van de Beek, W. Kremers, R. C. Daly et al., "Effect of neurologic complications on outcome after heart transplant," *Archives of Neurology*, vol. 65, no. 2, pp. 226–231, 2008.

[10] F. Pérez-Miralles, J. C. Sánchez-Manso, L. Almenar-Bonet, T. Sevilla-Mantecón, L. Martínez-Dolz, and J. J. Vílchez-Padilla, "Incidence of and risk factors for neurologic complications after heart transplantation," *Transplantation Proceedings*, vol. 37, no. 9, pp. 4067–4070, 2005.

[11] J. Hinchey, C. Chaves, B. Appignani et al., "A reversible posterior leukoencephalopathy syndrome," *The New England Journal of Medicine*, vol. 334, no. 8, pp. 494–500, 1996.

[12] W. Bartynski, "Posterior reversible encephalopathy syndrome, part 2: controversies surrounding pathophysiology of vasogenic edema," *AJNR. American Journal of Neuroradiology*, vol. 29, no. 6, pp. 1043–1049, 2008.

[13] A. S. Barbas, A. S. Rege, A. W. Castleberry et al., "Posterior reversible encephalopathy syndrome independently associated with tacrolimus and sirolimus after multivisceral transplantation," *American Journal of Transplantation*, vol. 13, no. 3, pp. 808–810, 2013.

[14] M. H. Harirchian, M. Ghaffarpour, M. Tabaeizadeh, and B. Siroos, "Immunosuppressive drugs, an emerging cause of posterior reversible encephalopathy syndrome: case series," *Journal of Stroke and Cerebrovascular Diseases*, vol. 24, no. 8, pp. e191–e195, 2015.

[15] A. B. Jain, J. J. Fung, S. Todo et al., "One thousand consecutive primary orthotopic liver transplants under FK 506: survival and adverse events," *Transplantation Proceedings*, vol. 27, no. 1, pp. 1099–1104, 1995.

[16] R. Wong, G. Z. Beguelin, M. de Lima et al., "Tacrolimus-associated posterior reversible encephalopathy syndrome after allogeneic haematopoietic stem cell transplantation," *British Journal of Haematology*, vol. 122, no. 1, pp. 128–134, 2003.

[17] J. E. Fugate and A. A. Rabinstein, "Posterior reversible encephalopathy syndrome: clinical and radiological manifestations, pathophysiology, and outstanding questions," *Lancet Neurology*, vol. 14, no. 9, pp. 914–925, 2015.

[18] B. Gao, C. Lyu, A. Lerner, and A. M. McKinney, "Controversy of posterior reversible encephalopathy syndrome: what have we learnt in the last 20 years?," *Journal of Neurology, Neurosurgery & Psychiatry*, vol. 89, no. 1, pp. 14–20, 2018.

[19] A. M. McKinney, J. Short, C. L. Truwit et al., "Posterior reversible encephalopathy syndrome: incidence of atypical regions of involvement and imaging findings," *American Journal of Roentgenology*, vol. 189, no. 4, pp. 904–912, 2007.

[20] N. Willard, J. M. Honce, and B. K. Kleinschmidt-DeMasters, "PRES: review of histological features," *Journal of Neuropathology and Experimental Neurology*, vol. 77, no. 2, pp. 100–118, 2018.

[21] Z. Chen, G. Zhang, A. Lerner, A. Wang, G. Bo, and J. Liu, "Risk factors for poor outcome in posterior reversible encephalopathy syndrome: systematic review and meta-analysis," *Quantitative Imaging in Medicine and Surgery*, vol. 8, no. 4, pp. 421–432, 2018.

[22] T. Song, Z. Rao, Q. Tan et al., "Calcineurin inhibitors associated posterior reversible encephalopathy syndrome in solid organ transplantation report of 2 cases and literature review," *Medicine*, vol. 95, no. 14, article e3173, 2016.

[23] M. M. Burnett, C. P. Hess, J. P. Roberts, N. M. Bass, V. C. Douglas, and S. A. Josephson, "Presentation of reversible posterior leukoencephalopathy syndrome in patients on calcineurin inhibitors," *Clinical Neurology and Neurosurgery*, vol. 112, no. 10, pp. 886–891, 2010.

[24] M. H. Ch, F. Alicia Núñez, L. Tomas Mesa, H. Raúl Escobar, C. Francisco Barriga, and L. Isidro Huete, "Leucoencefalopatía reversible posterior: cuatro casos clínicos," *Revista Médica de Chile*, vol. 136, pp. 93–98, 2008.

[25] Y. Kumai, O. Seguchi, T. Sato et al., "Reversible cerebral vasoconstriction syndrome after heart transplantation: a case report," *Transplantation Proceedings*, vol. 49, no. 10, pp. 2415–2418, 2017.

[26] A. Kapoor, E. Birks, A. Lenneman, and K. McCants, "Posterior reversible encephalopathy syndrome after heart transplantation: diagnosis and immunosuppressive therapy," *Texas Heart Institute Journal*, vol. 44, no. 3, pp. 205–208, 2017.

[27] R. Ramirez, P. R. Muskula, and M. P. Everley, "Posterior reversible encephalopathy. syndrome after orthotopic heart transplantation: a case report," *American Journal of Case Reports*, vol. 18, pp. 487–490, 2017.

[28] C. Roth and A. Ferbert, "Posterior reversible encephalopathy syndrome: long-term follow-up," *Journal of Neurology, Neurosurgery, and Psychiatry*, vol. 81, no. 7, pp. 773–777, 2010.

17

Left Bundle Branch Block Chest Pain Conundrum

Karthik Seetharam, Ayesha Cheema, Gary Friedman, and Roman Pachulski

Division of Cardiology, St. John's Episcopal Hospital-South Shore, New York, New York, USA

Correspondence should be addressed to Roman Pachulski; rpachuls@ehs.org

Academic Editor: Alfredo E. Rodriguez

Left bundle branch block is a pattern of altered ventricular depolarization and subsequently affects repolarization. These obscure patterns can affect the traditional ST segment shift criteria for the electrocardiographic detection of coronary insufficiency syndromes. Previously, patients with coronary ischemic pain and LBBB judged to be "new" (not previously documented) were considered to have ST elevation myocardial infarction (STEMI) warranting acute thrombolytic therapy. Current STEMI management favors emergent invasive angiography; however, recent data suggests the prevalence of coronary obstructive pathology may be as low as 50%. The application of more specific, less-sensitive Sgarbossa electrocardiographic criteria may reduce angiographic assessment in an otherwise high-risk population unlikely to tolerate further myocardial injury. We present a case that may facilitate a more nuanced EKG-based approach to distinguish those who may benefit from acute invasive angiography while reducing the frequency of unnecessary angiographic evaluation.

1. Introduction

In the era of thrombolysis, all patients with left bundle branch block (LBBB) (Figure 1) were felt to warrant acute thrombolytic reperfusion [1]. Previous percutaneous coronary intervention (PCI) reports suggest obstructive pathology in LBBB patients may be as low as 50% [1] resulting in diminished enthusiasm for routine urgent catheterization. The primary goal is to rapidly submit to angiography, only those who have the highest likelihood of obstructive pathology while not withholding reperfusion from a population that likely has advanced cardiac disease. These patients are less likely to tolerate additional insult. We present a case that may facilitate a more nuanced acute reperfusion strategy for chest pain patients with resting QRS abnormalities that obscure the acute electrocardiogram (EKG) diagnosis of coronary obstruction.

2. Case History

A 72-year-old male presented with exertional retrosternal chest pain, remote PCI, regional wall motion anomaly, and reduced left ventricular ejection fraction (LVEF) 29%. Initial troponin on presentation was 0.567 ($N < 0.036$). An electrocardiogram (EKG) (Figure 2) revealed QRS 122 ms, predominantly negative V1, but with terminal 80 ms negativity (S wave) in V6, and 3.5 mm horizontal ST elevation V1-V3. These findings were interpreted as left bundle branch block (LBBB) with insufficient ST shift by Sgarbossa [1] criteria, to infer acute coronary insufficiency, and the patient was treated conservatively with aspirin and sublingual nitroglycerin. After consultation by the cardiologists in our institution, this prompted a revised EKG diagnosis of left ventricular hypertrophy with QRS widening and STEMI (>2 mm ST elevation in 2 contiguous precordial leads). Treatment included dual antiplatelet therapy, heparin, and expeditious angiography. A proximal LAD 99% stenosis was successfully treated with drug eluting stent placement. On the following day, the peak troponin was 142. The patient did not experience clinical heart failure and recovered uneventfully.

3. Discussion

In this case, several clinical indicators suggested a high likelihood of acute coronary obstruction including prior PCI, regional wall motion anomaly, reduced LVEF, elevated

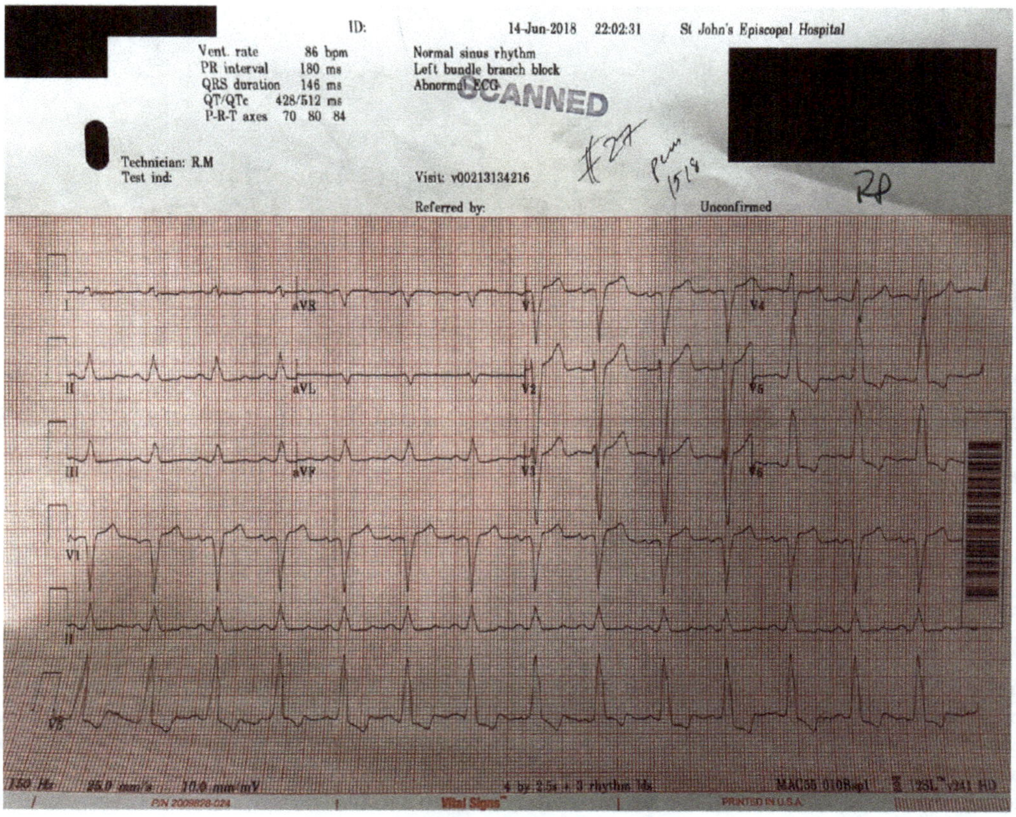

Figure 1: LBBB.

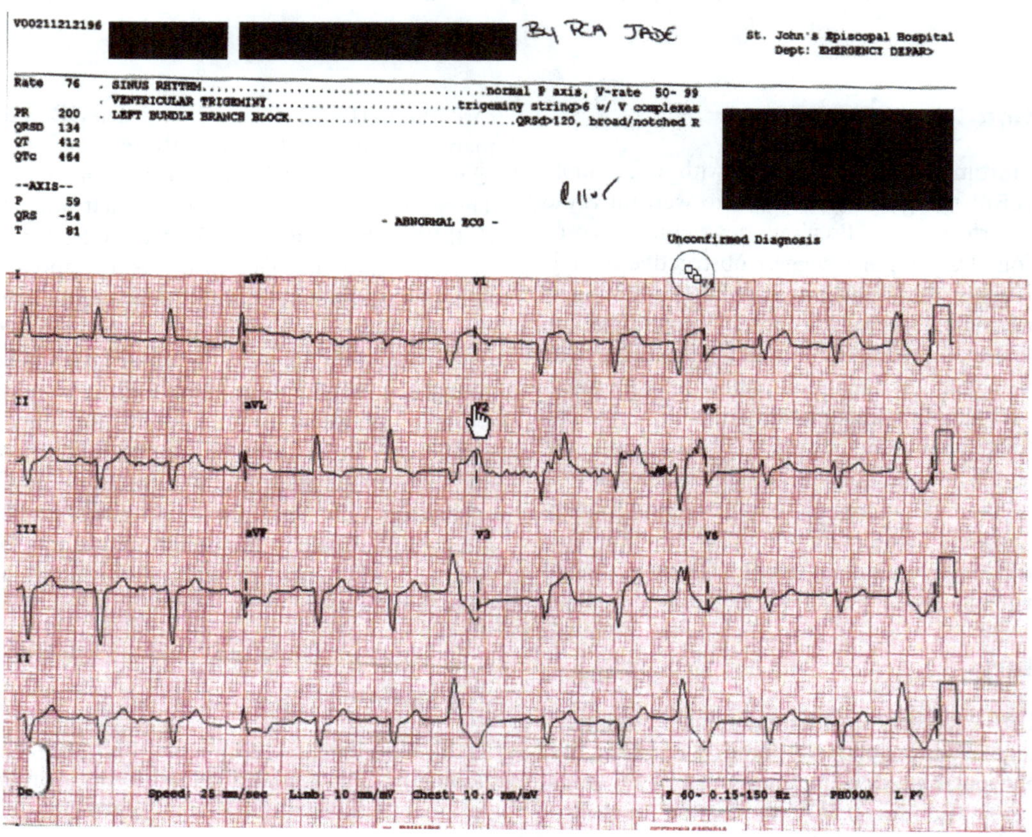

Figure 2: Patient EKG.

troponin, and ischemic chest pain. All prior EKG's showed minimal (<130 ms) QRS widening with leftward terminal negativity as expected with prolonged intraventricular conduction incurred by LV hypertrophy rather than LBBB. As a result, all late forces are leftward and delayed by non-Purkinje (left bundle) fiber conduction.

While LBBB is generally a marker of advanced cardiac disease rendering further myocardial decline [1], low coronary artery disease prevalence may incur unnecessary invasive intervention and cost. Many automated EKG algorithms assign a diagnosis of LBBB to QRS > 120 ms, predominantly negative in V1 regardless of V6 morphology [2, 3]. This may misidentify up to 1/3 of patients with prolonged conduction due to left ventricular hypertrophy (chronic hypertension or valvular disease) as having LBBB [2]. Patients with left ventricular hypertrophy have prolonged, rather than disordered, depolarization and should not be disqualified from traditional EKG STEMI criteria. With true block of the left bundle, all late forces are leftward and cannot manifest terminal QRS negativity (S wave) in leads I, AVL, V5, and V6 [4]. Patients with QRS > 110 ms (rarely >130 ms) and terminal QRS negativity (S wave) in leads I, AVL, V5, and V6 are more accurately described as having left ventricular hypertrophy with QRS widening [5].

4. Conclusion

True block of the left bundle alters ventricular repolarization and invalidates traditional ST segment shift criteria for infarction. However, conduction prolongation due to left ventricular hypertrophy does not. The latter should be diagnosed when the QRS is <140 ms and there is terminal leftward negativity (S wave in I, AVL, V5, and V6). Prospective evaluation of a strategy where Sgarbossa criteria is only applied if QRS > 140 ms or QRS > 120 ms without terminal V6 negativity, while utilizing traditional criteria for those with intermediate QRS duration 120-140 ms with terminal V6 negativity to verify intervention accuracy may prove useful. In addition, the more accurate modified Sgarbossa criteria with a fractional rather than absolute ST displacement criterion could be evaluated.

References

[1] P. T. O'Gara, F. G. Kushner, D. D. Ascheim et al., "2013 ACCF/AHA guideline for the management of ST-elevation myocardial infarction: a report of the American College of Cardiology Foundation/American Heart Association Task Force on Practice Guidelines," *Journal of the American College of Cardiology*, vol. 61, no. 4, article S0735109712055623, pp. e78–e140, 2013.

[2] R. Baranowski, L. Malek, D. Prokopowicz, M. Spiewak, and J. Misko, "Electrocardiographic diagnosis of the left ventricular hypertrophy in patients with left bundle branch block: is it necessary to verify old criteria?," *Cardiology Journal*, vol. 19, no. 6, pp. 591–596, 2012.

[3] L. Galeotti, P. M. van Dam, Z. Loring, D. Chan, and D. G. Strauss, "Evaluating strict and conventional left bundle branch block criteria using electrocardiographic simulations," *Europace*, vol. 15, no. 12, pp. 1816–1821, 2013.

[4] J. A. Vassallo, D. M. Cassidy, F. E. Marchlinski et al., "Endocardial activation of left bundle branch block," *Circulation*, vol. 69, no. 5, pp. 914–923, 1984.

[5] E. B. Sgarbossa, S. L. Pinski, A. Barbagelata et al., "Electrocardiographic diagnosis of evolving acute myocardial infarction in the presence of left bundle-branch block. GUSTO-1 (Global Utilization of Streptokinase and Tissue Plasminogen Activator for Occluded Coronary Arteries) Investigators," *The New England Journal of Medicine*, vol. 334, no. 8, pp. 481–487, 1996.

18

Epicardial Unipolar Lead Loss of Ventricular Capture during Radiofrequency Ablation of Atrial Fibrillation

Daniel J. Chu[1] **and Wilson W. Lam**[1,2]

[1]*Cardiology Section, Department of Medicine, Baylor College of Medicine, Houston, TX 77030, USA*
[2]*Texas Heart Institute, Baylor St. Luke's Medical Center, Houston. TX 77030, USA*

Correspondence should be addressed to Daniel J. Chu; daniel.chu@bcm.edu

Academic Editor: Assad Movahed

Introduction. Abnormal pacemaker behavior can occur during radiofrequency ablation. The behaviors are varied and include loss of capture. The mechanisms in this context have not been well described in the literature. We describe a case of epicardial unipolar lead loss of ventricular capture during pulmonary vein isolation. *Case History.* A 48-year-old man with an epicardial dual chamber pacemaker and persistent atrial fibrillation presented for radiofrequency ablation (RFA) of his abnormal rhythm. During RFA, intermittent loss of ventricular capture was witnessed. Review of the device settings prior to and after the procedure showed an increase in ventricular threshold after the procedure. Loss of capture was shown to be dependent on location and RF energy delivered. It was independent of QTc and independent of local cellular changes that would increase threshold. *Conclusion.* We hypothesize the mechanism of loss of ventricular capture in this patient with an epicardial pacemaker with unipolar leads is related to intermittent shunt of voltage from the pulse generator to the grounding pad rather than the unipolar lead.

1. Introduction

Since the inception of the wearable pacemaker in 1957, cardiac implantable electronic devices (CIEDs) have become increasingly common in medicine [1]. In the modern era of electrophysiology, devices, along with radiofrequency ablation (RFA), comprise two of the main therapeutic options available for treating arrhythmias [2–4]. Invariably, more patients with permanent pacemakers are needing RFA. Despite this, there is a paucity of literature on the topic to base recommendations.

Early experience of the effect of RF energy on implanted pacemaker behavior demonstrated unusual responses in more than 50% of cases [5]. These responses ranged from oversensing, inappropriate pacing, reversion to noise mode, and loss of ventricular capture. Thought to be due in part to the impact of RF energy on the pulse generator, the mechanism of dysfunction remains incompletely understood.

To date, there is only a single case report as part of a series from Sadoul et al. [6] to describe transient loss of capture during RFA in a patient with a permanent pacemaker [5]. We report this case of epicardial unipolar lead loss of ventricular capture during RFA in order to add to the existing literature on this subject and contribute to the process of better understanding the causes of these abnormal device behaviors.

2. Case Presentation

A 48-year-old man with a history of congenital ventricular septal defect (VSD), complete heart block, and atrial fibrillation presented for pulmonary vein isolation. He underwent VSD repair as a child; however, the surgery was complicated by complete heart block. As a result, the patient had an epicardial dual chamber pacemaker. The initial epicardial dual chamber system was implanted in 1973; however, it was completely replaced in 1995. Thus, his current unipolar leads were in place since 1995. Since then, he had undergone several generator changes. His present system consisted of an atrial unipolar lead (Medtronic 4965), a ventricular unipolar lead (Medtronic 4965), and pulse generator (Medtronic Adapta ADDR01, DDD).

On presentation, his baseline rhythm was atrial fibrillation with ventricular pacing. Prior to the procedure, the device was reprogrammed to VOO 70 to avoid inhibition from interference with ablation. Ventricular threshold was confirmed to be 1.25 V @ 1.5 ms and output was set at 2.5 V @ 1.5 ms. Grounding pads were placed on the patient's back between the sacrum and the level of the umbilicus.

During wide antral circumferential ablation of the right upper pulmonary vein (RUPV), most distant to the ventricular epicardial lead, however closest to the grounding pad, intermittent loss of ventricular capture for single beats was noted (Figure 1). This was not present with ablation of the left-sided veins, roof, or right lower pulmonary vein. During ablation with 45 W at the RUPV, ventricular threshold increased to 3 V @ 1.5 ms, prompting intermittent loss of ventricular capture. Subsequent delivery of ablations at 40 W, 30 W, and 20 W also had loss of ventricular capture, while delivery of 15 W did not. Notably, once RF energy was turned off, the device functioned well and there was no loss of capture.

We then moved the coronary sinus (CS) decapolar catheter to the right ventricular apex. A threshold of 1.4 mA @ 1 ms was determined, and the pacemaker was set to VVI 40. Ablation at 45 W power did not lead to loss of capture. However, the VVI pacemaker had ventricular pacing throughout suggesting a decrease in sensed R wave amplitude, which we observed. Of note, QTc was unchanged between loss of capture beats at the RUPV, nonloss of capture beats at the left sided veins, and nonablation beats around the RUPV.

The patient underwent successful pulmonary vein isolation, and his final rhythm was A-sensed, V-paced. His postop course was unfortunately complicated by a small right MCA stroke resulting in mild residual deficits.

3. Discussion

In this case, we noticed abnormal pacemaker behavior during pulmonary vein isolation in a patient with atrial fibrillation. Given our observations, we hypothesize that loss of ventricular capture in this patient with an epicardial unipolar lead is (1) location dependent —loss of ventricular capture occurred at the most posterior structure, furthest from the RV epicardial pacing lead, however closest in proximity to the arc to posterior-inferior grounding pad; and (2) energy dependent—thresholds increased for 20 W and higher but not for 15 W. Our findings support one hypothesis that abnormal pacemaker behaviors are related to the strength of the RF current delivered [5–7]. Additionally, they clarify the relationship of ventricular loss of capture with distance, suggesting that proximity to the electrical arc may result in this behavior, at least in unipolar leads. This mechanism is less likely to be the case in bipolar leads; however, which are tougher to drain as the energy is between two close points.

By moving the CS catheter to the RV apex, the objective was to see if the pacing energy was being stolen from the cardiac device to the grounding pad and therefore not reaching the unipolar lead, resulting in loss of capture. The bipolar pacing lead maintained capture throughout. Thus, if loss of capture were due to a metabolic issue throughout the myocardium resulting in increased thresholds, then the RV pacing would have had increased threshold while ablating at the RUPV which it did not.

Regarding the QTc, if there were local changes affecting repolarization, QT prolongation should have been observed, and it was not. If there was an autonomic effect that invoked an increase in threshold of all cells, then RV pacing threshold would have risen like the unipolar did. Since the RV captured with bipolar pacing but the unipolar did not, we suspect that current was stolen by the grounding pad.

Thus, we also demonstrated that loss of capture was (3) independent of cellular changes to increase threshold—as the RV decapolar threshold was unaffected during ablation and (4) independent of QTc interval—as QTc was unchanged at the same location when there was no loss of capture and at different locations with ablation.

3.1. Limitations. Generalizability of findings in this case is limited by the unique patient. Unipolar leads have become increasingly rare in patients as most leads today are bipolar. Similarly, epicardial leads are less common. Thus, these findings may only apply to a small population of people that is probably decreasing.

Additionally, we were not able to actually prove that energy was being shunted from the pulse generator to the grounding pad; however, we had a strong suspicion this was the case. This is therefore only a hypothesis of the mechanism of action, and additional studies can be done in the future to demonstrate this objectively.

Of note, ventricular pacing inhibition has been reported in the literature during VT ablation, and this is therefore not a completely novel topic. In that setting, it is more likely to occur with an endocardial as opposed to epicardial lead given proximity and the possibility of contact with the ablation catheter. In the case of our patient, however, the event occurred during pulmonary vein isolation with an epicardial dual chamber system. Additionally, the device was not inhibited. It was still pacing, but it needed more energy to capture as we suspect energy was being stolen.

4. Conclusion

In conclusion, just as ablation can lead to alterations in impedance and sensed R wave amplitude, we hypothesize the mechanism of loss of capture in this case is related to intermittent shunt of voltage from the generator to the grounding pad rather than the unipolar lead.

Though this mechanism only applies to unipolar leads which are increasingly uncommon, we believe the case expands on the current understanding of unusual pacemaker behavior due to RF energy and is therefore important. Future work should focus on collecting prospective data on abnormal pacemaker responses during delivery of RF current. In doing so, we may further define the underlying mechanism of abnormal CIED responses. Better understanding of these behaviors may ultimately contribute to the development of improved recommendations for these patients during these procedures.

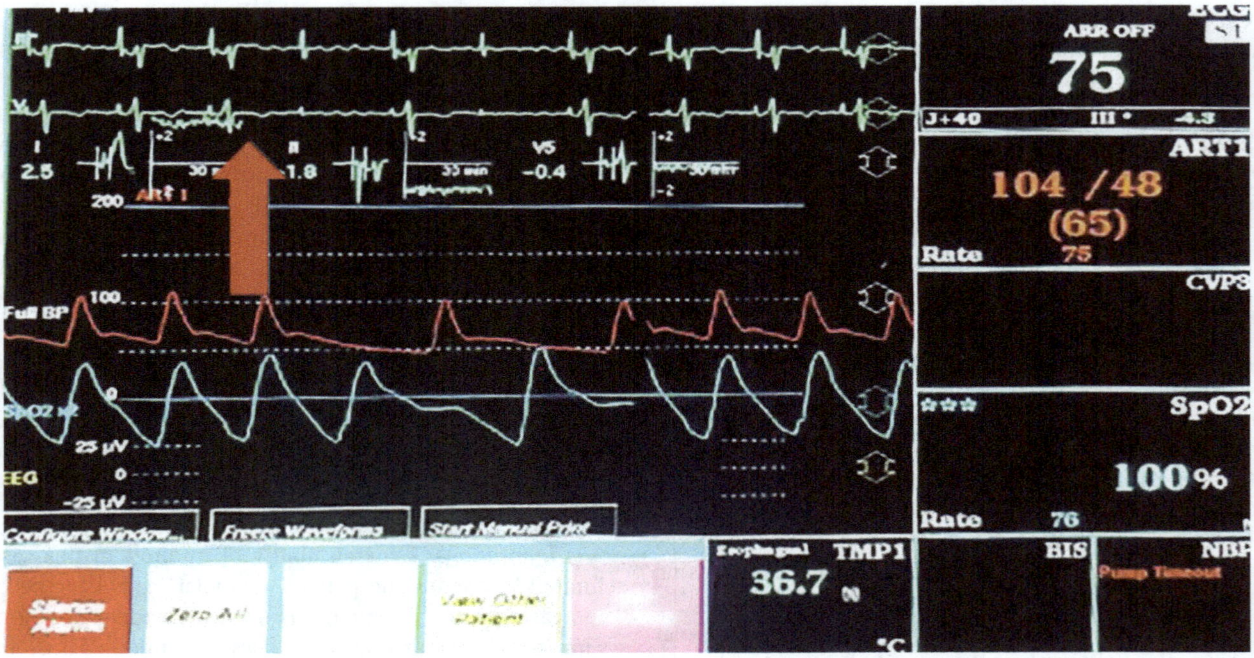

Figure 1: Monitor demonstrating intermittent loss of ventricular capture during RFA (arrow).

References

[1] H. G. Mond and A. Proclemer, "The 11th world survey of cardiac pacing and implantable cardioverter-defibrillators: calendar year 2009-a World Society of Arrhythmia's project," *Pacing and Clinical Electrophysiology*, vol. 34, no. 8, pp. 1013–1027, 2011.

[2] R. Cappato, H. Calkins, S. A. Chen et al., "Updated worldwide survey on the methods, efficacy, and safety of catheter ablation for human atrial fibrillation," *Circulation. Arrhythmia and Electrophysiology*, vol. 3, no. 1, pp. 32–38, 2010.

[3] A. J. Greenspon, J. D. Patel, E. Lau et al., "Trends in permanent pacemaker implantation in the United States from 1993 to 2009: increasing complexity of patients and procedures," *Journal of the American College of Cardiology*, vol. 60, no. 16, pp. 1540–1545, 2012.

[4] D. Lakkireddy, D. Patel, K. Ryschon et al., "Safety and efficacy of radiofrequency energy catheter ablation of atrial fibrillation in patients with pacemakers and implantable cardiac defibrillators," *Heart Rhythm*, vol. 2, no. 12, pp. 1309–1316, 2005.

[5] Y. H. Darrat, A. Agarwal, G. X. Morales et al., "Radiofrequency and cryo-ablation effect on transvenous pacing and defibrillatory lead integrity: an in vitro study," *Journal of Cardiovascular Electrophysiology*, vol. 27, no. 8, pp. 976–980, 2016.

[6] N. Sadoul, I. Blankoff, C. de Chillou et al., "Effects of radiofrequency catheter ablation on patients with permanent pacemakers," *Journal of Interventional Cardiac Electrophysiology*, vol. 1, no. 3, pp. 227–233, 1997.

[7] M. C. Chin, M. Rosenqvist, M. A. Lee, J. C. Griffin, and J. J. Langberg, "The effect of radiofrequency catheter ablation on permanent pacemakers: an experimental study," *Pacing and Clinical Electrophysiology*, vol. 13, no. 1, pp. 23–29, 1990.

Percutaneous Valvular Closure Followed by TAV-in-TAV Intervention during a Single Procedure in order to Treat a Severe Paravalvular Leak after Performing TAVI in a Bicuspid Aortic Stenosis

Georgios Tzimas,[1] Eric Eeckhout,[1] Panagiotis Antiochos,[1] Christan Roguelov,[1] Stephane Fournier,[1] Brahim Harbaoui,[2] Pierre Monney,[1] and Olivier Muller[1]

[1]*Department of Cardiology, University Hospital of Lausanne (CHUV), Rue du Bugnon 46, 1005 Lausanne, Switzerland*
[2]*Department of Cardiology, Hospices civils de Lyon, hôpital de la Croix-Rousse, 103 Grand Rue de la Crx Rousse, 69004 Lyon, France*

Correspondence should be addressed to Georgios Tzimas; georgios.tzimas@chuv.ch

Academic Editor: Adam Torbicki

In an era where transcatheter aortic valve implantation (TAVI) indications and utilization are expanding beyond high-risk patients, paravalvular leak remains the intervention's Achilles heel. Effective reduction of paravalvular leak is important in order to ensure an optimal clinical outcome. We present here the first case report in which percutaneous valvular closure using Amplatzer plugs followed by a TAV-in-TAV intervention during the same procedure managed to resolve a severe paravalvular leak with haemodynamic instability, after TAVI for a bicuspid aortic stenosis.

1. Introduction

As the indications for and utilization of TAVI are expanding beyond high-risk patients [1], paravalvular leak (PVL) remains the intervention's Achilles heel, as it has a negative impact on both short- and long-term prognoses [2–7]. Although several studies had demonstrated that TAVI constitutes a feasible safe intervention in patients with bicuspid aortic stenosis (AS), PVLs were described as one of the intervention's greatest weakness, as the total incidence of PVLs seems to be higher than in patients with tricuspid AS [8, 9]. Percutaneous closure as well as TAV-in-TAV intervention consists an effective procedure in order to improve PVL severity and symptoms. We present here the first case report of a severe PVL following TAVI, treated with percutaneous valvular closure using Amplatzer plugs and TAV-in-TAV intervention, both performed during a single procedure.

2. Case Report

A 79-year-old man with a medical history of hypertension, stage G3b chronic renal insufficiency, and interstitial lung disease presented with a four-month history of progressive dyspnoea (NYHA III).

Transthoracic echocardiography showed a bicuspid aortic valve (BAV) (Figures 1(a) and 1(b)) with severe, paradoxical, low-flow, low-gradient (mean gradient 26 mmHg) AS, a calculated aortic orifice area of 0.78 cm^2, and a preserved left ventricular ejection fraction of 55%. A coronary angiogram revealed no significant epicardial coronary stenosis. Aortic root assessment was completed by multidetector computed tomography (MDCT), which revealed severe aortic annular calcification, with an aortic valve calcium score of 10133 AV and a large aortic valve annulus (Figures 1(c) and 1(d)). After using the three multiplanar reformation planes, measurements were derived from the area as well as the

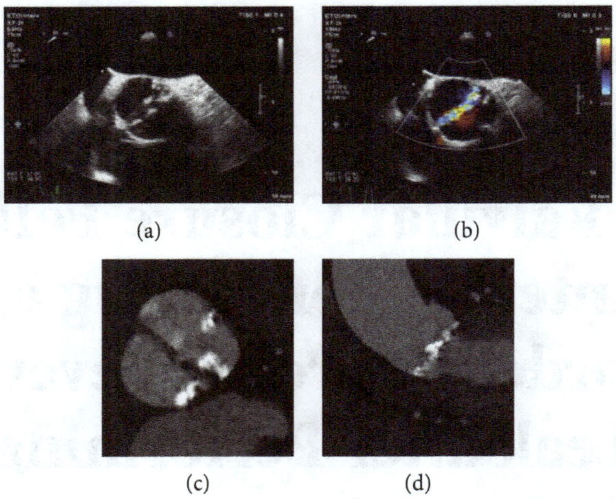

Figure 1: (a, b) Transthoracic echocardiography showing a bicuspid aortic valve. (c, d) Multidetector computed tomography scan revealing a large aortic valve annulus (annular area: 726.9 mm^2, perimeter: 93.38 mm, long axis: 33.9 mm, and short axis: 26.2 mm) with severe aortic annular calcification.

circumference of the virtual basal ring (mean diameter: 30.4 mm, annular area: 726.9 mm^2, perimeter: 93.38 mm, long axis: 33.9 mm, and short axis: 26.2 mm). MDCT did not reveal any calcification extending into the left ventricular outflow tract. Additional supra-annular measurement of the valve opening area at the level of the maximal calcification did not show a significant mismatch compared with the initial measurements. Based on his severe comorbidities, characteristics of frailty, and refusal of surgery, the heart team decided to perform a TAVI via a femoral approach.

Balloon aortic valvuloplasty was performed using a 28 mm × 4 cm Nucleus balloon (NuMED, NY). Given the aspect of the valve marked by a large annulus with severe annular calcification and the eventual benefit of a valve resheathing and optimised repositioning, a CoreValve Evolut R 34 mm (Medtronic Inc., MN, USA) was implanted. After valve deployment, fluoroscopy and transoesophageal echocardiography (TEE) (Figures 2(a) and 2(b)) revealed a PVL due to (i) suboptimal valve expansion because of interference with the valvular ring by nodular calcifications and (ii) low positioning of the aortic valve prosthesis. The patient showed signs of haemodynamic instability, necessitating the initiation of inotropic support.

Our initial approach included postdilatation with the largest balloon available in our catheterization laboratory (28 mm × 4 cm Nucleus balloon (NuMED, NY)), attempting a better valve expansion and sealing the paravalvular space. However, fluoroscopy and TEE showed no improvement to the PVL (Supplementary 1). Among the possible strategies, percutaneous valvular closure using Amplatzer plugs constitutes a viable alternative in patients developing a PVL after TAVI [10, 11]. After an urgent discussion, the heart team decided to proceed with paravalvular implantation of a cardiac plug in an attempt to seal the PVL and improve the patient's haemodynamic status. After measuring the size of the leak by TEE, a Terumo wire (Terumo Interventional Systems, Somerset, New Jersey) was easily pushed through the aortic prosthesis struts, and the first 12 mm Amplatzer Vascular Plug II (AVPII) (AGA Medical Corp., Plymouth,

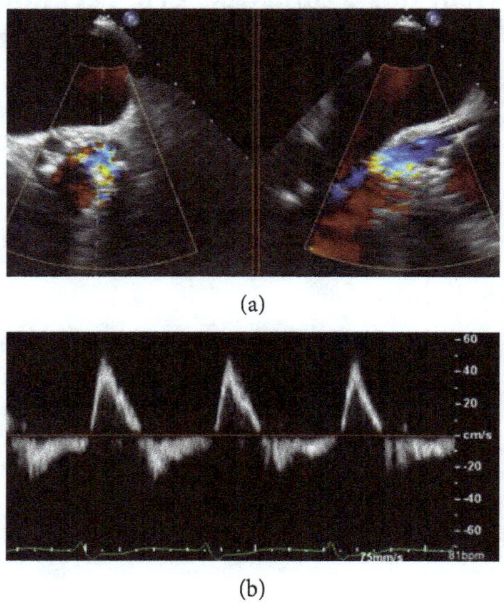

Figure 2: (a) Transoesophageal echocardiography showing a severe paravalvular leak after deployment of a CoreValve Evolut R 34 mm. (b) Pulsed wave Doppler in the descending aorta showing the presence of a consistent holodiastolic retrograde flow.

Minnesota) was successfully implanted. Before detachment, coronary permeability was verified by coronary angiography. However, this failed to reduce the severity of the PVL. Following the same procedure as previously, we decided to implant a second 10 mm AVPII (Figures 3(a) and 3(b)) (AGA Medical Corp., Plymouth, Minnesota), which was positioned parallel to the first one. Again, fluoroscopy and TEE did not show any significant reduction in the PVL (Supplementary 2), and the patient remained haemodynamically unstable requiring continuous inotropic therapy.

We decided to proceed with a TAV-in-TAV implantation as a rescue procedure, using a second aortic prosthesis (29 mm EDWARDS Sapien 3, Edwards Lifesciences, Irvine,

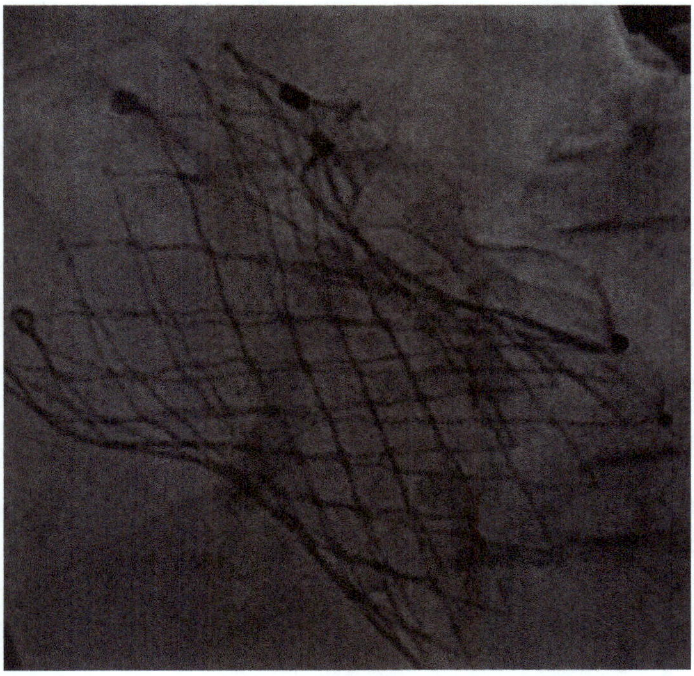

(a)

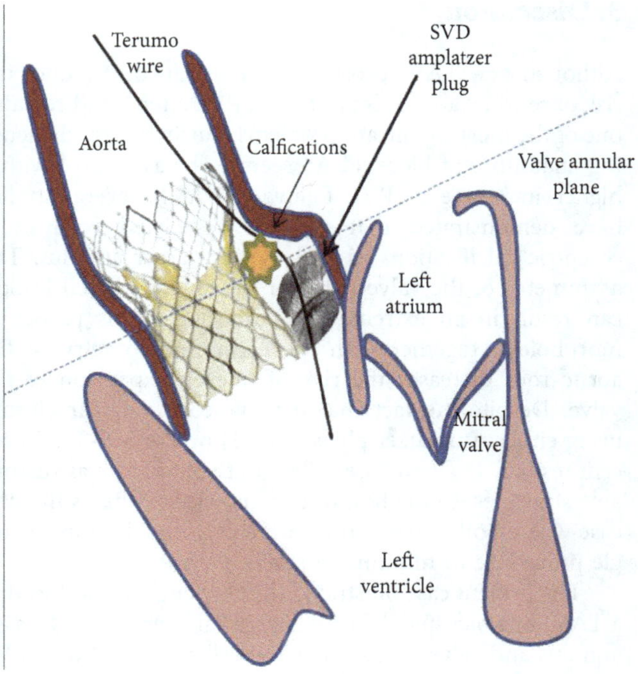

(b)

Figure 3: (a) Fluoroscopy with complete deployment of the two Amplatzer plugs. (b) A PVL was caused by the aortic prosthesis being set too low and its poor apposition against the heavily calcified commissure of the native aortic valve. A Terumo wire was pushed through the Evolut R valve's struts and then two SVD Amplatzer plugs were implanted. Due to persistent PVL after plug implantation, a further TAV-in-TAV intervention was performed. PVL: paravalvular leak; TAV: transcatheter aortic valve.

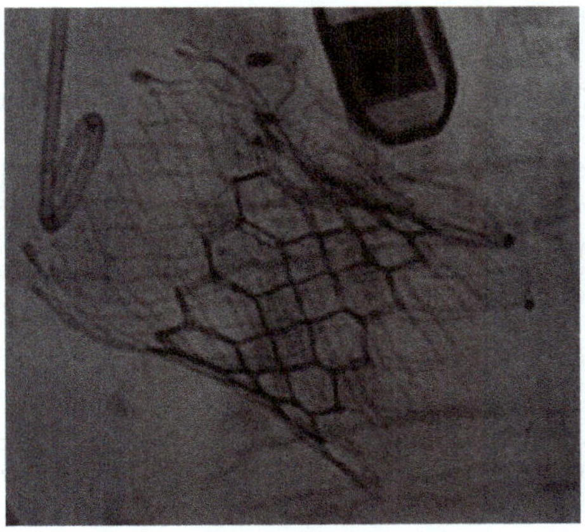

Figure 4: Fluoroscopy after complete deployment of the two Amplatzer plugs and the 29 mm EDWARDS Sapien 3.

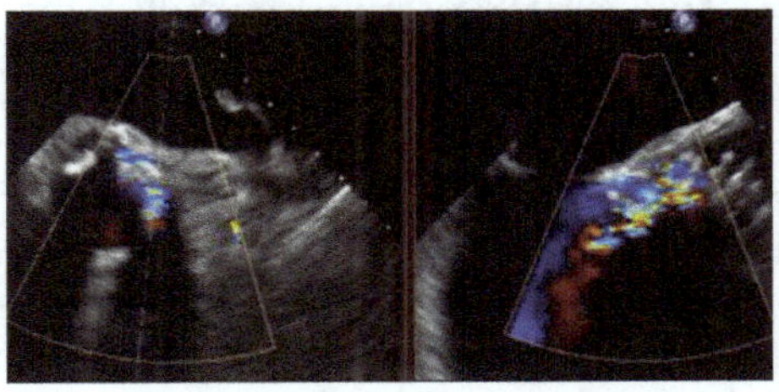

(a)

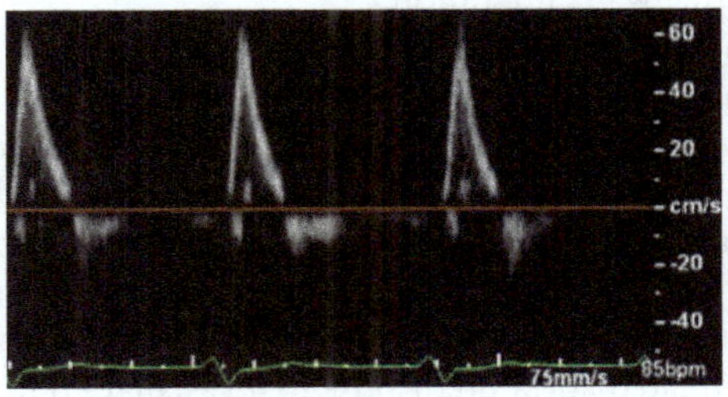

(b)

Figure 5: (a) Transoesophageal echocardiography revealing the sealing of the paravalvular leak and the presence of a mild residual aortic regurgitation after the deployment of a 29 mm EDWARDS Sapien 3. (b) Pulsed wave Doppler in the descending aorta showing an antegrade flow without diastolic flow reversal.

California). This was deployed within the first valve (Figure 4), and the final outcome was the elimination of the AS, the sealing of the PVL, and the presence of a mild residual aortic regurgitation (Figures 5(a) and 5(b), Supplementary 3).

Nevertheless, a final aortic root angiography revealed a type A aortic dissection arising in the aortic sinuses and extending into the ascending aorta. The permeability of the coronary arteries was intact, and no pericardial infusion was observed. After a multidisciplinary discussion, a conventional surgical intervention was proposed to the family, but they refused this option. Continuation of all resuscitation therapy was abandoned, and the patient died three days later.

3. Discussion

Although new TAVI prostheses are designed to reduce the risk of residual aortic regurgitation, PVL after TAVI remains one of the most significant problems. Furthermore, challenging anatomies of bicuspid AS seem to be associated with a higher incidence of PVL following TAVI. Several studies have demonstrated that BAV is associated with more eccentric calcifications as well as with larger annulus. The asymmetry of the valve made of two unequal-sized leaflets can result in an extreme elliptical shape. This particular morphology together with the eccentric geometry of the aortic root increases the risk of uneven expansion of the valve. Despite the fact that percutaneous valvular closure using either Amplatzer plugs [10, 11] or TAV-in-TAV procedures [12, 13] is well described in the literature as reasonable strategies, to the best of our knowledge, this is the first case where both interventions were performed during a single procedure to minimise a severe PVL.

The present case illustrated the challenges of performing a TAVI in a bicuspid AS with a large valvular annulus. Large annulus and valve undersizing are well associated with PVL and prosthesis migration [14]. A recent study conducted by Attizzani et al. [15] showed a lower rate of procedural and device success, as well as longer procedural durations, among patients treated with a 31 mm CoreValve rather than other valve sizes (23, 26, and 29 mm). Higher rates of TAV-in-TAV bail-out procedures were also reported. The adoption of a sizing strategy based on a multimodal imaging assessment (CT, TEE) therefore seems crucial in order to avoid subsequent prosthesis migration due to the lack of anchoring support. In the present case, we believe that BAV morphology characterized by the fusion of two leaflets results in a potentially suboptimal valve sizing due to the difficulty to accurately identify the true annular plane. The valve undersizing as well as the bicuspid anatomy marked by an elliptic shape and affected by extreme and asymmetric calcification led to a suboptimal expansion of the first aortic prosthesis and its downward migration.

Unfortunately, the final stage of the procedure was further complicated by the presence of a type A aortic dissection which eventually led to patient death. Although the precise pathological mechanisms are not completely understood, the dilatation of the ascending aorta in BAV seems to be due to genetic as well as haemodynamic factors. The presence of a severe calcified aorta or a sharply angulated aortic arc as well as a dilated aorta predispose to a vascular complication. The probability increases when repeated endovascular gestures are performed during the intervention. Even though the latest studies have shown excellent results in treating bicuspid AS, especially with the use of new-generation devices, this category of patients was traditionally excluded from the large RCT due to the increased risk of PVL and vascular complications. Thus, these outcomes could further be improved by increased experience and the use of dedicated imaging modalities in the selection of patients.

In conclusion, this case demonstrated that a combined approach involving paravalvular Amplatzer plug implantation and a TAV-in-TAV intervention during the same procedure could be a potential option in order to reduce severe PVL associated with haemodynamic instability. However, we cannot exclude that a TAV-in-TAV implantation, as the sole intervention, might have been sufficient to seal the PVL.

Supplementary Materials

Supplementary 1. Video 1: fluoroscopy showing a severe paravalvular leak after postdilatation of the CoreValve Evolut R 34 mm.

Supplementary 2. Video 2: fluoroscopy showing a persistent paravalvular leak despite the deployment of the two Amplatzer plugs.

Supplementary 3. Video 3: fluoroscopy revealing the sealing of the paravalvular leak and the presence of a mild residual aortic regurgitation after the deployment of a 29 mm EDWARDS Sapien 3.

References

[1] H. Baumgartner, V. Falk, J. J. Bax et al., "2017 ESC/EACTS Guidelines for the management of valvular heart disease," *European Heart Journal*, vol. 38, no. 36, pp. 2739–2791, 2017.

[2] H. Takagi, T. Umemoto, and ALICE (All-Literature Investigation of Cardiovascular Evidence) Group, "Impact of paravalvular aortic regurgitation after transcatheter aortic valve implantation on survival," *International Journal of Cardiology*, vol. 221, pp. 46–51, 2016.

[3] P. Kleczyński, W. Zasada, M. Bagieński et al., "Paravalvular leak after transcatheter aortic valve implantation (TAVI): short-term results. Data from Polish national POL-TAVI registry," *Cardiology Journal*, vol. 23, no. 2, pp. 163–168, 2016.

[4] M. Abdel-Wahab, R. Zahn, M. Horack et al., "Aortic regurgitation after transcatheter aortic valve implantation: incidence and early outcome. Results from the German transcatheter aortic valve interventions registry," *Heart*, vol. 97, no. 11, pp. 899–906, 2011.

[5] S. K. Kodali, M. R. Williams, C. R. Smith et al., "Two-year outcomes after transcatheter or surgical aortic-valve replacement," *New England Journal of Medicine*, vol. 366, no. 18, pp. 1686–1695, 2012.

[6] N. E. Moat, P. Ludman, M. A. de Belder et al., "Long-term outcomes after transcatheter aortic valve implantation in high-risk patients with severe aortic stenosis: the U.K. TAVI (United Kingdom Transcatheter Aortic Valve Implantation) Registry," *Journal of the American College of Cardiology*, vol. 58, no. 20, pp. 2130–2138, 2011.

[7] C. Tamburino, D. Capodanno, A. Ramondo et al., "Incidence and predictors of early and late mortality after transcatheter aortic valve implantation in 663 patients with severe aortic stenosis," *Circulation*, vol. 123, no. 3, pp. 299–308, 2011.

[8] T. Bauer, A. Linke, H. Sievert et al., "Comparison of the effectiveness of transcatheter aortic valve implantation in patients with stenotic bicuspid versus tricuspid aortic valves (from the German TAVI Registry)," *The American Journal of Cardiology*, vol. 113, no. 3, pp. 518–521, 2014.

[9] A. Yousef, T. Simard, A. Pourdjabbar et al., "Performance of transcatheter aortic valve implantation in patients with bicuspid aortic valve: systematic review," *International Journal of Cardiology*, vol. 176, no. 2, pp. 562–564, 2014.

[10] P. Sorajja, R. Bae, J. A. Lesser, and W. A. Pedersen, "Percutaneous repair of paravalvular prosthetic regurgitation: patient selection, techniques and outcomes," *Heart*, vol. 101, no. 9, pp. 665–673, 2015.

[11] R. A. Nishimura, C. M. Otto, R. O. Bonow et al., "2014 AHA/ACC guideline for the management of patients with valvular heart disease: executive summary: a report of the American College of Cardiology/American Heart Association Task Force on Practice Guidelines," *Journal of the American College of Cardiology*, vol. 63, no. 22, pp. 2438–2488, 2014.

[12] S. Toggweiler, D. A. Wood, J. Rodés-Cabau et al., "Transcatheter valve-in-valve implantation for failed balloon-expandable transcatheter aortic valves," *JACC: Cardiovascular Interventions*, vol. 5, no. 5, pp. 571–577, 2012.

[13] R. R. Makkar, H. Jilaihawi, T. Chakravarty et al., "Determinants and outcomes of acute transcatheter valve-in-valve therapy or embolization: a study of multiple valve implants in the U.S. PARTNER trial (Placement of AoRTic TraNscathetER Valve Trial Edwards SAPIEN Transcatheter Heart Valve)," *Journal of the American College of Cardiology*, vol. 62, no. 5, pp. 418–430, 2013.

[14] J. M. Sinning, C. Hammerstingl, M. Vasa-Nicotera et al., "Aortic regurgitation index defines severity of peri-prosthetic regurgitation and predicts outcome in patients after transcatheter aortic valve implantation," *Journal of the American College of Cardiology*, vol. 59, no. 13, pp. 1134–1141, 2012.

[15] G. F. Attizzani, Y. Ohno, A. Latib et al., "Acute and long-term (2-years) clinical outcomes of the CoreValve 31mm in large aortic annuli: a multicenter study," *International Journal of Cardiology*, vol. 227, pp. 543–549, 2017.

20

Master of the Masquerade: An Atypical Presentation of Acute Aortic Dissection

Ramy Mando[1] **Daniel Tim,**[2,3] **Anthony DeCicco,**[2,3] **Justin Trivax,**[2,3] **and Ivan Hanson**[2,3]

[1]*Department of Internal Medicine, Beaumont Health System, Royal Oak, MI, USA*
[2]*Department of Cardiovascular Medicine, Beaumont Health System, Royal Oak, MI, USA*
[3]*Oakland University William Beaumont School of Medicine, Auburn Hills, MI, USA*

Correspondence should be addressed to Ivan Hanson; ivan.hanson@beaumont.org

Academic Editor: Assad Movahed

Acute aortic dissection (AAD) is associated with unacceptably high mortality rate. As such, early diagnosis and aggressive management are essential in order to avoid life-threatening complications. Herein, we report an atypical presentation of AAD and clinical sequelae.

1. Introduction

The incidence of AAD is ~2.3 per 100,000 person-years with mortality rates greater than 50% within 30 days of diagnosis [1]. Furthermore, for every hour that AAD involving the ascending aorta (Sanford type A) is left untreated, mortality rate increases by 1% [2–4]. It is for these reasons that this devastating condition requires a high index of suspicion to make the diagnosis and implement treatment strategies as quickly as possible.

The International Registry of Aortic Dissection (IRAD) was established in 1996 to raise awareness and provide guidance in the diagnosis and treatment of this condition. Overall, type A dissection constitutes 67% of AAD. The most common risk factors for AAD include hypertension (76.6%), atherosclerotic disease (27%), prior cardiac surgery (16%), and Marfan syndrome (5%) [5]. A study utilizing the IRAD with a focus on younger patients (<40 years of age) revealed that this population constituted 7% of patients who suffered AAD. Furthermore, the study identified unique risk factors in this population including Marfan syndrome, bicuspid aortic valves, and larger aortic dimensions [6].

Abrupt and severe chest and back pain are the most common presenting signs and symptoms for type A (79% vs. 43%, respectively) and type B (63% vs. 64%, respectively) aortic dissection. In general, anterior chest pain is more consistent with type A dissection while back pain was found to be more consistent with type B dissection [7]. Acute abdominal pain was the main presenting symptoms in only 4.6% of cases in the IRAD and was associated with increased mortality [8].

Herein, we present a case of AAD that presented with atypical chest pain, abdominal pain, scrotal edema, seizure, pericardial tamponade, and death. Unfortunately, AAD was not suspected until the patient developed refractory cardiac arrest. We hope that our case raises awareness of these atypical features so that future patients may be diagnosed and treated earlier.

2. Case Description

A 33-year-old male with no past medical history presented to the emergency department (ED) for atypical chest pain described as pleuritic and positional. He described associated nausea, vomiting, diarrhea, epigastric pain, and myalgia. He also reported decreased oral intake for 2-3 days prior to presentation. On examination, blood pressure (BP) was 127/56 mmHg, heart rate (HR) was 94 bpm, and he was afebrile. He was 180 cm tall and weighed 70 kg. He appeared to be in mild distress, exhibited bilateral anterior chest wall and epigastric tenderness. A 12-lead electrocardiogram (ECG) revealed normal sinus rhythm with a rate of 92 bpm, normal axis with no ST or T-wave abnormalities (Figure 1(a)). Initial

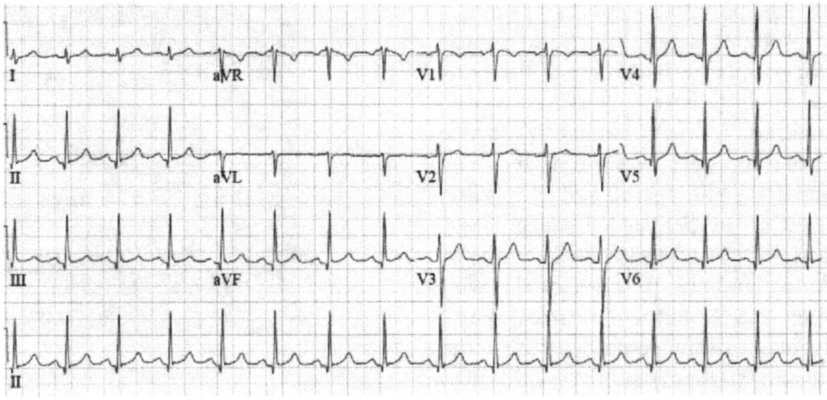

(a)

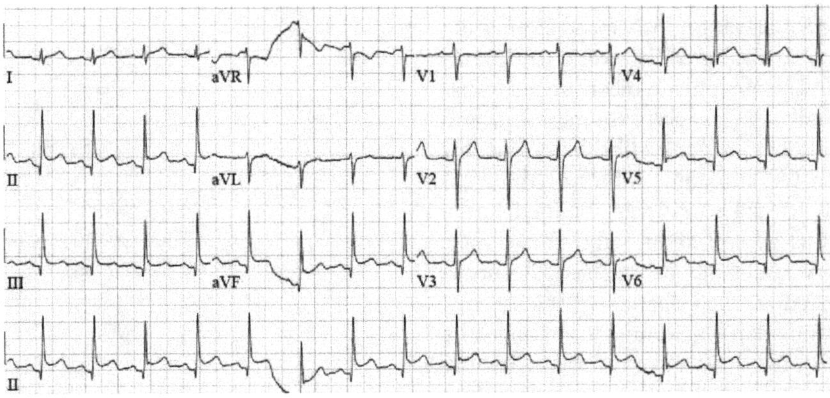

(b)

FIGURE 1: (a) EKG at the initial presentation revealing normal sinus rhythm and no significant ST or T-wave abnormalities. HR 92 bpm. (b) EKG obtained at the time of the second presentation. Notable changes include diffuse ST-elevation. HR 96 bpm.

labs were notable for leukocyte count of 17,200 bil/L, serum creatinine 1.42 mg/dL, and presence of hyaline casts in the urine. Acute abdominal series was unremarkable with the exception of a single mildly dilated small bowel loop consistent with ileus versus enteritis. He was treated with intravenous hydration, antiemetics, morphine, and ketorolac for pain control. On reevaluation, he reported significant symptomatic improvement and was discharged home with close follow-up with his primary care physician. The following day, he presented to the ED with persistent nausea, vomiting, diarrhea, and abdominal pain. He also developed scrotal pain and swelling. Physical examination revealed BP of 117/73 mmHg and HR of 104 bpm. He exhibited continued chest wall tenderness and epigastric pain as well as scrotal swelling and tenderness. 12-lead ECG revealed sinus tachycardia with a rate of 100 bpm, early repolarization changes with ST elevation in the lateral leads (Figure 1(b)). Troponin was mildly elevated at 0.11 ng/mL (elevated from 0.01 ng/mL the day prior). Other labs were notable for an improving leukocytosis (11K bil/L), a new normocytic anemia (12.9 g/dL compared to 14.1 g/dL the day prior), and stable renal function. Liver panel revealed an AST of 33 U/L, ALT of 23 U/L, and total bilirubin of 0.8 mg/dL. Ultrasound of the scrotum revealed right-sided hydrocele and left-sided varicocele. Computed tomography (CT) of the chest, abdomen, and pelvis revealed a moderate pericardial effusion with complex-appearing fluid concerning for hemopericardium. The CT was also notable for periportal edema, perihepatic ascites, bilateral pleural effusion, and scattered free fluid throughout the abdomen and pelvis. He was managed with hydration, morphine, and ketorolac and transferred to our hospital for further management.

During transport, he was noted to have had sudden loss of consciousness associated with clonic jerking, followed by rapid and complete recovery of normal neurologic function. On arrival to the ED, BP was 116/64 mmHg, HR was 96 bpm, and the patient was in no acute distress. Laboratory evaluation was significant for an increase in AST (99 U/L), ALT (101 U/L), and total bilirubin (1.6 mg/dL). A bedside echocardiogram was done and revealed a normal ejection fraction, normal right ventricular diameter, and a moderate pericardial effusion. He was admitted to the inpatient unit with consultations placed to general surgery for abdominal pain and rheumatology for evaluation of serositis. Five hours later, the patient became tachycardic with HR ranging from 140 to 150 bpm and hypotensive with systolic BP around 70 mmHg. Phenylephrine was started immediately with improvement in blood pressure. A bedside echocardiogram revealed a large pericardial effusion, with evidence of diastolic compression of the right ventricle, consistent with pericardial tamponade. He was taken to the catheterization laboratory for emergent pericardiocentesis.

In the catheterization lab, pericardiocentesis via apical approach was attempted. Agitated saline injection through a microcatheter was performed, but a large part of the pericardial space was occupied by echo-dense material and saline bubbles were not visualized in the pericardial space (Figure 2). Next, subxiphoid approach was attempted. The pericardial space was entered, but again, agitated saline bubbles were not visualized in the pericardial space. However, the wire was successfully passed through the catheter under fluoroscopic guidance, and the position of the wire appeared to be appropriately located in the pericardial space. While attempting to advance a drainage catheter over the wire, the patient had recurrent, sudden loss of consciousness and clonic activity. Subsequently, there was a rapid decline in heart rate and a 12-lead ECG revealed marked sinus bradycardia with inferior ST-elevation. Advanced cardiac life support (ACLS) protocol was initiated including cardiopulmonary resuscitation (CPR), epinephrine/bicarbonate, transvenous pacemaker placement (via right femoral vein), and cardioversion for intermittent ventricular fibrillation. At this point, there was concern for iatrogenic injury of the right coronary artery. Femoral arterial access was obtained, and a right Judkins catheter was advanced into the aortic root. The right coronary artery could not be engaged. A supravalvular aortogram revealed marked dilation of the ascending aorta with a dissection flap beginning just above the sinotubular junction along the outer curve of the ascending aorta, involving the arch and extending to the descending aorta. The right coronary and innominate arteries were occluded (Figure 3). Efforts to stabilize the patient for emergent dissection repair were unsuccessful, and he expired immediately after CPR was stopped. Autopsy revealed extension of aortic dissection from the aortic root to bilateral iliac arteries. The root was dilated, and the aortic valve was tricuspid. Histopathology is pending at the time of this report.

3. Discussion

This case is unique and illustrates several points. (1) The presentation of AAD may include atypical chest pain and signs/symptoms of heart failure. (2) Presence of a complex effusion on CT or echocardiogram should raise the possibility of hemopericardium caused by extension of aortic dissection in the appropriate clinical setting. (3) Seizure activity may be a manifestation of AAD due to acute cerebral ischemia.

Patients younger than 40 years of age often do not present with the "typical" risk factors and characteristics [6, 7]. Moreover, the 4.6% patients who present with abdominal pain as their primary complaint have higher mortality rates, likely related to less clinician awareness of this manifestation of AAD. This, unfortunately, may have contributed to the demise of our patient. There are no reports describing nausea, vomiting, and diarrhea as symptoms associated with AAD; however, stimulation of cardiac vagal afferent nerves associated with inferior myocardial infarction may trigger these symptoms [9].

Acute onset testicular swelling and pain was the second atypical feature of AAD. Few cases describing this as the predominant symptom have been published. In one case, a

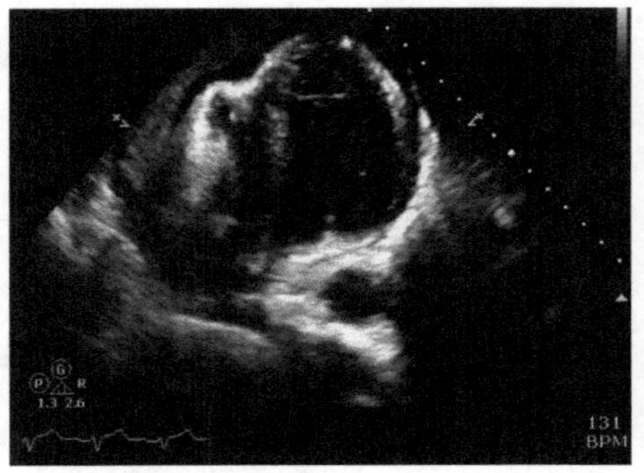

Figure 2: Transesophageal echocardiogram revealing a large pericardial effusion with diastolic compression of the right ventricle.

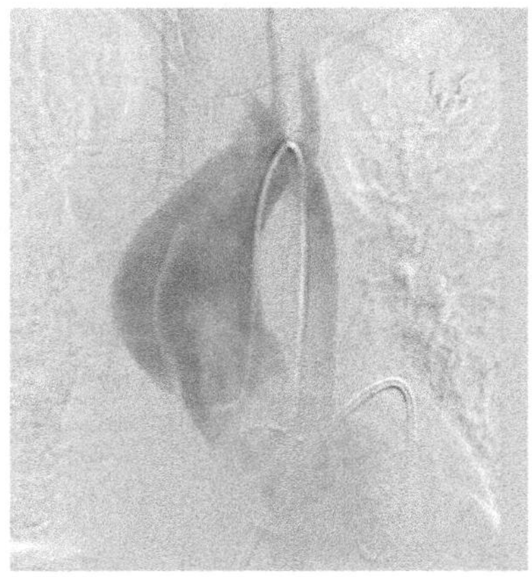

Figure 3: Supravalvular aortography revealing marked dilation of the ascending aorta with a dissection flap beginning just above the right sinus of Valsalva extending to at least the aortic arch.

77-year-old male presented with 2 days of sharp testicular pain. Diagnostic studies were largely unremarkable, and he was admitted for observation. Hours later, he suffered from cardiac arrest and autopsy revealed extensive type A dissection [10]. Another case highlighted a 49-year-old male who presented with sudden onset testicular pain. His physical examination was notable for a significantly reduced BP in the right leg compared to the left leg [11]. In our patient, evidence of scrotal swelling, elevated transaminases, and ascites may have indicated acute right ventricular failure due to ischemic right ventricular dysfunction and/or cardiac tamponade. Alternatively, it is possible that extension of the dissection flap led to acute arterial insufficiency of the mesenteric vasculature.

The presence of enteritis on the initial abdominal X-ray with symptoms of abdominal pain, nausea, vomiting, and diarrhea would be consistent with viral gastroenteritis. The following day, a CT was obtained which revealed a pericardial effusion that "does not measure at simple fluid density," concerning for hemopericardium. Initially, the patient's symptoms in the first 8 hours were largely attributed to viral pericarditis. However, it should be noted on CT that attenuation values can be obtained with high accuracy. Attenuations greater than those of water are consistent with complex effusions most commonly related to hemopericardium, malignancy, or purulent exudates. As such, CT allows for the differentiation of simple pericardial effusions from chylous, malignant, and hemorrhagic effusions with a high degree of certainty [12, 13]. In this case, despite the misleading symptoms at presentation, our patient should have been immediately referred for a more specific diagnostic examination to further characterize the effusion. Immediate diagnosis and management are critical in the treatment of this catastrophic pathology. The consideration of AAD should be made in patients with evidence of hemopericardium, in the appropriate clinical setting.

The final atypical presentation of AAD manifested in our patient was his seizure-like activity. This was initially observed during his transport to our facility by EMS and prior to his cardiac arrest in the catheterization lab. This is may have been due to global cerebral ischemia in the setting of impending hemodynamic collapse and propagation of the dissection. Neurologic symptoms in the setting of AAD are well described and can be seen in as many as one-third of cases. Symptoms may include seizures, aphasia, unconsciousness, syncope, Horner syndrome, paraparesis, anterior spinal cord syndrome, Brown-Sequard syndrome, ischemic neuropathy, and plexopathy [14].

4. Conclusion

AAD is a devastating diagnosis with a high mortality rate that requires a low threshold for making the diagnosis, as earlier intervention leads to reduced mortality. This case illustrates that AAD can masquerade as other, more benign, conditions when signs and symptoms are atypical. We hope this report improves clinician awareness of the less common manifestations of AAD.

References

[1] I. H. Melvinsdottir, S. H. Lund, B. A. Agnarsson, K. Sigvaldason, T. Gudbjartsson, and A. Geirsson, "The incidence and mortality of acute thoracic aortic dissection: results from a whole nation study," *European Journal of Cardio-Thoracic Surgery*, vol. 50, no. 6, pp. 1111–1117, 2016.

[2] M. A. Coady, J. A. Rizzo, L. J. Goldstein, and J. A. Elefteriades, "Natural history, pathogenesis, and etiology of thoracic aortic aneurysms and dissections," *Cardiology Clinics*, vol. 17, no. 4, pp. 615–35; vii, 1999, vii.

[3] J. Lindsay Jr. and J. W. Hurst, "Clinical features and prognosis in dissecting aneurysm of the aorta. A re-appraisal," *Circulation*, vol. 35, no. 5, pp. 880–888, 1967.

[4] T. P. Tran and A. Khoynezhad, "Current management of type B aortic dissection," *Vascular Health and Risk Management*, vol. 5, no. 1, pp. 53–63, 2009.

[5] A. Evangelista, E. M. Isselbacher, E. Bossone et al., "Insights from the International Registry of Acute Aortic Dissection: a 20-year experience of collaborative clinical research," *Circulation*, vol. 137, no. 17, pp. 1846–1860, 2018.

[6] J. L. Januzzi, E. M. Isselbacher, R. Fattori et al., "Characterizing the young patient with aortic dissection: results from the International Registry of Aortic Dissection (IRAD)," *Journal of the American College of Cardiology*, vol. 43, no. 4, pp. 665–669, 2004.

[7] P. G. Hagan, C. A. Nienaber, E. M. Isselbacher et al., "The International Registry of Acute Aortic Dissection (IRAD): new insights into an old disease," *JAMA*, vol. 283, no. 7, pp. 897–903, 2000.

[8] G. R. Upchurch Jr., C. Nienaber, R. Fattori et al., "Acute aortic dissection presenting with primarily abdominal pain: a rare manifestation of a deadly disease," *Annals of Vascular Surgery*, vol. 19, no. 3, pp. 367–373, 2005.

[9] T. Kawasaki, Y. Akakabe, M. Yamano et al., "Vagal enhancement as evidence of residual ischemia after inferior myocardial infarction," *Pacing and Clinical Electrophysiology*, vol. 32, no. 1, pp. 52–58, 2009.

[10] K. M. Chan-Tack, "Aortic dissection presenting as bilateral testicular pain," *The New England Journal of Medicine*, vol. 343, no. 16, p. 1199, 2000.

[11] G. M. Guarín-Loaiza, L. C. Nocua-Báez, and G. Alfonso-Hernández, "Bilateral testicular pain as an acute aortic dissection symptom," *Revista de la Facultad de Medicina*, vol. 64, no. 3, pp. 571–574, 2016.

[12] S. M. O'Leary, P. L. Williams, M. P. Williams et al., "Imaging the pericardium: appearances on ECG-gated 64-detector row cardiac computed tomography," *The British Journal of Radiology*, vol. 83, no. 987, pp. 194–205, 2010.

[13] J. Bogaert and M. Francone, "Pericardial disease: value of CT and MR imaging," *Radiology*, vol. 267, no. 2, pp. 340–356, 2013.

[14] C. Gaul, W. Dietrich, and F. J. Erbguth, "Neurological symptoms in aortic dissection: a challenge for neurologists," *Cerebrovascular Diseases*, vol. 26, no. 1, pp. 1–8, 2008.

Successful Resolution of a Large Left Atrial and Left Atrial Appendage Thrombus with Rivaroxaban

Safwan Gaznabi,[1] Ashraf Abugroun,[1] Hasan Mahbub,[2] and Enrique Campos[3]

[1]*Department of Internal Medicine, Advocate Illinois Masonic Medical Center, 836 W Wellington Ave., Chicago, IL 60657, USA*
[2]*Department of Internal Medicine, Flushing Hospital Medical Center, 4500 Parsons Blvd, Flushing, NY 11355, USA*
[3]*Department of Cardiology, Advocate Illinois Masonic Medical Center, 836 W Wellington Ave, Chicago, IL 60657, USA*

Correspondence should be addressed to Safwan Gaznabi; sgaznabi@gmail.com

Academic Editor: Aiden Abidov

A 79-year-old male was admitted to the hospital for acute exacerbation of heart failure. The patient had history of atrial fibrillation and was planned for cardioversion. Preprocedure transesophageal echocardiogram (TEE) revealed a large multilobulated mobile thrombus in the left atrial appendage. The patient refused warfarin therapy and instead chose to take rivaroxaban. Upon outpatient follow-up, 3 months later, no visible thrombus was appreciated on repeat TEE. This case demonstrates successful resolution of left atrial and left atrial appendage thrombi with the use of rivaroxaban. At present time, limited data is available to support the use of rivaroxaban for treatment of intracardiac thrombi. This case highlights the need for further studies to investigate the outcomes and relative efficiency of use of direct oral anticoagulants (DOACs) in lysis of intracardiac thrombus. The benefits of DOACs compared to the standard of therapy could increase patient compliance, reduce length of stay, and improve treatment efficacy.

1. Introduction

Atrial fibrillation is an ever-growing global problem, with an estimated 2.7-6.1 million affected in the United States and roughly 33.5 million affected worldwide [1]. Left atrial abnormalities, such as dilated left atrium and reduced left atrial and/or left atrial appendage blood flow, are independent risk factors for development of thromboembolism [2, 3]. In order to estimate the annual minimal risk of a thromboembolic event in these patients, we use the CHA2DS2-VASc scoring tool. Anticoagulation therapy helps to mitigate the risks of thromboembolic events and specifically in cases of nonvalvular atrial fibrillation (NVAF) [4, 5]. In cases of left atrial or left atrial appendage (LA/LAA) thrombus, current guidelines recommend vitamin K antagonist (VKA) therapy [6–10]. Here, we describe a successful resolution of left atrial and left atrial appendage thrombus with use of rivaroxaban.

2. Case Report

A 79-year-old male with past medical history of hypertension, atrial fibrillation (CHA2DS2-VASc score = 4, only on Aspirin), type 2 diabetes mellitus, and right lower extremity leiomyosarcoma with lymphedema of the affected limb treated with surgical resection and radiotherapy presented to the emergency department with exertional dyspnea, worsening of lower extremity edema, and weight gain. On arrival vitals shows blood pressure 140/95, heart rate 80, and SpO_2 98. Physical examination was remarkable for irregular heartbeat, decreased bilateral lung sounds, and bilateral grade 3+ lower extremity edema up to the sacrum. Electrocardiogram (EKG) showed atrial fibrillation with new left bundle branch block (LBBB) (Figure 1). The laboratory workup was significant for brain natriuretic peptide (BNP) 2,233 pg/ml, troponin 0.38 ng/ml, and d-dimer 1.81 mg/l. Otherwise, he had normal basic metabolic panel

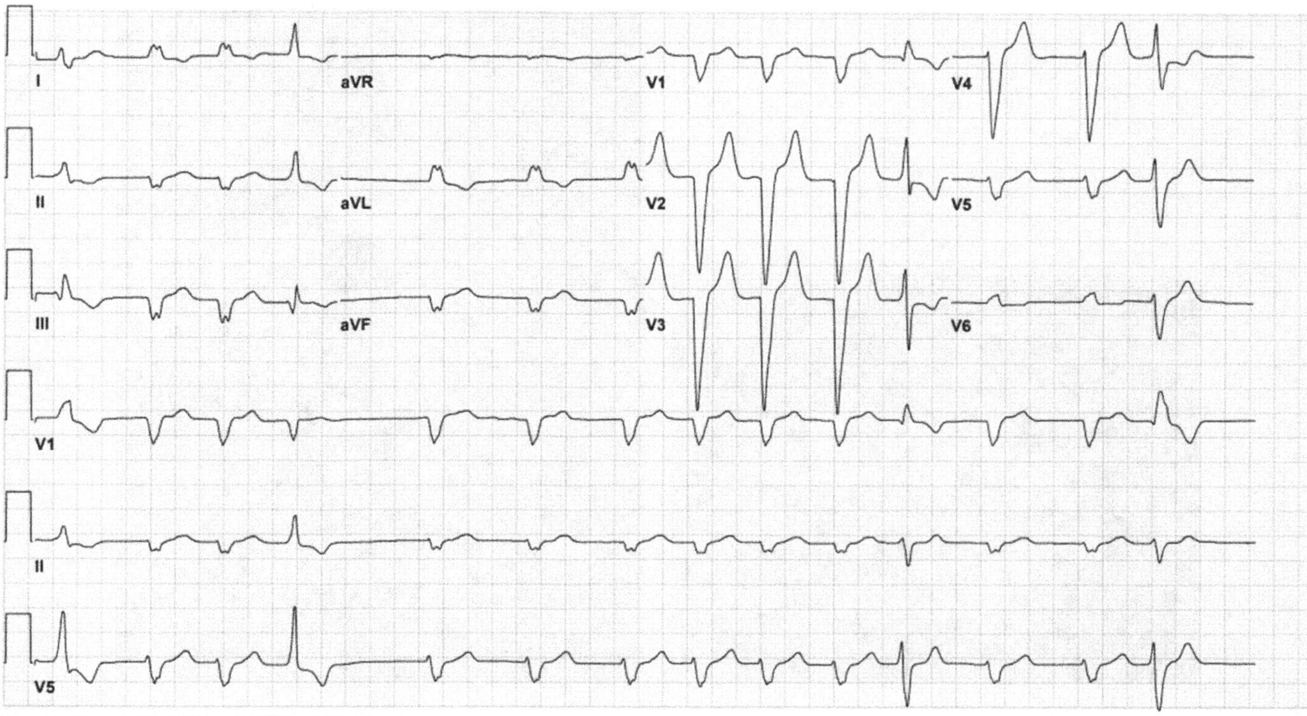

Figure 1: EKG shows atrial fibrillation and LBBB.

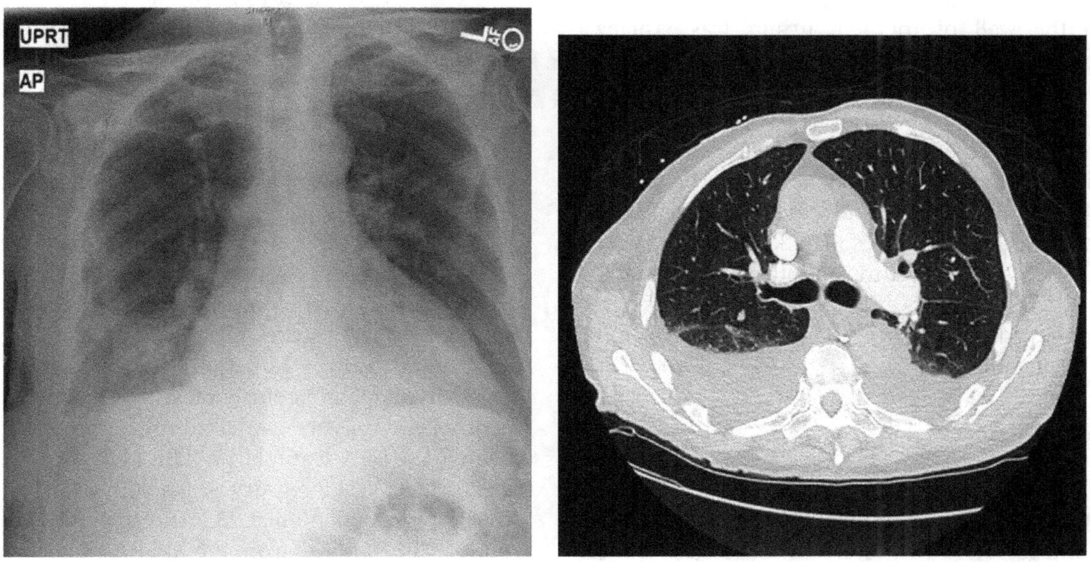

(a) (b)

Figure 2: (a) CXR showed cardiomegaly with pulmonary congestion and bilateral pleural effusion. (b) CT chest with contrast showed moderately large bilateral pleural effusions, right greater than left, with cardiomegaly and reflux of IV contrast into the IVC, consistent with cardiogenic pulmonary vascular congestion.

(BMP) and complete blood count (CBC). Chest X-ray (CXR) and computed tomography (CT) of the chest showed cardiomegaly and moderate pleural effusion in bilateral lung fields (Figure 2).

Transthoracic echocardiogram (TTE) showed left ventricular ejection fraction of 20% and severe global hypokinesis. Coronary angiogram revealed minimal coronary artery disease. The patient was diagnosed with nonischemic cardiomyopathy and was treated with lisinopril, metoprolol, spironolactone, diuretics, and enoxaparin. Despite medical management, he remained in atrial fibrillation for which he was scheduled for rhythm restoration with transesophageal echocardiogram- (TEE-) guided DC cardioversion (DCCV). TEE revealed a large multilobulated mobile thrombus in the

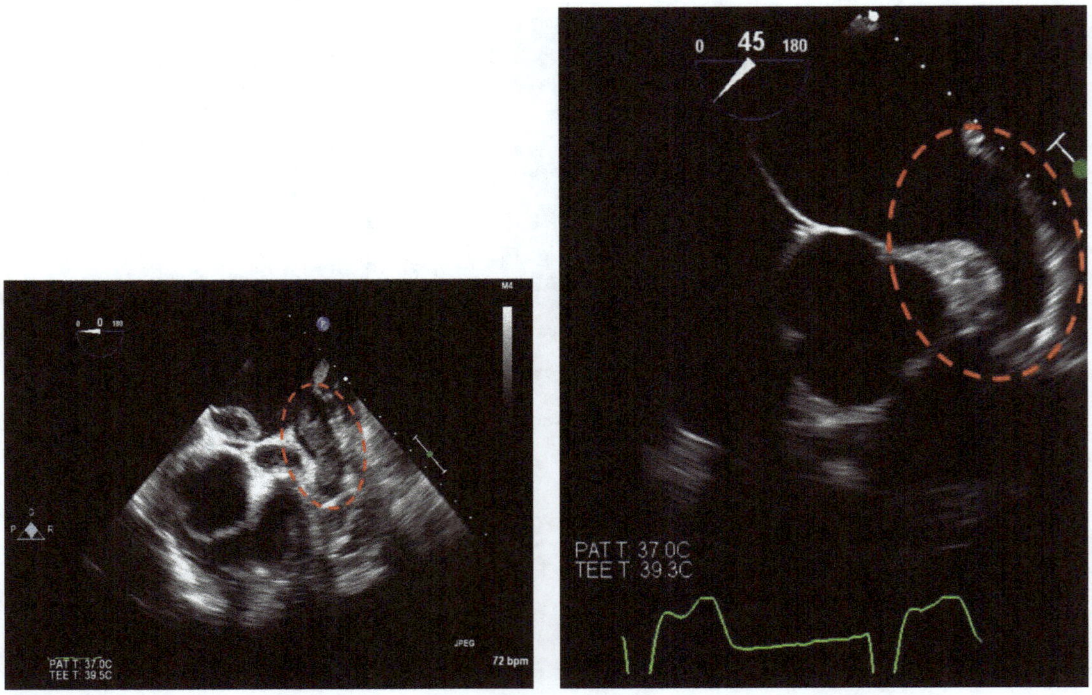

(a) (b)

FIGURE 3: (a) The TEE transesophageal short axis view shows a large multilobulated mobile thrombus in the left atrial appendage. (b) TEE done 3 months later shows resolution of the thrombus.

left atrial appendage, and sessile irregular echogenic material attached to the wall of the left atrium was visualized (Figure 3(a)). Accordingly, cardioversion was aborted. The patient refused anticoagulation with Coumadin therapy and instead opted for rivaroxaban, aware of risks of possible anticoagulation failure or adverse events, as he would not be on standard of therapy. The patient was discharged with guideline-directed management for coronary artery disease and heart failure as well as rivaroxaban 20 mg daily. On subsequent outpatient follow-up three months later, repeat TEE showed no visible thrombus (Figure 3(b)). No evidence of clinical thromboembolic events was noted between initial and follow-up encounters.

3. Discussion

Standard of therapy for stroke prophylaxis in setting of LA/LAA/intracardiac thrombus in patients with NVAF is vitamin K antagonist (VKA) oral anticoagulation [6–10]; however, there is limited data regarding the use and clinical outcomes of direct thrombin inhibitors (DOACs) for diagnosed thrombus in LA/LAA. The ROCKET-AF trial evaluated the treatment of nonvalvular atrial fibrillation (NVAF) with the direct oral factor Xa inhibitor (rivaroxaban) compared with warfarin. Rivaroxaban was noninferior to warfarin in preventing stroke or systemic embolism in NVAF patients [11]. Among patients excluded were those with mitral valve stenosis, prosthetic valves, and left ventricular thrombus; however, there is no specific mention of inclusion or exclusion of LA/LAA thrombus. Investigators commented that patients in the warfarin group were in the therapeutic INR range, a mean of 55% of the time [11].

According to the 2018 European Heart Rhythm Association Practical Guide on the use of nonvitamin K antagonist oral anticoagulants in patients with atrial fibrillation [12], in patients with atrial fibrilation ≥ 48-hour duration (or unknown) provided TEE negative for thrombi, the initiation of DOACs can be considered with at least a single DOAC dose ≥ 4 hours before electrical or pharmacological cardioversion. Otherwise, an alternative strategy would be initiating DOAC therapy for at least 3 weeks prior to cardioversion. After cardioversion, continuous oral anticoagulation is mandatory for at least another 4 weeks, irrespective of the CHA2DS2-VASc score [7]. One prospective open-label multicenter study by Lip et al. (X-TRA study) explored the use of vitamin K antagonist oral anticoagulation for the treatment of nonvalvular atrial fibrillation/flutter with documented LA/LAA thrombi on TEE [13]. This was based on the 2015 CLOT AF registry which with a total of 156 sample sizes in ITT population at 23 institutions among 7 European country [14] findings from the X-TRA showed that resolved or reduced thrombus after rivaroxaban treatment was evident and consistent with LA/LAA thrombus resolution with VKA therapy, suggesting that rivaroxaban maybe a potential treatment option for LA/LAA thrombi in patients with NVAF or atrial flutter [13].

Warfarin inhibits the hepatic synthesis of the vitamin K-dependent coagulation factors by preventing extension of existing thrombi and de novo thrombosis [8]. Limitations for use of warfarin among cardiac patients who require anticoagulation therapy include a narrow therapeutic range, food and drug interactions, and unpredictable pharmacokinetics requiring regular and frequent International Normalized Ratio (INR) checks [15]. Failure of adequate anticoagulation can lead to progression of thromboembolism, hemorrhage, repeated hospital admissions, necessitation of more invasive procedures such as placement of a left atrial appendage closure device, increased cost burden, and increased risks of morbidity and mortality [9, 16, 17].

Rivaroxaban is approved for the reduction in risk of stroke for NVAF, primary and secondary venous thromboembolism (VTE) prophylaxes, and treatment of VTE; however, limited data and literature have been reported to establish the use or efficacy of DOACs on established left-sided intracardiac thrombus and its outcomes. This case demonstrates successful resolution of LA/LAA thrombi on DOAC therapy, specifically rivaroxaban. If enough clinical data supports DOAC relative efficacy in lysis of LA/LAA/intracardiac thrombus, the benefits of DOAC compared to the standard of therapy could increase patient compliance, reduce length of stay, and improve treatment efficacy.

4. Conclusion

At present time, there is limited data on DOACs or factor Xa inhibitors in cases of diagnosed left atrial/left atrial appendage/intracardiac thrombi. Ideally, a well-designed randomized clinical trial to provide meaningful data and guidance as to the use of DOACs for such cases.

References

[1] S. S. Chugh, R. Havmoeller, K. Narayanan et al., "Worldwide epidemiology of atrial fibrillation: a Global Burden of Disease 2010 Study," *Circulation*, vol. 129, no. 8, pp. 837–847, 2014.

[2] M. E. Brickner, D. B. Friedman, C. G. Cigarroa, and P. A. Grayburn, "Relation of thrombus in the left atrial appendage by transesophageal echocardiography to clinical risk factors for thrombus formation," *The American Journal of Cardiology*, vol. 74, no. 4, pp. 391–393, 1994.

[3] O. Kamp, "Importance of left atrial appendage flow as a predictor of thromboembolic events in patients with atrial fibrillation," *European Heart Journal*, vol. 20, no. 13, pp. 979–985, 1999.

[4] C. T. Ruff, R. P. Giugliano, E. Braunwald et al., "Comparison of the efficacy and safety of new oral anticoagulants with warfarin in patients with atrial fibrillation: a metaanalysis of randomised trials," *The Lancet*, vol. 383, no. 9921, pp. 955–962, 2014.

[5] C. A. Salazar, D. D. Aguila, and E. G. Cordova, "Direct thrombin inhibitors versus vitamin K antagonists for preventing cerebral or systemic embolism in patients with non-valvular atrial fibrillation," *Cochrane Database of Systematic Reviews*, no. 3, 2014.

[6] Developed with the special contribution of the European Heart Rhythm Association (EHRA), Endorsed by the European Association for Cardio-Thoracic Surgery (EACTS), Authors/Task Force Members et al., "Guidelines for the management of atrial fibrillation: The Task Force for the Management of Atrial Fibrillation of the European Society of Cardiology (ESC)," *European Heart Journal*, vol. 31, no. 19, pp. 2369–2429, 2010.

[7] P. Kirchhof, S. Benussi, D. Kotecha et al., "2016 ESC Guidelines for the management of atrial fibrillation developed in collaboration with EACTS," *European Heart Journal*, vol. 37, no. 38, pp. 2893–2962, 2016.

[8] G. Corrado, G. Tadeo, S. Beretta et al., "Atrial thrombi resolution after prolonged anticoagulation in patients with atrial fibrillation," *Chest*, vol. 115, no. 1, pp. 140–143, 1999.

[9] U. O. Egolum, D. G. Stover, D. Lenihan et al., "Intracardiac thrombus: diagnosis, complications and management," *The American Journal of the Medical Sciences*, vol. 345, no. 5, pp. 391–395, 2013.

[10] R. Delewi, F. Zijlstra, and J. J. Piek, "Left ventricular thrombus formation after acute myocardial infarction," *Heart*, vol. 98, no. 23, pp. 1743–1749, 2012.

[11] M. R. Patel, K. W. Mahaffey, J. Garg et al., "Rivaroxaban versus warfarin in nonvalvular atrial fibrillation," *New England Journal of Medicine*, vol. 365, no. 10, pp. 883–891, 2011.

[12] J. Steffel, P. Verhamme, T. S. Potpara et al., "The 2018 European Heart Rhythm Association Practical Guide on the use of non-vitamin K antagonist oral anticoagulants in patients with atrial fibrillation," *European Heart Journal*, vol. 39, no. 16, pp. 1330–1393, 2018.

[13] G. Y. Lip, C. Hammerstingl, F. Marin et al., "Left atrial thrombus resolution in atrial fibrillation or flutter: results of a prospective study with rivaroxaban (X-TRA) and a retrospective observational registry providing baseline data (CLOT-AF)," *American Heart Journal*, vol. 178, pp. 126–134, 2016.

[14] G. Y. H. Lip, C. Hammerstingl, F. Marin et al., "Rationale and design of a study exploring the efficacy of once-daily oral rivaroxaban (X-TRA) on the outcome of left atrial/left atrial appendage thrombus in nonvalvular atrial fibrillation or atrial flutter and a retrospective observational registry providing baseline data (CLOT-AF)," *American Heart Journal*, vol. 169, no. 4, pp. 464–471.e2, 2015.

[15] S. Dobashi, T. Fujino, and T. Ikeda, "Use of apixaban for an elderly patient with left atrial thrombus," *BMJ Case Reports*, vol. 2014, no. 1, article bcr2014203870, 2014.

[16] S. Agarwal, R. Hachamovitch, and V. Menon, "Current trial-associated outcomes with warfarin in prevention of stroke in patients with nonvalvular atrial fibrillation: a meta-analysis," *Archives of Internal Medicine*, vol. 172, no. 8, pp. 623–631, 2012.

[17] E. S. Mearns, C. M. White, C. G. Kohn et al., "Quality of vitamin K antagonist control and outcomes in atrial fibrillation patients: a meta-analysis and meta-regression," *Thrombosis Journal*, vol. 12, no. 1, p. 14, 2014.

22

Transvenous Extraction and Removal of Pacing Leads Placed after Cardiac Transplantation

Caleb Norton,[1] **Benjamin Holmes**,[2] **Asad Al Aboud**,[2] **Eun-Jeong Kim**,[2] **Holly Gonzales**,[2] **Christopher Ellis**,[2] **Roy John**,[2] **George H. Crossley III**,[2] **and Jay Montgomery**[2]

[1]*Department of Medicine, Vanderbilt University Medical Center, Nashville, TN, USA*
[2]*Division of Cardiovascular Medicine, Vanderbilt University Medical Center, Nashville, TN, USA*

Correspondence should be addressed to Jay Montgomery; jay.a.montgomery@vumc.org

Academic Editor: Tayfun Sahin

There is an increasing prevalence of cardiac implantable electronic devices (CIEDs) due to expanding adoption and availability of these evidence-based therapies. With the increased prevalence of these life-saving devices, there has also been an increased demand for lead removal and lead extraction. Understanding the specific subgroups of patients at high risk for complications during and after lead extraction has become imperative to properly manage endovascular CIED leads. There have been multiple published studies describing clinical variables that predict adverse outcomes in CIED system extractions; however, the risk of complications in leads placed after cardiac transplantation has not specifically been addressed to date. We present four cases of transvenous extraction and removal of pacing leads placed after cardiac transplantation. There were no major complications related to extraction in these four cases; however, three of the four patients died within one year after the procedure. While the etiology of death in these cases seemed to be unrelated to the extraction procedure, the indications for extraction (infection in the setting of immunosuppression and calcineurin-associated ESRD and poor sensing/capture possibly secondary to chronic rejection and/or frequent right heart biopsies) likely contributed at least indirectly to the subsequent death.

1. Introduction

There is an increasing prevalence of cardiac implantable electronic devices (CIEDs) due to expanding adoption and availability of these evidence-based therapies [1–3]. From 1993 to 2006, it is estimated that index pacemaker and implantable cardioverter-defibrillator (ICD) implants in the U.S. increased from 46.7 to 61.6 and 6.1 to 46.2 per 100,000, respectively [4]. With the increased prevalence of these life-saving devices, there has also been an increased demand for lead removal and lead extraction (defined as removal of a lead implanted for >12 months or requiring specialized tools) [5]. Understanding the specific subgroups of patients at high risk for complications during and after lead extraction has become imperative to properly manage endovascular CIED leads. There have been multiple published studies describing clinical variables that predict adverse outcomes in CIED system extractions [6–9]. In review of these large retrospective registries, the risk of complications in the cardiac transplant population has not been specifically addressed to date. Based on Organ Procurement and Transplantation Network data as of November 25, 2018, there were 3,242 cardiac transplants performed in the United States in 2017. It is estimated that 10.9% of transplant recipients develop bradyarrhythmias requiring pacemaker implantation, with the most common indication being sinoatrial dysfunction [10, 11]. We present four cases of transvenous extraction and removal of pacing leads implanted after cardiac transplantation.

2. Case One

A 75-year-old man with a past medical history of ischemic cardiomyopathy who underwent orthotopic heart transplantation (OHT) in 1997 (biatrial anastomosis) was referred for pacemaker system extraction. His initial posttransplant course had been complicated by sinus node dysfunction with a slow junctional escape rhythm, and he underwent implantation of a single chamber AAI Medtronic 8088B pacemaker with a Medtronic 4068 lead placed in the right atrium shortly after his transplantation. In 2007, the atrial lead had low impedance and impending failure, so a Medtronic 3830 lead was added in the right atrial appendage at the time of generator change.

He developed end-stage renal disease (ESRD) secondary to calcineurin inhibitor toxicity, and hemodialysis was started in 2012. He developed recurrent infections in his left upper extremity fistula site (initially methicillin-sensitive *Staphylococcus aureus* but later polymicrobial) in 2016 with eventual pacemaker pocket infection requiring full CIED system extraction.

The Medtronic 3830 lead, which had been indwelling for nine years, was extracted using laser energy application along the proximal portion of the lead. The older Medtronic 4068 lead, indwelling for 19 years, required extensive application of laser energy at multiple points along the lead for removal. The pocket was debrided, and the incision was closed using vertical mattress sutures. There was no temporary pacemaker placed, as he was not pacemaker-dependent. The patient was readmitted within 30 days due to concern that the pacemaker pocket site infection had not been fully cleared. This was ultimately treated by drainage of a complex fluid collection associated with the previous pacemaker site. The patient was admitted six months later due to sepsis secondary to disseminated histoplasmosis and ultimately died secondary to multiorgan failure.

3. Case Two

A 59-year-old man with a past medical history of nonischemic cardiomyopathy who initially underwent OHT in 1994 (biatrial anastomosis) was referred for pacemaker lead revision. His posttransplant course had been complicated by transplant vasculopathy, and he ultimately required a second heart transplant in 2002 (bicaval anastomosis). He also developed ESRD and underwent deceased donor kidney transplantation in 2004. He developed ehrlichiosis in 2011 in addition to cryptococcal pneumonia and histoplasmosis requiring chronic treatment with antifungals. In 2013, he had syncope leading to a subarachnoid hemorrhage and was diagnosed with sinus node dysfunction in the setting of intermittent sinus bradycardia to less than 20 beats per minute. He underwent dual chamber pacemaker placement in 2013 (Medtronic ADDRL1) with a Medtronic 5076 lead in the ventricular position and a Medtronic 5592 lead placed in the right atrial appendage after an active fixation lead was deemed to be unstable.

He was admitted for volume overload three years later, and pacemaker interrogation revealed undersensing on the atrial channel due to a gradual P wave amplitude decrease from 4.7 mV at implant to ~0.4 mV, leading to asynchronous ventricular pacing and failure to recognize atrial arrhythmias. No change in lead position was detectable on chest X-ray. An atrial lead addition was planned. However, the left subclavian vein was occluded. He underwent extraction of the atrial lead to obtain venous access. A 12 French Spectranetics SLS II laser sheath was advanced over the lead, and minimal application of laser energy was used to free adhesions. Countertraction using a snare was also employed from the femoral vein. The lead was removed, and subclavian access was retained. A Medtronic 3830 lead was implanted in the right atrium. The patient tolerated the procedure well, and he had no complications within the next 30 days. However, he was admitted with cryptogenic encephalopathy two months later which was thought to be at least partially related to subclinical cirrhosis. He was ultimately discharged to inpatient hospice and died shortly thereafter.

4. Case Three

A 60-year-old man with a past medical history of nonischemic cardiomyopathy who underwent OHT in 1994 was referred for pacemaker extraction (biatrial anastomosis). His posttransplant course was complicated by sinus node dysfunction, and he underwent dual chamber pacemaker placement (Medtronic P1501) in 2008 with Medtronic 3830 leads in the right atrium and right ventricle. He also developed ESRD secondary to calcineurin inhibitor toxicity and underwent deceased donor kidney transplant in 2008. He was admitted with sepsis secondary to *Escherichia coli* in 2014, and a TEE during this admission demonstrated vegetations involving the pacemaker leads. He underwent extraction of the six-year-old system with manual traction alone. His hospital course was complicated by worsening renal graft function thought to be secondary to sepsis, which ultimately required reinitiation of dialysis. He was discharged to a rehabilitation facility with a plan for four weeks of intravenous ceftriaxone but was subsequently readmitted with recurrent sepsis secondary to *Escherichia coli* within 30 days. He was found to have a left atrial appendage thrombus (despite sinus rhythm). The source of his persistent *E. coli* bacteremia was unknown; however, it was hypothesized that the left atrial appendage thrombus could have been a nidus for recurrent infection. He was discharged on a 6-week course of meropenem with eventual clearance of the bacteremia and reimplantation of a dual chamber pacemaker 10 months later. He ultimately died three years later after a prolonged hospital stay related to ascending cholangitis and septic shock as well as hemorrhagic shock related to a spontaneous retroperitoneal hemorrhage.

5. Case Four

A 68-year-old man with a past medical history of ischemic cardiomyopathy who underwent OHT in 1991 (biatrial anastomosis) was referred for pacemaker lead revision. His course had been notable for paroxysmal atrial fibrillation and sinus node dysfunction developing 25 years after transplantation. He underwent dual chamber pacemaker placement in 2017 (Medtronic A2DR01) with a Medtronic 3830 atrial lead and Medtronic 5076 ventricular lead.

He was admitted for management of atrial fibrillation with rapid ventricular response four months after device implantation. Device interrogation during the admission showed undersensing on the atrial channel. He underwent revision of the atrial lead 8 months after the initial implantation with lead removal via manual traction and new lead placement on the posterior right atrial septum due to poor sensing and pacing thresholds elsewhere. He had no immediate complications and was discharged home the same day. He had no complications within 30 days after discharge. However, he died from complications of recurrent aspiration pneumonia unrelated to the procedure two months after lead revision.

6. Discussion

We present four cases of transvenous extraction/removal of CIED leads placed after cardiac transplantation. All four of these patients underwent extraction for reasons that are plausibly related to their posttransplant status: two related to infection and two due to poor sensing on the atrial channel. Overall, these patients seemed to have a similar or slightly reduced degree of lead binding and tissue in-growth, with a 19-year-old lead requiring significant manual sheath dissection and laser-assisted dissection. More recent leads were removed more easily, often with manual traction. The average procedure duration was 92 minutes (longest 120 minutes, shortest 72 minutes), in comparison to estimated average procedure duration of 135 minutes in the largest single-center registry (though this comparison is clearly confounded) [8]. While no conclusions can be made based on the limitations of this small case series, this does suggest that there is likely no major increase in procedural duration related to prior transplantation status. In addition, three out of four patients died within seven months of the procedure (the fourth lived 44 months), though none had a major complication from the procedure itself. Overall, this may suggest that nonprocedural factors predict high mortality in patients requiring lead extraction after heart transplant.

Several attempts have been made to identify high-risk groups for developing adverse outcomes after lead extraction [6–9]. Brunner et al. analyzed more than 5000 cases of transvenous lead extraction in a single center and identified multivariable predictors of major complications [8]. The risk factors for major periprocedural complications were cerebrovascular disease, ejection fraction less than or equal to 15%, lower platelet count, INR greater than or equal to 1.2, use of mechanical sheaths, and use of powered sheaths. This study also identified predictors of all-cause mortality within 30 days of lead extraction, including body mass index less than 25, ESRD, advanced NYHA functional class, lower hemoglobin, higher INR, lead extraction for infection, and extraction of a dual coil ICD lead. Cardiac transplantation was not considered in the patient characteristics in this study, nor was it considered in other studies that attempted to identify high-risk populations [6–9].

Several prior studies have shown longer lead implant duration to be associated with an increased need for powered or mechanical sheaths as well as an increase in procedural failure [12–15]. In our series, increased lead dwell time (up to 19 years) seemed to be associated with a proportional increase in lead adhesions, as would be expected in a nontransplant population. Of note, case 4 was the only patient that had leads removed within 12 months of initial implantation. The other extractions ranged between 3 and 19 years after initial implantation.

Lead extraction for infection has previously been cited as a risk factor for mortality at 30 days and at one year after lead extraction [8, 16]. In our series, we present two patients who required system extraction secondary to infections (one case due to pocket infection; the other due to lead vegetations and bacteremia). *Staphylococcus aureus* (as seen in case one) is a relatively frequent pathogen in CIED-related infections [17]. The presence of ESRD with an arteriovenous fistula that became infected seemed to be the initial inciting event for this patient. Gram-negative *Escherichia coli* bacteremia (as seen in case three) is a relatively uncommon cause of lead-related endocarditis, and it is likely that it was related to underlying immunosuppression [17]. Case one required readmission within 30 days due to sepsis secondary to a persistent fluid collection at the site of the previous pacing system. Case three had readmission for sepsis and *E. coli* bacteremia of unclear etiology. Pocket site infection after extraction is an uncommon scenario after extraction for infection and is presumably related to the posttransplant immunosuppressed state.

In theory, chronic rejection leading to progressive fibrosis after cardiac transplantation could be a mechanism of poor sensing and capture over time after CIED implantation. In addition, partial or complete dislodgement may occur over time due to frequent right heart catheterization and endomyocardial biopsy with unintentional force placed on endocardial leads. In the two patients without infection, the initial procedural plan for lead failure was for lead addition rather than extraction and replacement. Given the relatively short lifespan of the patients in our cohort, this seems like a reasonable strategy when feasible. However, given the increased incidence of superior vena cava syndrome in some OHT populations (younger patients, bicaval anastomosis), procedural decision-making should be individualized as increased lead burden is thought to be a risk factor for this entity [18–20].

The predominant surgical technique used for cardiac transplantation has changed over time from primarily biatrial to bicaval anastomosis. While this series is too small to detect any difference in safety, it is plausible that surgical technique may affect the likelihood of major perioperative complications. In addition, it is thought that patients with prior cardiac surgery (including transplant) may be protected against some major adverse events, such as hemodynamically significant venous lacerations, due to the presence of adhesions, though the largest available dataset did not detect a significant difference [8].

7. Conclusions

We describe four patients who underwent transvenous extraction/removal of CIED leads placed after cardiac transplantation. There were no major complications related to extraction in these four cases. However, in three of the four cases in our series, the patients died within one year of extraction (2, 3, 7, and 44 months, respectively). Small numbers and the retrospective nature of this series preclude a comparison of the degree of lead binding and procedural complexity. For the same reason, a determination cannot be made regarding the appropriateness and safety of lead extraction for various indications in the transplant population. While the etiology of death in these cases seemed to be unrelated to the extraction procedure, the indications for extraction (infection in the setting of immunosuppression and calcineurin-associated ESRD and poor sensing/capture possibly related to chronic rejection) likely contributed at least indirectly to the subsequent death.

References

[1] C. Zhan, W. B. Baine, A. Sedrakyan, and C. Steiner, "Cardiac device implantation in the United States from 1997 through 2004: a population-based analysis," *Journal of General Internal Medicine*, vol. 23, Suppl 1, pp. 13–19, 2008.

[2] A. E. Epstein, J. P. DiMarco, K. A. Ellenbogen et al., "ACC/AHA/HRS 2008 guidelines for device-based therapy of cardiac rhythm abnormalities: a report of the American College of Cardiology/American Heart Association Task Force on practice guidelines (writing committee to revise the ACC/AHA/NASPE 2002 guideline update for implantation of cardiac pacemakers and antiarrhythmia devices) developed in collaboration with the American Association for Thoracic Surgery and Society of Thoracic Surgeons," *Journal of the American College of Cardiology*, vol. 51, no. 21, pp. e1–e62, 2008.

[3] J. A. Ezekowitz, B. H. Rowe, D. M. Dryden et al., "Systematic review: implantable cardioverter defibrillators for adults with left ventricular systolic dysfunction," *Annals of Internal Medicine*, vol. 147, no. 4, pp. 251–262, 2007.

[4] S. M. Kurtz, J. A. Ochoa, E. Lau et al., "Implantation trends and patient profiles for pacemakers and implantable cardioverter defibrillators in the United States: 1993–2006," *Pacing and Clinical Electrophysiology*, vol. 33, no. 6, pp. 705–711, 2010.

[5] B. L. Wilkoff, C. J. Love, C. L. Byrd et al., "Transvenous lead extraction: Heart Rhythm Society expert consensus on facilities, training, indications, and patient management: this document was endorsed by the American Heart Association (AHA)," *Heart Rhythm*, vol. 6, no. 7, pp. 1085–1104, 2009.

[6] S. K. Agarwal, S. Kamireddy, J. Nemec, A. Voigt, and S. Saba, "Predictors of complications of endovascular chronic lead extractions from pacemakers and defibrillators: a single-operator experience," *Journal of Cardiovascular Electrophysiology*, vol. 20, no. 2, pp. 171–175, 2009.

[7] M. Maytin, S. O. Jones, and L. M. Epstein, "Long-term mortality after transvenous lead extraction," *Circulation: Arrhythmia and Electrophysiology*, vol. 5, no. 2, pp. 252–257, 2012.

[8] M. P. Brunner, E. M. Cronin, V. E. Duarte et al., "Clinical predictors of adverse patient outcomes in an experience of more than 5000 chronic endovascular pacemaker and defibrillator lead extractions," *Heart Rhythm*, vol. 11, no. 5, pp. 799–805, 2014.

[9] M. P. Brunner, C. Yu, A. A. Hussein et al., "Nomogram for predicting 30-day all-cause mortality after transvenous pacemaker and defibrillator lead extraction," *Heart Rhythm*, vol. 12, no. 12, pp. 2381–2386, 2015.

[10] D. J. Cantillon, K. G. Tarakji, T. Hu et al., "Long-term outcomes and clinical predictors for pacemaker-requiring bradyarrhythmias after cardiac transplantation: analysis of the UNOS/OPTN cardiac transplant database," *Heart Rhythm*, vol. 7, no. 11, pp. 1567–1571, 2010.

[11] D. J. Cantillon, E. Z. Gorodeski, M. Caccamo et al., "Long-term outcomes and clinical predictors for pacing after cardiac transplantation," *The Journal of Heart and Lung Transplantation*, vol. 28, no. 8, pp. 791–798, 2009.

[12] O. Wazni, L. M. Epstein, R. G. Carrillo et al., "Lead extraction in the contemporary setting: the LExICon study: an observational retrospective study of consecutive laser lead extractions," *Journal of the American College of Cardiology*, vol. 55, no. 6, pp. 579–586, 2010.

[13] M. Maytin, C. J. Love, A. Fischer et al., "Multicenter experience with extraction of the Sprint Fidelis implantable cardioverter-defibrillator lead," *Journal of the American College of Cardiology*, vol. 56, no. 8, pp. 646–650, 2010.

[14] L. Segreti, A. di Cori, E. Soldati et al., "Major predictors of fibrous adherences in transvenous implantable cardioverter-defibrillator lead extraction," *Heart Rhythm*, vol. 11, no. 12, pp. 2196–2201, 2014.

[15] M. Maytin, B. L. Wilkoff, M. Brunner et al., "Multicenter experience with extraction of the Riata/Riata ST ICD lead," *Heart Rhythm*, vol. 11, no. 9, pp. 1613–1618, 2014.

[16] K. G. Tarakji, O. M. Wazni, S. Harb, A. Hsu, W. Saliba, and B. L. Wilkoff, "Risk factors for 1-year mortality among patients with cardiac implantable electronic device infection undergoing transvenous lead extraction: the impact of the infection type and the presence of vegetation on survival," *Europace*, vol. 16, no. 10, pp. 1490–1495, 2014.

[17] M. R. Sohail, D. Z. Uslan, A. H. Khan et al., "Management and outcome of permanent pacemaker and implantable cardioverter-defibrillator infections," *Journal of the American College of Cardiology*, vol. 49, no. 18, pp. 1851–1859, 2007.

[18] G. S. Morchi, B. Pietra, M. M. Boucek, and K. C. Chan, "Interventional cardiac catheterization procedures in pediatric cardiac transplant patients: transplant surgery is not the end of the road," *Catheterization and Cardiovascular Interventions*, vol. 72, no. 6, pp. 831–836, 2008.

[19] O. Aldoss, N. I. Arain, J. M. Vinocur et al., "Frequency of superior vena cava obstruction in pediatric heart transplant recipients and its relation to previous superior cavopulmonary anastomosis," *The American Journal of Cardiology*, vol. 112, no. 2, pp. 286–291, 2013.

[20] F. M. Kusumoto, M. H. Schoenfeld, B. L. Wilkoff et al., "2017 HRS expert consensus statement on cardiovascular implantable electronic device lead management and extraction," *Heart Rhythm*, vol. 14, no. 12, pp. e503–e551, 2017.

23

An Asymptomatic Patient with an Additional Cardiac Chamber Giant Left Atrial Appendage

Alexandros P. Evangeliou,[1] Evangelia Sotiroglou,[1] Nikolaos Charitakis,[1] Georgios Loufopoulos,[1] Christos Varassas,[1] Spiridon Papadopoulos,[2] Stergios Tzikas,[1] and Vassilios Vassilikos[1]

[1]*3rd Department of Cardiology, Ippokratio Hospital, Aristotle University of Thessaloniki, Thessaloniki, Greece*
[2]*Department of Radiology, Ippokratio Hospital, Thessaloniki, Greece*

Correspondence should be addressed to Stergios Tzikas; tzikas@gmail.com

Academic Editor: Kathleen Ngu

We present the case of an asymptomatic 54-year-old male, referred to our department for a follow-up cardiological consultation. Echocardiography assessment showed an unknown cavity adjacent to the lateral wall of the left ventricle. A large left atrial appendage was revealed in further investigations, and the treatment option was proved to be an impasse.

1. Introduction

Giant LAA or left atrial appendage aneurysm (LAAA) is an uncommon finding, and it either has a congenital origin or is acquired due to valvular dysfunction such as mitral regurgitation. Most of the cases are asymptomatic, but systemic thromboembolic events and supraventricular tachycardias (SVTs) may also be complications of untreated patients.

2. History of Presentation

A 54-year-old male presented at our department for follow-up consultation a year after percutaneous coronary intervention for an acute coronary syndrome involving the right coronary artery. The patient was asymptomatic, denying angina, palpitations, or other cardiac symptoms. The clinical examination, as well as the laboratory blood measurements, showed no abnormality.

3. Past Medical History

The past medical history of the patient comprises arterial hypertension, an acute myocardial infarction due to the right coronary artery obstruction, managed with interventional implantation of a drug-eluting stent in the culprit lesion, and a hospitalization due to a pleural empyema following a pulmonary infection a decade ago.

4. Investigations

Twelve-lead electrocardiogram confirmed sinus rhythm, atrioventricular conduction was normal, QRS complex width was narrow, the repolarization was typical, and the absence of supraventricular arrhythmia or other structural heart diseases is appreciated.

The transthoracic echocardiography (TTE) assessment unveiled normal functional features and no valvular dysfunction, and a cavity without contractility adjacent to the basal lateral wall of the left ventricle was notable (Figure 1(a), video (available here)). Due to the inability to accurately characterize this echocardiographically depicted abnormality, further medical investigations were performed. A transesophageal echocardiography (TEE) assessment (Figures 1(b)–1(d)) showed communication of the cavity with the left atrium with slow blood flow within the LAA without thrombi; thus, the diagnosis of the giant LAA was established. The LAA was undiagnosed in the TTE assessment which was performed

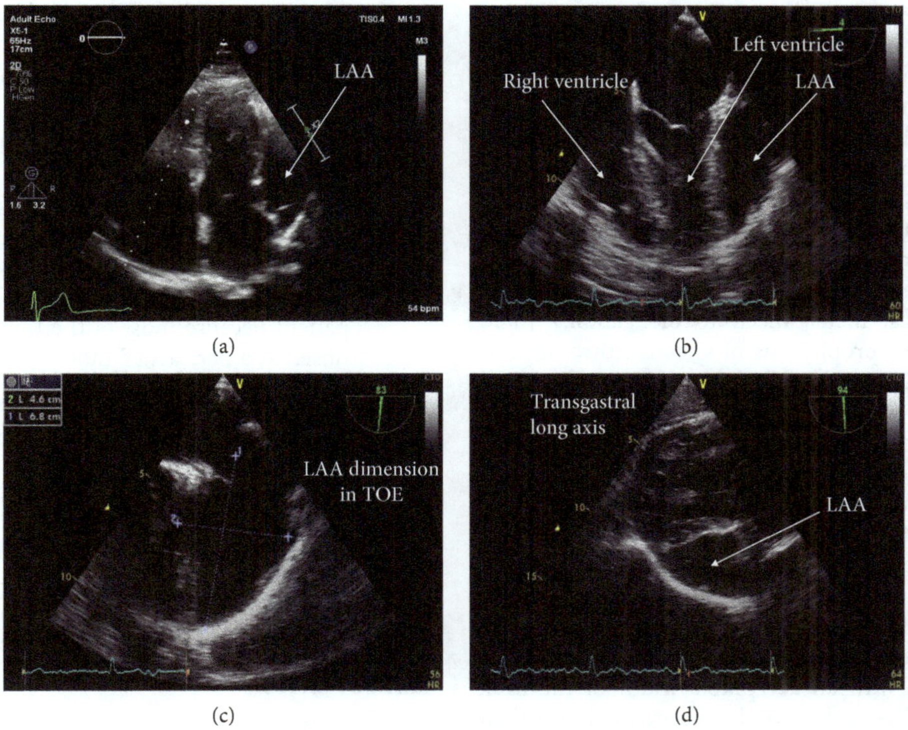

Figure 1: Echocardiographic views of the LAA.

one year ago, since it is an entity which cannot be easily revealed and further investigation is required.

Cardiac computed tomography (CT) was performed to evaluate the size, the relation of LAA with around organs, and the communication with the left atrium. CT revealed an abnormal left border of cardiac silhouette and enlargement of LAA (Figure 2). The enhancement with the contrast agent confirmed the presence of a LAA (4.6×6.8 cm in size).

In order to assess the possible systemic thromboembolic risk, considering the size of the LAA, a brain magnetic resonance imaging (MRI) was performed. T2 and fluid-attenuated inversion recovery (FLAIR) brain MRI revealed white matter hyperintensity (WMH) lesions in both cerebral hemispheres, without enrichment of lesions after the contrast agent administration as a sign of prior cerebral embolisms.

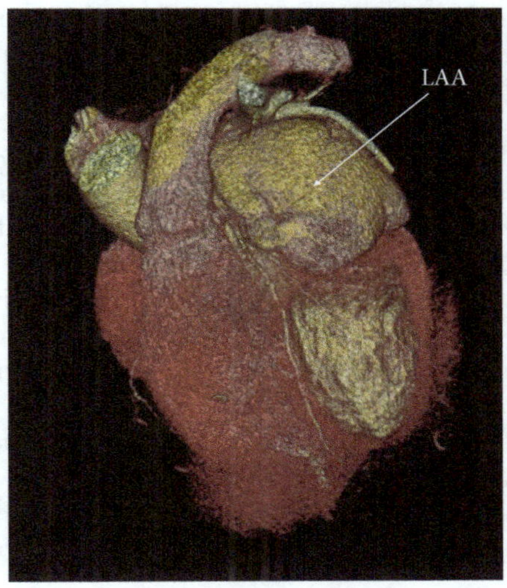

Figure 2: Cardiac CT depicting the LAA. Angiographic "shadow" of the LAA.

5. Differential Diagnosis

The differential diagnosis comprises pleural effusion, pericardial effusion, giant LAA, and LAAA with an acquired origin.

6. Management

Due to the lack of evidence-based guidelines for the management of such cases, our prime consideration was to assess the thromboembolic risk of this congenital abnormality. The idea to interventionally seal the LAA, in order to minimize the thromboembolic risk, is futile due to the large LAA neck (7.5 cm^2, maximal diameter > 40 mm). The available occluders with a maximum diameter of 33 mm are inappropriate in this case. Moreover, the absence of symptoms or echo contrast inside the LAA also excludes surgical treatment. However, after the MRI findings, oral anticoagulation was proposed as a possible management, and the patient accepted this option of treatment.

7. Discussion

Giant LAA or LAAA is an uncommon finding, and only a few cases are reported on the published literature. There is no consensus about these two medical terms, and most of the time, an extensive misunderstanding exists, concerning the description of a huge LAA in echocardiography assessment. It either has a congenital origin or is acquired due to valvular dysfunction such as mitral regurgitation [1]. Congenital LAA is mostly asymptomatic, but systemic thromboembolic events and SVTs due to atrial enlargement may also be complications of untreated patients [2]. LAA is the most likely site of thrombus formation in patients with atrial fibrillation (AF), indicating a clinically significant early diagnosis.

The treatment armamentarium for patients with giant LAA includes surgical aneurysmectomy or ligation [3] and oral anticoagulant for prophylaxis of systemic thromboembolic events as well as antiarrhythmic therapy for atrial tachyarrhythmias when indicated [4, 5]. Recommendation of surgical occlusion in symptomatic patients is based only on nonrandomized or observational cohort studies [6], as it can prevent thromboembolic complications and atrial arrhythmias associated with the LA enlargement.

Transcatheter device occlusion [7] has also been reported for the occlusion of narrow neck LAAs, with a high rate of success, in patients with anticoagulant contraindication [8]. All the published case reports are referred to the occlusion of atrial appendage with an acceptable width of the neck while the available sizes of these occluders are not larger than 33 mm. So, there is no report of device occlusion in really giant LAA treatment.

There is a gap of evidence in the management of asymptomatic and uncomplicated patients with normal sinus rhythm and huge LAA. Some authors favor surgery even in asymptomatic patients to prevent possible morbid and fatal complications associated with AF and systemic embolization [9]. In addition, there is no evidence that treatment of asymptomatic patients with oral anticoagulant agents can lead to stroke prevention, overwhelming the adverse events of such treatment. Interventional LAA occlusion is not an option in the majority of cases, due to device LAA orifice mismatch.

As far as our patient is concerned, despite being asymptomatic, his brain MRI demonstrated WMH lesions in both cerebral hemispheres, showing an increased risk of future systemic thromboembolic events [10]. However, the absence of arrhythmia, symptomatic stroke, or transient ischemic attack could not empower the choice of surgical excision, thus leaving anticoagulation as the only reasonable alternative.

8. Follow-Up

The patient remains asymptomatic and uncomplicated during the 3-month follow-up period. There are no signs of cardiac arrhythmias or systemic embolization, he remains in sinus rhythm, and no additional hospitalizations have occurred.

9. Conclusion

Giant LAAs can be initially depicted as an additional cardiac chamber. Further imaging can reveal the complete anatomy of this mostly congenital anomaly. In asymptomatic patients with giant LAAs, surgical occlusion is not recommended, and no evidence-based guidelines exist so far. After assessing the individual thromboembolic and bleeding risk of the patient, an appropriate treatment option might be oral anticoagulation therapy.

10. Learning Objectives

The following are the learning objectives:

(1) To be able to recognize the presence of a LAA with TTE or TEE examination in the asymptomatic patient because most of the times they are misdiagnosed as a pericardial fluid

(2) To be able to define the right treatment option for this patient if the transcatheter or surgical occlusion is indicated

(3) To be able to determine the appropriate treatment option, depending on the existence and the progression of clinical symptoms of the patient during the follow-up period

Abbreviations

LAA: Left atrial appendage
LAAA: Left atrial appendage aneurysm
SVTs: Supraventricular tachycardias
TTE: Transthoracic echocardiography
TEE: Transesophageal echocardiography
CT: Computed tomography
MRI: Magnetic resonance imaging
FLAIR: Fluid-attenuated inversion recovery
WMH: White matter hyperintensity
AF: Atrial fibrillation.

Consent

Informed consent has been obtained from the patient.

References

[1] H. Terada, Y. Tanaka, K. Kashima, K. Sannou, and T. Arima, "Left atrial diverticulum associated with severe mitral regurgitation," *Japanese Circulation Journal*, vol. 64, no. 6, pp. 474–476, 2000.

[2] W. M. M. Kuiten, L. M. de Heer, E. van Aarnhem, K. Onsea, and L. A. van Herwerden, "Giant left atrial appendage: a rare anomaly," *The Annals of Thoracic Surgery*, vol. 96, no. 4, pp. 1478–1480, 2013.

[3] M. R. Aryal, F. A. Hakim, S. Ghimire et al., "Left atrial appendage aneurysm: a systematic review of 82 cases," *Echocardiography*, vol. 31, no. 10, pp. 1312–1318, 2014.

[4] H. S. Yong, E. J. Kim, and C. U. Choi, "Giant left atrial appendage aneurysm," *European Heart Journal*, vol. 28, no. 18, p. 2207, 2007.

[5] E. Plonska-Gosciniak, B. Larysz, K. Jurczyk, and J. D. Kasprzak, "Five-chambered heart: a 20-year story of left atrial appendage aneurysm," *European Heart Journal*, vol. 30, no. 8, p. 1014, 2009.

[6] A. S. Kanderian, A. M. Gillinov, G. B. Pettersson, E. Blackstone, and A. L. Klein, "Success of surgical left atrial appendage closure: assessment by transesophageal echocardiography," *Journal of the American College of Cardiology*, vol. 52, no. 11, pp. 924–929, 2008.

[7] P. B. Sick, G. Schuler, K. E. Hauptmann et al., "Initial worldwide experience with the WATCHMAN left atrial appendage system for stroke prevention in atrial fibrillation," *Journal of the American College of Cardiology*, vol. 49, no. 13, pp. 1490–1495, 2007.

[8] V. Y. Reddy, S. K. Doshi, S. Kar et al., "5-year outcomes after left atrial appendage closure: from the PREVAIL and PROTECT AF trials," *Journal of the American College of Cardiology*, vol. 70, no. 24, pp. 2964–2975, 2017.

[9] Y. Nakai, M. Asano, N. Nomura, and A. Mishima, "Surgical management of an aneurysm of the left atrial appendage to prevent potential sequelae," *Interactive Cardiovascular and Thoracic Surgery*, vol. 17, no. 3, pp. 586-587, 2013.

[10] F. Moroni, E. Ammirati, M. A. Rocca, M. Filippi, M. Magnoni, and P. G. Camici, "Cardiovascular disease and brain health: focus on white matter hyperintensities," *International Journal of Cardiology: Heart & Vasculature*, vol. 19, pp. 63–69, 2018.

24

Resistant Ventricular Arrhythmia and the Role of Overdrive Pacing in the Suppression of the Electrical Storm

Mohamed Magdi, Mahmood Mubasher, Hakam Alzaeem, and Tahir Hamid

Hamad Medical Corporation, Qatar

Correspondence should be addressed to Mahmood Mubasher; dr.mahmood357@gmail.com

Academic Editor: Christopher S. Snyder

Ventricular arrhythmia storm is a state of cardiac instability characterized by multiple ventricular arrhythmias or multiple ICD therapies within a 24-hour duration. Management of this life-threatening state depends on the reversal of the cause besides either electrical or medical management of the arrhythmia. We report a case of a 54-year-old male who underwent a percutaneous coronary intervention following massive acute myocardial infarction. Afterwards, he developed frequent life-threatening ventricular arrhythmias that required multiple shocks and antiarrhythmic medications. Despite all these interventions, it was very difficult to control the electrical instability, but after overdrive ventricular pacing, the storm subsided and within a few days the case was stabilized. Overdrive pacing is an easy temporary modality to control the resistant arrhythmia following myocardial infarction.

1. Introduction

Electrical storm is a life-threatening arrhythmia that might occur after myocardial infarction. In severe cases, arrhythmias are resistant to medications and the direct current (DC) shock. Repeated shocks are also injurious to the heart and lead to progressive myocardial inflammation and fibrosis [1–4]. The management is usually difficult and challenging with poor prognosis and high mortality. In our case, we found that temporary overdrive pacing gives a safer method to abort the arrhythmia and to avoid progressive myocardial damage with repeated electrical shocks.

2. Case History

A 54-year-old diabetic and hypertensive male patient presented with a central chest pain while sleeping that lasted for an hour. On the ambulance, he became drowsy and developed ventricular tachycardia that was reverted to sinus rhythm by DC shock.

On admission to ED (3 hours after the pain), he was in pain and in the physical exam and he was fully conscious and oriented and in distress. Vitals were within the normal limits except for a slightly elevated blood pressure of 150/90. ECG showed normal sinus rhythm and ST elevation in leads V1 to V6 with deep Q waves in the same leads (Figure 1).

In the coronary catheterization lab (30 minutes after admission to ED), coronary angiography showed total proximal left anterior descending (LAD) artery occlusion and midleft circumflex (LCX) 80% lesion. The LAD lesion was stented with a DES.

After the procedure, he was stable with residual chest pain. Then, 2 hours later, he was found unresponsive with pulseless ventricular tachycardia, and after a single DC shock, he regained his consciousness and his sinus rhythm again (Figure 2).

The next morning, he developed asymptomatic sustained ventricular tachycardia that reverted spontaneously to sinus rhythm; then, the telemetry showed multiple premature ventricular complexes (PVCs) and nonsustained ventricular tachycardia (NSVT) (Figure 3). Amiodarone 150 mg IV bolus was given followed by 1 mg/minute IV infusion for 6 hours and then 0.5 mg/minute IV infusion for 18 hours. Serum electrolytes were within normal limits.

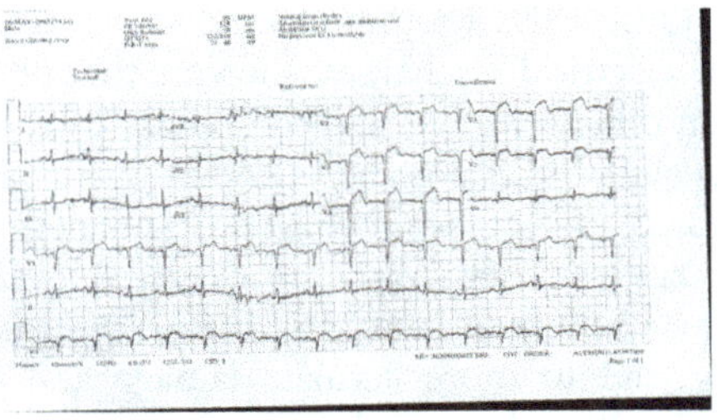

Figure 1: Normal sinus rhythm, ST elevation, and Q waves in leads V1, V2, V3, V4, V5, and V6.

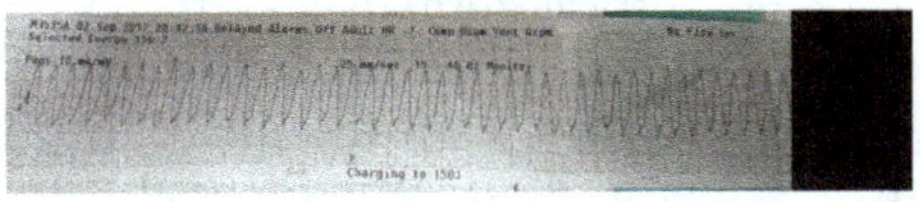

Figure 2: Ventricular tachycardia.

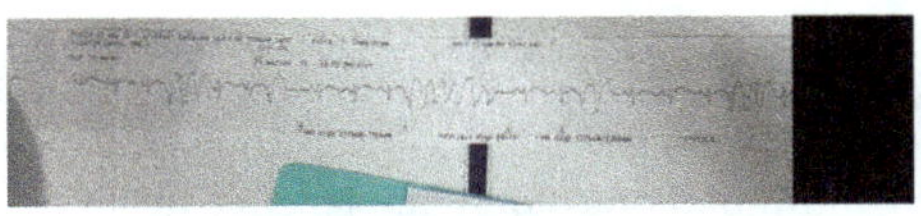

Figure 3: Multiple PVCs and NSVT.

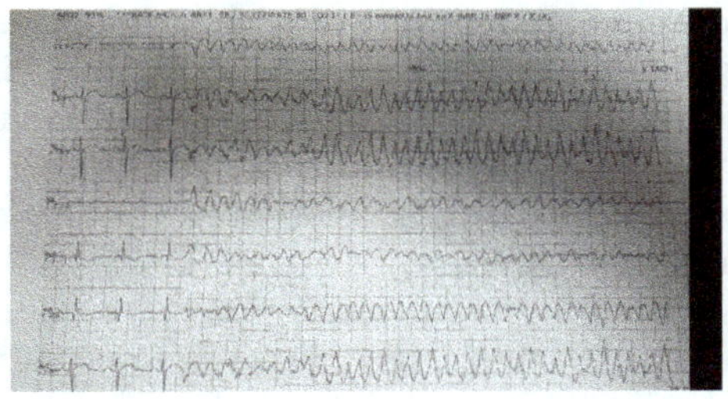

Figure 4: Ventricular tachycardia.

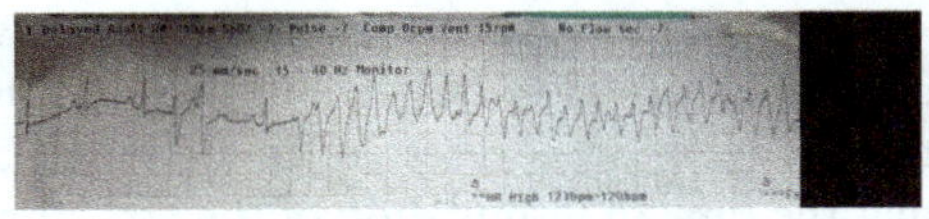

Figure 5: Ventricular tachycardia preceded by PVCs.

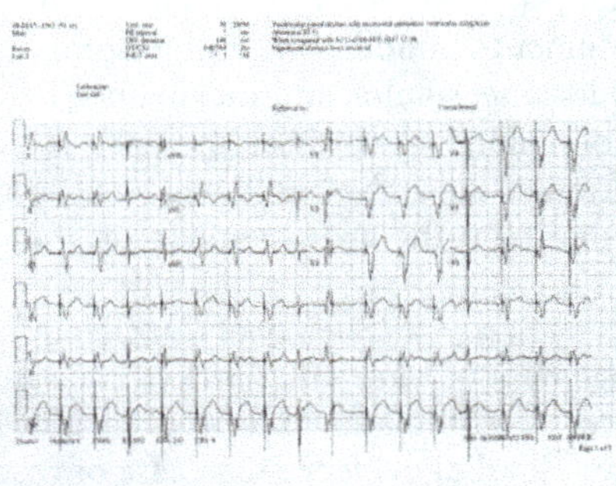

Figure 6: Ventricular paced rhythm at rate of 100.

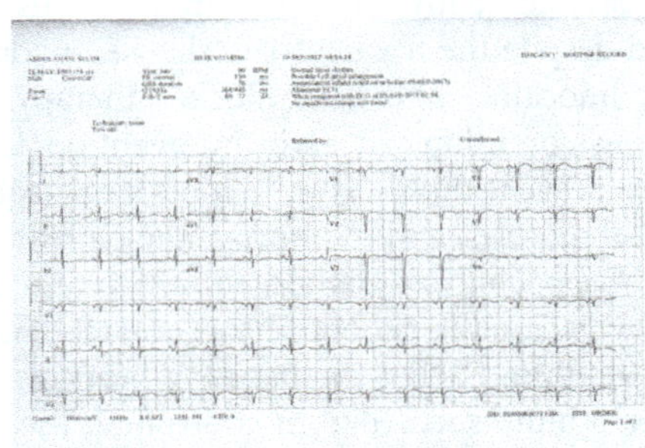

Figure 7: Sinus rhythm after pacemaker removal.

After two hours, he developed again asymptomatic ventricular tachycardia and IV lidocaine 70 mg bolus was given. Then, relook coronary angiography showed patent LAD stent and small ostial LCX clot that was aspirated.

In the evening, he had ventricular tachycardia (Figure 4) with hypotension, so the situation required the suppression of the arrhythmia by a DC shock, endotracheal intubation, and sedation (midazolam 0.1 mg/kg/hour). An intra-aortic balloon pump (IABP) and norepinephrine infusion 0.1 mcg/kg/minute were initiated to support his cardiogenic shock state.

The next day, clusters of ventricular tachycardia triggered by ventricular premature contractions occurred (Figure 5) and required multiple electrical defibrillations. Consequently, the patient was transferred to the catheterization lab, and a transcutaneous pacemaker was inserted.

After overdrive pacing with a rate of 100, his rhythm was stable with complete suppression of PVCs and no further attacks of ventricular arrhythmias (Figure 6).

In the next day, gradual weaning of inotropes and sedations started until it is completely stopped. His rhythm was stable on oral amiodarone 400 mg twice daily and metoprolol 25 mg twice daily in addition to the pacing.

After another 24 hours of stable rhythm, the pacemaker was removed and close observation showed no any ventricular arrhythmias (Figure 7). The next day, the patient was weaned from the mechanical ventilator.

He was observed in the coronary care unit for 2 days showing hemodynamic and electrical stability. After 2 weeks of discharge, he was seen in the clinic in a good state of health.

3. Discussion

Electrical storm (ES) indicates a state of life-threatening cardiac electrical instability characterized by clusters of ventricular arrhythmias in a short amount of time. It is defined as the presence of at least 3 distinct episodes of sustained ventricular tachycardia or VF in the last 24 hours. In the patients with an ICD, the most widely accepted definition of the electrical storm is three or more appropriate therapies for ventricular tachyarrhythmias, including antitachycardia pacing or shocks, within 24 hours [5].

Studies have shown that in only 10-25% of patients with the electrical storm, clear precipitating causes were identified

[6]. Some important causes are reversible, and their management can facilitate the control of the arrhythmias like acute myocardial ischemia, new or worsening heart failure, drug intoxication, or electrolyte disturbances.

ES is a clinical emergency that needs appropriate early management. Initially, antiarrhythmic drugs such as beta blocker and amiodarone are usually used [7, 8]. The drug of choice to start is amiodarone 150 mg IV over 10 minutes, followed by 1 mg/minute IV infusion for 6 hours and then by 0.5 mg/minute IV infusion for 18 additional hours.

Then, beta blockers are very important in the suppression of the sympathetic discharges after the arrhythmias and DC shocks. Propranolol (40 mg every 6 hours) has shown superior efficacy to metoprolol in a trial performed on 60 patients with electrical storm who received amiodarone, and this showed that the time to termination of the arrhythmias was earlier in the propranolol group in addition to lower rate of tachycardia recurrence or ICD discharges and shorter stay in the hospital [9]. There are other medications that can be used as an adjunct to amiodarone and propranolol like procainamide, lidocaine, sotalol, and mexiletine [10–12].

In case of failure of medical therapy, radiofrequency catheter ablation of the arrhythmogenic focus is a promising effective method for the management of the ventricular arrhythmia [13].

In the recent European Society of Cardiology's guidelines for the management of ventricular arrhythmias, transvenous catheter overdrive stimulation received a class IIa recommendation, and level of evidence C in case of recurrent ventricular arrhythmia despite the use of drug therapy and catheter ablation is not possible [14].

In our case, we report a state of severe electrical storm following a massive acute myocardial infarction. This arrhythmia persisted despite the frequent DC shocks in addition to amiodarone, lidocaine, and beta blocker therapy. In this life-threatening condition, an early intervention is needed to save life, to prevent the short- and long-term sequelae on the myocardial muscles, and to improve the patient's quality of life. Overdrive pacing is a method utilized to terminate the tachycardia by pacing the patient's heart at a rate faster than the intrinsic rhythm. Pacing the patient's heart at a rate of 100 beats per minute succeeded in controlling the arrhythmia without the need of multiple DC shocks.

Kurisu et al. [15] reported a similar case, but the electrical storm developed after 7 days of the myocardial infarction that was resistant to the conventional antiarrhythmic medications, and overdrive pacing was a feasible easy way to stabilize the case. Yoshida et al. [16] achieved an excellent suppression of the arrhythmia by overdrive pacing in a patient with multiple myeloma and coronary artery disease after coronary artery bypass grafting.

Additionally, in the management of the ES, there were other reported management plans. Mulpuru et al. [17] found that sedation with propofol was helpful in controlling the ventricular arrhythmias in a patient who presented with multiple ICD discharges and showed a poor response to oral antiarrhythmic medications. Tsagalou et al. [18] reported a case of an electrical storm that was refractory to amiodarone, metoprolol, and lignocaine, but after substitution of metoprolol with the nonselective propranolol, he achieved a good control of the electrical discharges, showing that propranolol is better than other selective beta blockers in treating ES.

ES usually reflects a poor prognosis with higher mortality, increased rate of hospitalization, and negative impact on the quality of life. Also, the electrical cardiac shocks besides their beneficial control of the arrhythmia and their frequency lead to more cardiac damage and progressive inflammation that later end up with cardiac fibrosis and worsening cardiac function [3, 4].

4. Conclusions

In severe cases of electrical storm that is refractory to the initial management, overdrive pacing is a helpful temporary method in the stabilization of the case and it could be a very important early tool to decrease the mortality in resistant arrhythmia after myocardial infarction.

References

[1] A. E. Epstein, G. N. Kay, V. J. Plumb, S. M. Dailey, and P. G. Anderson, "Gross and microscopic pathological changes associated with nonthoracotomy implantable defibrillator leads," *Circulation*, vol. 98, no. 15, pp. 1517–1524, 1998.

[2] J. A. Joglar, D. J. Kessler, P. J. Welch et al., "Effects of repeated electrical defibrillations on cardiac troponin I levels," *The American Journal of Cardiology*, vol. 83, no. 2, pp. 270–272, 1999.

[3] K. Gatzoulis, G. Andrikopoulos, T. Apostolopoulos et al., "Electrical storm is an independent predictor of adverse long-term outcome in the era of implantable defibrillator therapy," *Europace*, vol. 7, no. 2, pp. 184–192, 2005.

[4] A. Verma, F. Kilicaslan, N. F. Marrouche et al., "Prevalence, predictors, and mortality significance of the causative arrhythmia in patients with electrical storm," *Journal of Cardiovascular Electrophysiology*, vol. 15, no. 11, pp. 1265–1270, 2004.

[5] S. H. Hohnloser, H. R. Al-Khalidi, C. M. Pratt et al., "Electrical storm in patients with an implantable defibrillator: incidence, features, and preventive therapy: insights from a randomized trial," *European Heart Journal*, vol. 27, no. 24, pp. 3027–3032, 2006.

[6] C. T. Pedersen, G. N. Kay, J. Kalman et al., "EHRA/HRS/APHRS expert consensus on ventricular arrhythmias," *EP Europace*, vol. 16, no. 9, pp. 1257–1283, 2014.

[7] W. N. Brodine, R. T. Tung, J. K. Lee et al., "Effects of beta-blockers on implantable cardioverter defibrillator therapy and survival in the patients with ischemic cardiomyopathy (from the Multicenter Automatic Defibrillator Implantation Trial-II)," *The American Journal of Cardiology*, vol. 96, no. 5, pp. 691–695, 2005.

[8] D. Muser, P. Santangeli, and J. J. Liang, "Management of ventricular tachycardia storm in patients with structural heart disease," *World Journal of Cardiology*, vol. 9, no. 6, pp. 521–530, 2017.

[9] S. Chatzidou, C. Kontogiannis, D. I. Tsilimigras et al., "Propranolol versus metoprolol for treatment of electrical storm in patients with implantable cardioverter-defibrillator," *Journal of the American College of Cardiology*, vol. 71, no. 17, pp. 1897–1906, 2018.

[10] A. P. M. Gorgels, A. van den Dool, A. Hofs et al., "Comparison of procainamide and lidocaine in terminating sustained monomorphic ventricular tachycardia," *The American Journal of Cardiology*, vol. 78, no. 1, pp. 43–46, 1996.

[11] A. Pacifico, S. H. Hohnloser, J. H. Williams et al., "Prevention of implantable-defibrillator shocks by treatment with sotalol," *The New England Journal of Medicine*, vol. 340, no. 24, pp. 1855–1862, 1999.

[12] D. Gao, H. van Herendael, L. Alshengeiti et al., "Mexiletine as an adjunctive therapy to amiodarone reduces the frequency of ventricular tachyarrhythmia events in patients with an implantable defibrillator," *Journal of Cardiovascular Pharmacology*, vol. 62, no. 2, pp. 199–204, 2013.

[13] H. Tanner, G. Hindricks, M. Volkmer et al., "Catheter ablation of recurrent scar-related ventricular tachycardia using electroanatomical mapping and irrigated ablation technology: results of the prospective multicenter Euro-VT-study," *Journal of Cardiovascular Electrophysiology*, vol. 21, no. 1, pp. 47–53, 2010.

[14] S. G. Priori, C. Blomström-Lundqvist, A. Mazzanti et al., "2015 ESC guidelines for the management of patients with ventricular arrhythmias and the prevention of sudden cardiac death: the Task Force for the Management of Patients with Ventricular Arrhythmias and the Prevention of Sudden Cardiac Death of the European Society of Cardiology (ESC) Endorsed by: Association for European Pediatrics and Congenital Cardiology (AEPC)," *European Heart Journal*, vol. 36, no. 41, pp. 2793–2867, 2015.

[15] S. Kurisu, I. Inoue, T. Kawagoe et al., "Temporary overdriving pacing as an adjunct to antiarrhythmic drug therapy for electrical storm in acute myocardial infarction," *Circulation Journal*, vol. 69, no. 5, pp. 613–616, 2005.

[16] T. Yoshida, Y. Naito, and K. Nishimura, "Temporary ventricular overdrive pacing for electrical storm after coronary artery bypass grafting," *General Thoracic and Cardiovascular Surgery*, vol. 59, no. 11, pp. 756–759, 2011.

[17] S. K. Mulpuru, D. V. Patel, S. L. Wilbur, B. C. Vasavada, and T. Furqan, "Electrical storm and termination with propofol therapy: a case report," *International Journal of Cardiology*, vol. 128, no. 1, pp. e6–e8, 2008.

[18] E. P. Tsagalou, J. Kanakakis, S. Rokas, and M. I. Anastasiou-Nana, "Suppression by propranolol and amiodarone of an electrical storm refractory to metoprolol and amiodarone," *International Journal of Cardiology*, vol. 99, no. 2, pp. 341-342, 2005.

25

Anterior Papillary Muscle Rupture due to Acute Myocardial Microinfarction of the Small High Lateral Branch

Takanori Kono, Kazuyoshi Takagi, Shinya Negoto, and Eiki Tayama

Department of Surgery, Division of Cardiovascular Surgery, Kurume University School of Medicine, 67 Asahi-machi, Kurume City, Fukuoka, Japan

Correspondence should be addressed to Takanori Kono; kono_takanori@med.kurume-u.ac.jp

Academic Editor: Manabu Shirotani

Papillary muscle rupture is a catastrophic condition, of which most cases manifest posterior papillary muscle rupture. Anterior papillary muscle rupture is a rare condition. Particularly, anterior papillary muscle rupture due to acute myocardial microinfarction of the small high lateral branch is extremely rare. Since papillary muscle rupture can occur even in such a small branch or small area due to myocardial infarction, echocardiographic and/or ventriculographic confirmation is essential in cases of sudden worsening of heart failure. Herein, we report the case of anterior papillary muscle rupture with a good outcome. A 61-year-old man was admitted to our hospital with cardiogenic shock. Echocardiography revealed severe mitral regurgitation due to papillary muscle rupture. Coronary angiography demonstrated high-grade stenosis in the high lateral branch. However, no other significant stenoses were found. Emergency mitral valve replacement was performed. The patient was discharged 19 days after surgery without any complications.

1. Introduction

The incidence of papillary muscle rupture (PMR) in cases of acute myocardial infarction (AMI) is approximately 1%–5% [1]. Most of these cases are posterior PMR, and anterior PMR is a very rare condition [2, 3]. Cardiogenic shock in patients with PMR occurred in about 85% of hospitalized cases of AMI, often requiring mechanical circulatory support (MCS) devices [4]. Surgical outcomes of PMR remain poor with a reported early mortality rate of 25–40% [1, 5]. Herein, we report the case of anterior PMR with good outcomes. This case was diagnosed using transthoracic and transesophageal echocardiography and managed with preoperative extracorporeal membrane oxygenation (ECMO), Impella (Abiomed, Danvers, MA, USA), and prompt mitral valve replacement (MVR).

2. Case Presentation

A 61-year-old man was transferred to our hospital with complaints of fever and chills. His condition progressed to a state of shock during examination and was transported to our emergency center due to cardiogenic shock and septic shock. The patient had low systolic blood pressure, 40 mmHg; fast heart rate, 143 beats/min; and high temperature, 40.6°C. A late systolic murmur was heard at the cardiac apex. Arterial blood gas analysis during oxygen ventilation at 10 L/min revealed the following: pH, 6.952; PaO_2, 59.8 mmHg; $PaCO_2$, 80.9 mmHg; HCO^{3-}, 17.0 mEq/L; and lactic acid, 12.4 mmol/L. ECMO was immediately established. Electrocardiogram revealed ST-segment elevation in leads I, aVL, and aVR (Figure 1(a)). Chest radiographs showed severe bilateral pulmonary congestion (Figure 1(b)). Laboratory tests of the blood revealed the following: white blood cell count, 20,200/μL; C-reactive protein, 4.27 mg/dL; creatine phosphokinase/creatine phosphokinase-MB isozyme, 687/54 IU/L; aspartate transaminase/alanine transaminase, 121/36 IU/L; lactate dehydrogenase, 616 IU/L; and N-terminal (NT) prohormone B-type natriuretic peptide, 5249.3 ng/L. Results of nasopharyngeal swab tests for coronavirus disease 2019 (COVID-19) and flu were negative. Transthoracic and transesophageal echocardiography demonstrated severe mitral regurgitation due to PMR (Figures 1(c) and 1(d), Videos 1 and 2). Coronary

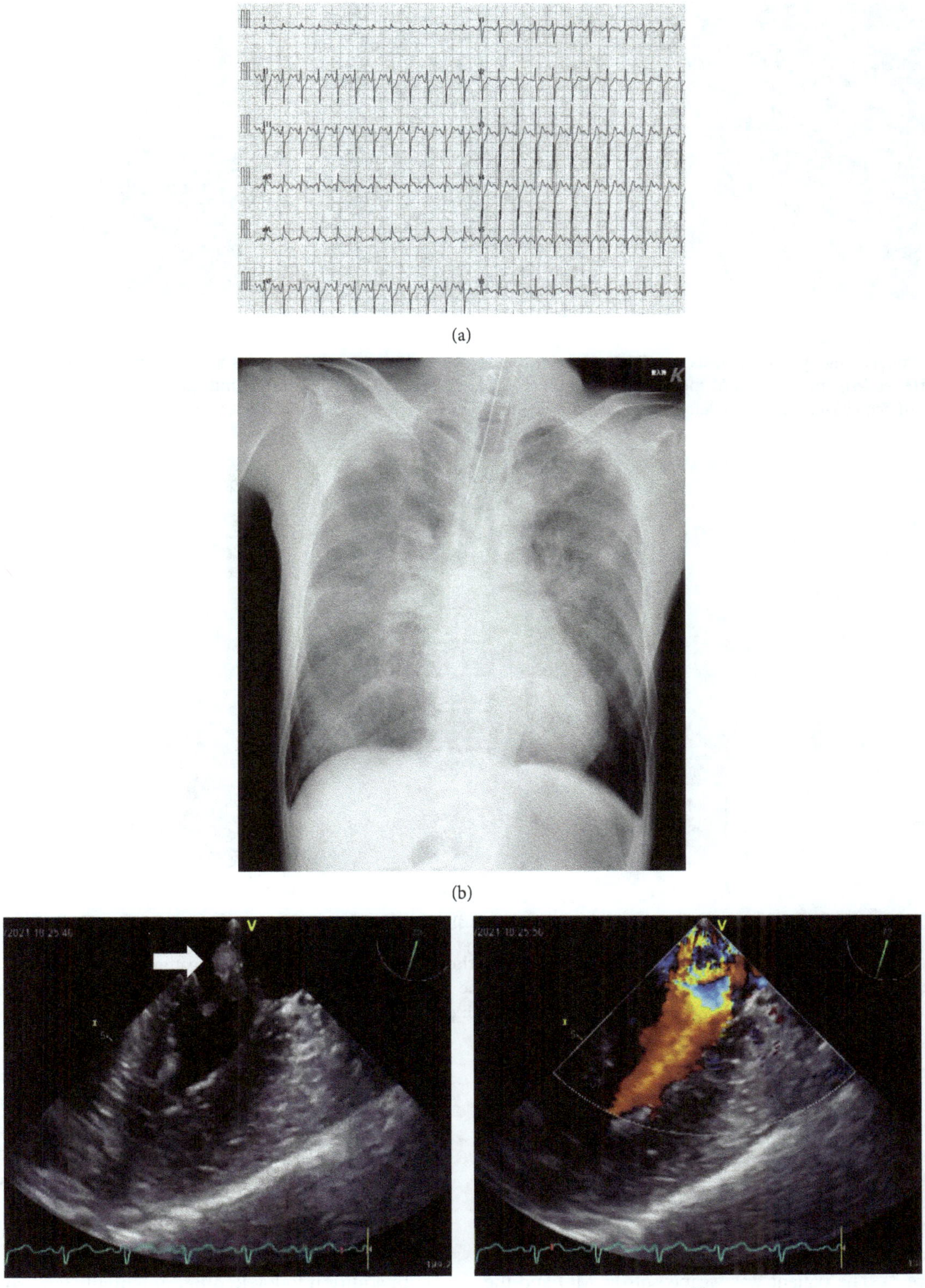

Figure 1: Preoperative electrocardiogram reveals ST-segment elevation in leads I, aVL, and aVR (a). Preoperative chest radiographs reveal severe pulmonary congestion (b). Preoperative transesophageal echocardiography reveals severe mitral regurgitation due to papillary muscle rupture (c, d). The white arrow indicates the ruptured anterior papillary muscle.

angiography was performed after Impella CP was placed via the left femoral artery for further hemodynamic support and left ventricle unloading (ECMO flow, 2.5 L/min; Impella performance level, P6). Activated clotting time was maintained around 200 seconds. A high-grade stenosis (99%) was noted in the high lateral branch (HL). However, no other lesions with significant stenosis were noted (Figure 2, Video 3). Emergency surgery was performed. Although lateral wall infarction

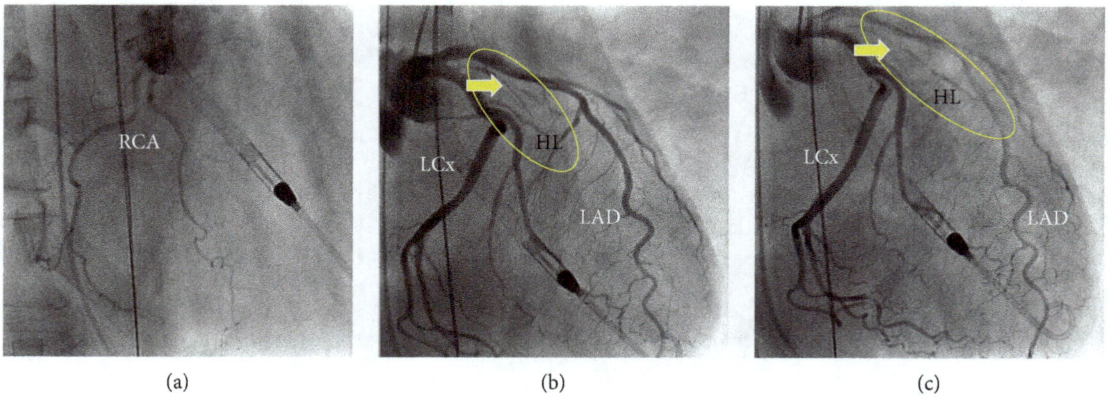

FIGURE 2: Coronary angiography reveals no significant stenosis in the right coronary artery (a) and left anterior descending artery and circumflex arteries (b), and stenosis of the high lateral branch (c) is observed. The yellow circle indicates the high lateral branch, and the yellow arrow indicates stenosis. LAD: left anterior descending artery; LCx: left circumflex artery; RCA: right coronary artery.

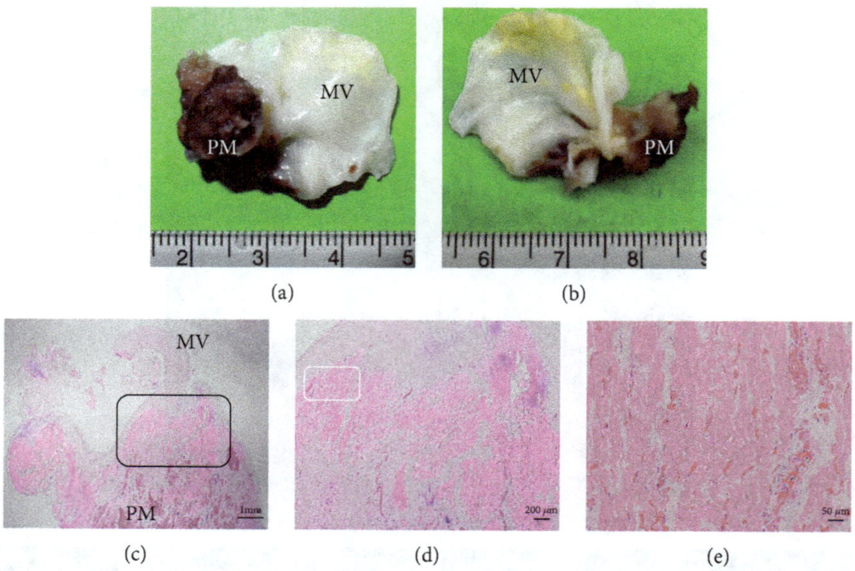

FIGURE 3: Resected specimen reveals complete rupture of the anterior papillary muscle (a, b). The pathological findings of the resected anterior papillary muscle reveal ischemic changes and necrosis of the myocytes (c–e). The black quadrangle indicates the area of (d), and the white quadrangle indicates the area of (e). MV: mitral valve; PM: papillary muscle.

was suspected, gross ischemic changes were not observed intraoperatively. The anterior leaflet of the mitral valve (A1-2) and the posterior leaflet (P1) with the ruptured anterior papillary muscle (PM) had prolapsed into the left atrium. MVR was performed using a 27 mm mechanical valve (St. Jude Medical, St Paul, MN, USA). Pathological examination of the resected PM revealed ischemic changes and necrosis of the myocytes almost entirely with features such as wavy fibers, loss of nuclei, and striations (Figure 3). The patient was weaned off ECMO and the Impella after MVR and returned to the intensive care unit on intra-aortic balloon pumping (IABP) support. IABP was removed on postoperative day (POD) 3, and the patient was discharged on POD19 without any complications.

3. Discussion

PMR is a rare but catastrophic complication. Its reported incidence is 1%–5% of all cases of AMI with an onset of 2–7 days after AMI [1, 6]. More than 80% of patients with PMR develop cardiogenic shock and die within 24 hours [7]. The consequent estimated mortality has been reported to be approximately 80%–90% with medical treatment and 19%–30% with emergency surgery [2, 8]. The poor preoperative conditions in such patients may contribute to poor surgical outcomes. Therefore, early diagnosis and adequate preoperative management are important.

In addition to PMR, other potentially fatal complications of myocardial infarction (MI) include left ventricular rupture and ventricular septum perforation. In this case, we were able to diagnose the patient with PMR using transthoracic and transesophageal echocardiography. Otherwise, the sensitivity of echocardiography for diagnosing complications after AMI showed marked variation [9]. Some reports indicated that left ventriculography (LVG) was useful for identifying mechanical complications after AMI [10]. Performing LVG along with coronary angiography can provide immediate information of complications in the catheter laboratory and is important for preoperative patient assessment to consider additional surgical procedures. We better might have considered performing LVG to rule out other complications in this case.

Since overall incidence of cardiogenic shock in patients with PMR is extremely high, appropriate MCS device use is needed. Although IABP is easy to insert and reported to be used in more than 90% of PMR cases [4], the effect of single use of IABP is not sufficient in these severely ill patients. Despite ECMO being a good treatment option, it might worsen mitral regurgitation due to increased afterload [4]. Impella is a reasonable option for left ventricular unloading and reduction in mitral regurgitation. However, using Impella alone cannot improve hypoxia due to pulmonary edema. The usefulness of ECMO and Impella in preoperative management has been reported [7], and the prompt introduction of Impella in addition to ECMO, in this case, is thought to have contributed to the good outcome. Although there have been reports of good results of combined ECMO and Impella following elective surgery, we suggest that prompt introduction of MCS soon after diagnosis and emergency surgery may improve the outcomes. Furthermore, MCS is useful for left ventricular unloading in the perioperative period after PMR repair. However, due to the high risk of bleeding with Impella, IABP is better for postoperative management if cardiac function is adequate.

PMR is 6–12 times more common in the posterior papillary muscle (PM) compared with the anterior PM because the posterior PM typically has a single blood supply from the right coronary artery or left circumflex artery (LCx). The anterior PM has dual blood supply from the left anterior descending artery and LCx [2, 3]. However, on rare occasions, the anterior PM may have a single blood supply, which can result in anterior PMR. Furthermore, PMs are located on the most endocardial part of the heart. Therefore, PMR can occur even in subendocardial MI and small-sized MI [2, 3]. Nishimura et al. reported that PMR was more likely to occur in smaller infarctions because a relatively good ventricular function may result in a greater shearing force at the site of potential rupture [3]. In the present patient, MI of the HL was not visible macroscopically because the patient had a microinfarction on the small HL branch. However, pathological findings revealed PMR due to MI. To the best of our knowledge, anterior PMR is rare, and anterior PMR due to acute myocardial microinfarction of the small HL is extremely rare. Kuwata et al. reviewed previous reports of 15 cases of anterior PMR in Japan. They reported that the responsible lesions were in the LCx in 10 cases, high lateral branch in 3 cases (two-vessel disease in 1 case), and diagonal branch in 2 cases [11]. Since PMR can occur even in such a small branch or small area of MI, echocardiographic confirmation is essential in cases of sudden worsening of heart failure.

We chose MVR as our surgical strategy. Mitral valve repair has been reported to yield good results in selected cases with an operative mortality rate of 0%, 15 years freedom from moderate or severe mitral regurgitation [12]. On the other hand, repair of necrotic PMs is often difficult. In addition, there is a concern that the extent of necrosis may lead to recurrence of MR. The fact that valve replacement is actually chosen in many reported PMR cases may indicate that MVR is a reasonable option, given that the patient's goal for improving hemodynamics by eliminating mitral regurgitation [13].

In conclusion, we observed good outcomes in our patient with anterior PMR due to AMI of the HL due to rapid diagnosis, immediate introduction of MCS, and appropriate timing of surgery.

Consent

Written informed consent was obtained from the patient for the publication of this case report and any accompanying data and images.

Supplementary Materials

Videos 1 and 2: preoperative transthoracic (Video 1) and transesophageal (Video 2) echocardiography reveals severe mitral regurgitation due to papillary muscle rupture. Video 3: coronary angiography reveals a high-grade stenosis of the high lateral branch. However, no other lesions with significant stenosis were noted. *(Supplementary Materials)*

References

[1] W. Bouma, I. J. Wijdh-den Hamer, B. M. Koene et al., "Predictors of in-hospital mortality after mitral valve surgery for post-myocardial infarction papillary muscle rupture," *Journal of Cardiothoracic Surgery*, vol. 9, no. 1, 2014.

[2] J. Y. Wei, G. M. Hutchins, and B. H. Bulkley, "Papillary muscle rupture in fatal acute myocardial infarction," *Annals of Internal Medicine*, vol. 90, no. 2, pp. 149–152, 1979.

[3] R. A. Nishimura, H. V. Schaff, C. Shub, B. J. Gersh, W. D. Edwards, and A. J. Tajik, "Papillary muscle rupture complicating acute myocardial infarction: analysis of 17 patients," *The American Journal of Cardiology*, vol. 51, no. 3, pp. 373–377, 1983.

[4] M. Pauja, S. Ranka, K. Chauhan et al., "Rupture of papillary muscle and chordae tendinae Complicating STEMI," *ASAIO Journal*, vol. 67, no. 8, pp. 907–916, 2020.

[5] C. R. Thompson, C. E. Buller, L. A. Sleeper et al., "Cardiogenic shock due to acute severe mitral regurgitation complicating acute myocardial infarction: a report from the SHOCK trial registry. Should we use emergently revascularize occluded coronaries in cardiogenic shock?," *Journal of the American College of Cardiology*, vol. 36, Supplement A, pp. 1104–1109, 2000.

[6] B. Jalil, K. El-Kersh, J. Frizzell, and S. Ahmed, "Impella percutaneous left ventricular assist device for severe acute ischaemic mitral regurgitation as a bridge to surgery," *BMJ Case Reports*, vol. 2017, article bcr2017219749, 2017.

[7] K. Sugiyama, M. Kano, S. Takahashi, N. Koizumi, and H. Ogino, "Rupture of the anterolateral papillary muscle caused by a high lateral branch occlusion," *Open Journal of Thoracic Surgery*, vol. 8, no. 1, pp. 6–12, 2018.

[8] Y. Kishon, J. K. Oh, H. V. Schaff, C. J. Mullany, A. J. Tajik, and B. J. Gersh, "Mitral valve operation in postinfarction rupture of a papillary muscle: immediate results and long-term follow-up of 22 patients," *Mayo Clinic Proceedings*, vol. 67, no. 11, pp. 1023–1030, 1992.

[9] S. Leavey, J. Galvin, H. McCann, and D. Sugrue, "Post-myocardial infarction ventricular septal defect: an angiographic study," *Irish Journal of Medical Science*, vol. 163, no. 4, pp. 182-183, 1994.

[10] I. Krakau, H. Lapp, J. Wolfertz, and H. Gülker, "Direct visualization of left ventricular free wall rupture by levocardiography," *Cathet Cardiovasc Intervent*, vol. 56, no. 2, pp. 238–242, 2002.

[11] T. Kuwata, K. Mizuguchi, Y. Kameda, and T. Mori, "Acute anterolateral papillary muscle rupture following successful percutaneous coronary intervention and emergent mitral valve replacement," *Japanese Journal of Cardiovascular Surgery*, vol. 34, no. 2, pp. 144–147, 2005.

[12] W. Bouma, I. J. Wijdh-den Hamer, T. J. Klinkenberg et al., "Mitral valve repair for post-myocardial infarction papillary muscle rupture," *European Journal of Cardio-Thoracic Surgery*, vol. 44, no. 6, pp. 1063–1069, 2013.

[13] A. Kilic, I. Sultan, D. Chu, Y. Wamg, and T. G. Gleason, "Mitral valve surgery for papillary muscle rupture: outcomes in 1342 patients from the Society of Thoracic Surgeons database," *The Annals of Thoracic Surgery*, vol. 110, no. 6, pp. 1975–1981, 2020.

26

Pembrolizumab-Induced Mobitz Type 2 Second-Degree Atrioventricular Block

Alisha Khan,[1] **Sana Riaz**,[1] **and Robert Carhart Jr.**[2]

[1]*Department of Medicine, SUNY Upstate Medical University, USA*
[2]*Department of Cardiology, SUNY Upstate Medical University, USA*

Correspondence should be addressed to Alisha Khan; khanali@upstate.edu

Academic Editor: Kathleen Ngu

Pembrolizumab is a monoclonal antibody directed towards programmed cell death protein 1 (PD-1) and is an antineoplastic drug which has a growing variety of oncologic uses. Pembrolizumab is commonly associated with immune-related adverse events (IRAEs) but is infrequently noted to cause cardiotoxicities such as myocarditis, arrhythmias, and heart failure. The following case report illustrates the clinical course of a 67-year-old female patient with stage IV non-small-cell lung cancer who developed Mobitz type 2 second-degree atrioventricular block three weeks after receiving her first infusion of pembrolizumab. Within a few hours of presentation, she progressed to symptomatic complete heart block requiring emergent placement of a temporary transvenous pacemaker. The article further discusses proposed mechanisms to explain IRAEs and management of IRAEs. We conclude by recommending a higher degree of caution and awareness among all physicians when treating patients on immunotherapy and a multidisciplinary approach when considering resumption of immune checkpoint inhibitor therapy.

1. Introduction

Since its initial approval by the Food and Drug Administration in the United States in 2014, the indications for the use of the antineoplastic drug pembrolizumab have steadily continued to increase in the world of oncology. The drug is an immune checkpoint inhibitor most commonly used in the treatment of melanoma and non-small-cell lung cancer (NSCLC).

Pembrolizumab is an IgG4-kappa humanized monoclonal antibody directed towards programmed cell death protein 1 (PD-1). PD-1, also known as CD 274 or B7-H1, is a costimulation receptor expressed by activated T cells. Binding of pembrolizumab to the PD-1 receptor prevents two immune-suppressing ligands, PD-L1 and PD-L2, from interacting with PD-1. Blocking of the PD-1 receptor by pembrolizumab thereby leads to inhibition of effector T cell proliferation, reduces cytotoxic activity, and induces apoptosis in tumor-infiltrating T cells and regulatory T cell expression [1].

This immunotherapy may now be used as a first-line agent for patients whose malignant cells have a PD-L1 expression or tumor proportion score (TPS) ≥ 1% and who do not harbor EGFR (epidermal growth factor receptor) or ALK (anaplastic lymphoma kinase) mutations [2]. Overall survival with the use of pembrolizumab correlates with increasing levels of PD-L1 expression [2].

Despite its survival benefits, it is also known for its immune-related adverse events, which affect various organ systems. Immune-related cardiotoxicity is a rare but often fatal complication. Cardiotoxicities associated with pembrolizumab include myocarditis, heart failure, sick sinus syndrome, cardiomyopathy, cardiac fibrosis, and cardiac arrest [3–7]. The following case describes a patient who developed complete heart block which appears to be temporally related to the use of the anti-PD-1 antibody, pembrolizumab.

2. Case Presentation

We provided care for a 67-year-old female with a past medical history of stage IV NSCLC metastatic to the adrenal

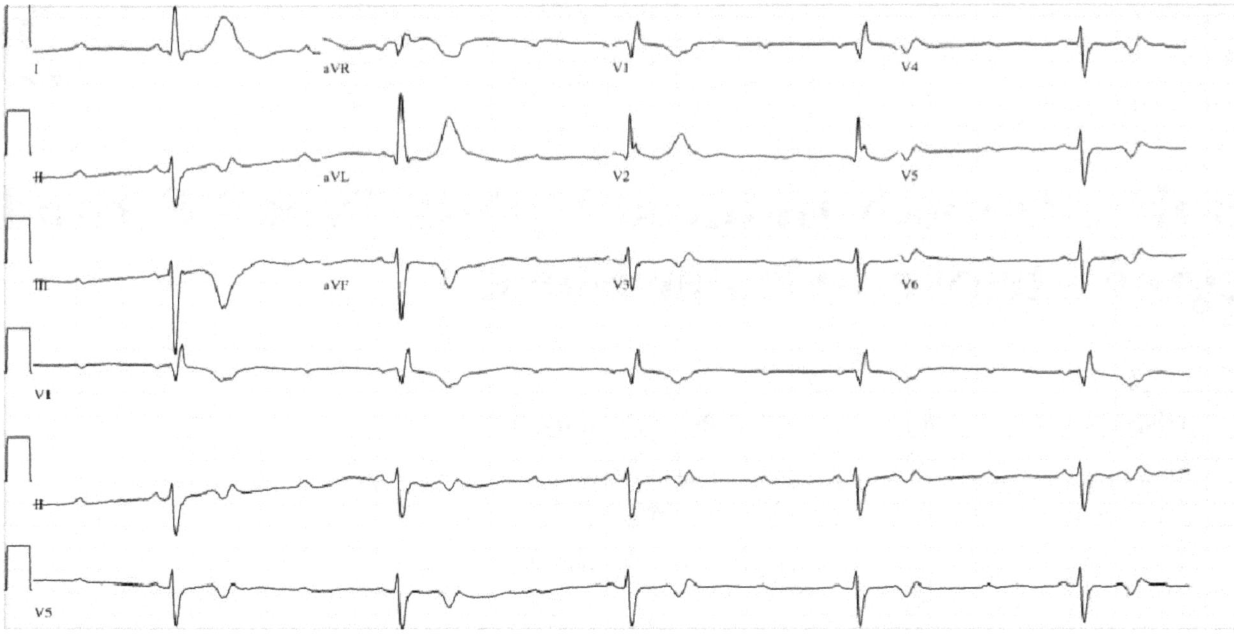

Figure 1: Progression of electrocardiogram tracings from the time of admission to immediately prior to transvenous pacer wire placement. Our patient was noted to have a heart rate of 31 bpm on admission, with initial EKG showing 2nd-degree AV block.

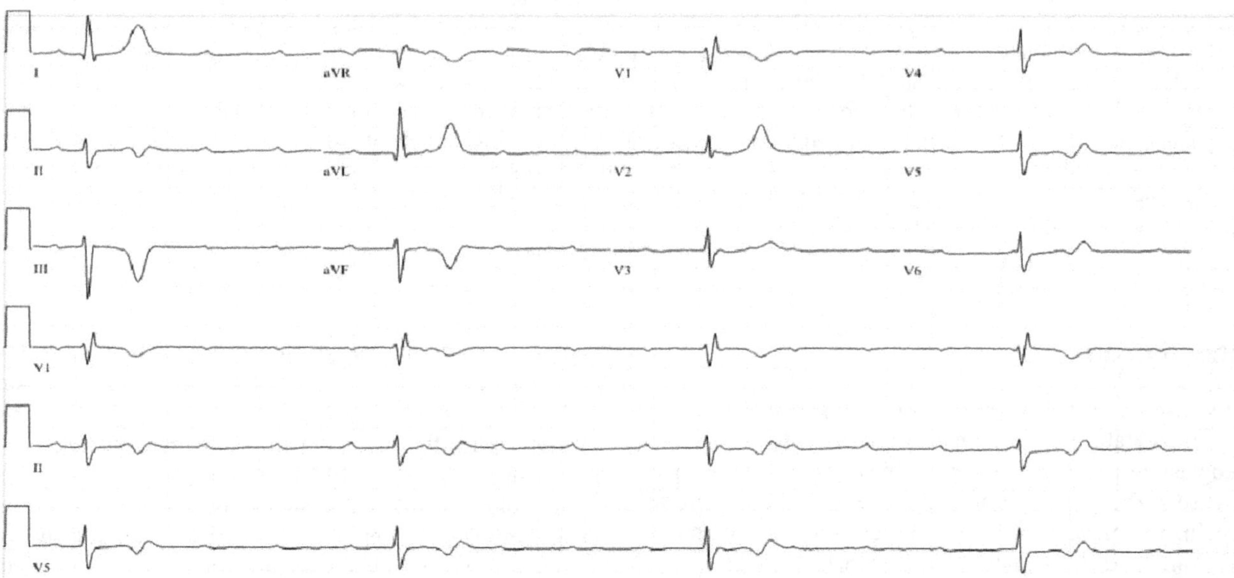

Figure 2: Progression of electrocardiogram tracings from the time of admission to immediately prior to transvenous pacer wire placement. Approximately three hours later, repeat EKG revealed complete heart block with ventricular rate of 22 bpm.

gland, lymph nodes, and brain, complicated by a prior seizure for which she was on levetiracetam, hypertension on amlodipine, hyperlipidemia on simvastatin, hypothyroidism on levothyroxine, and depression on trazodone who presented to our Emergency Department as a transfer from the Cancer Center for bradycardia which was noted on routine vital sign assessment as she was about to get her second immunotherapy dose.

Her recent PET scan showed progression of her cancer in the mediastinum and supraclavicular area. Lymph node biopsy revealed a PD-L1 expression of 90%, and hence, she received her first infusion of pembrolizumab 200 mg intravenously three weeks prior to our encounter, as it is usually administered.

In the Emergency Department, she was initially asymptomatic with a heart rate of 30 beats per minute (bpm) as noted on telemetry monitoring and blood pressure of 121/63 mmHg. On admission, her EKG depicted Mobitz type 2 second-degree atrioventricular block (Figure 1). The electrophysiologist was immediately consulted with plans to place a permanent pacemaker the following morning. However, approximately three hours later, as she shifted in bed

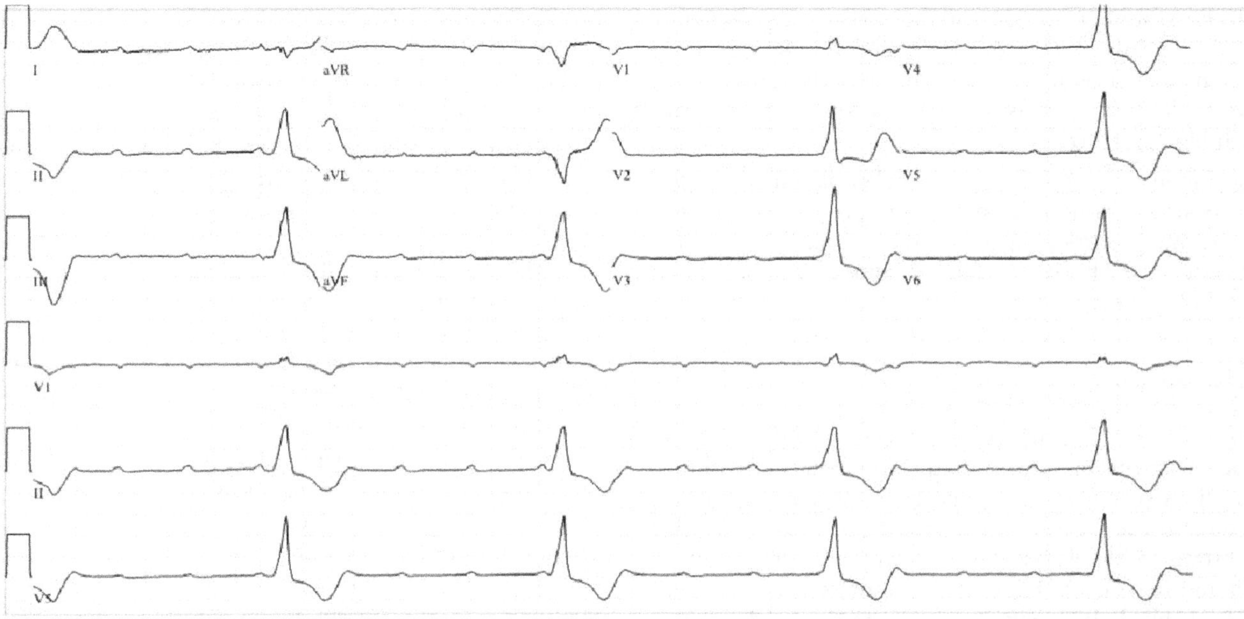

Figure 3: Progression of electrocardiogram tracings from the time of admission to immediately prior to transvenous pacer wire placement. EKG was repeated a few minutes later, showing complete heart block and idioventricular rhythm with a heart rate of 25 bmp immediately after starting a dobutamine infusion, at which point a transvenous pacer wire was emergently placed.

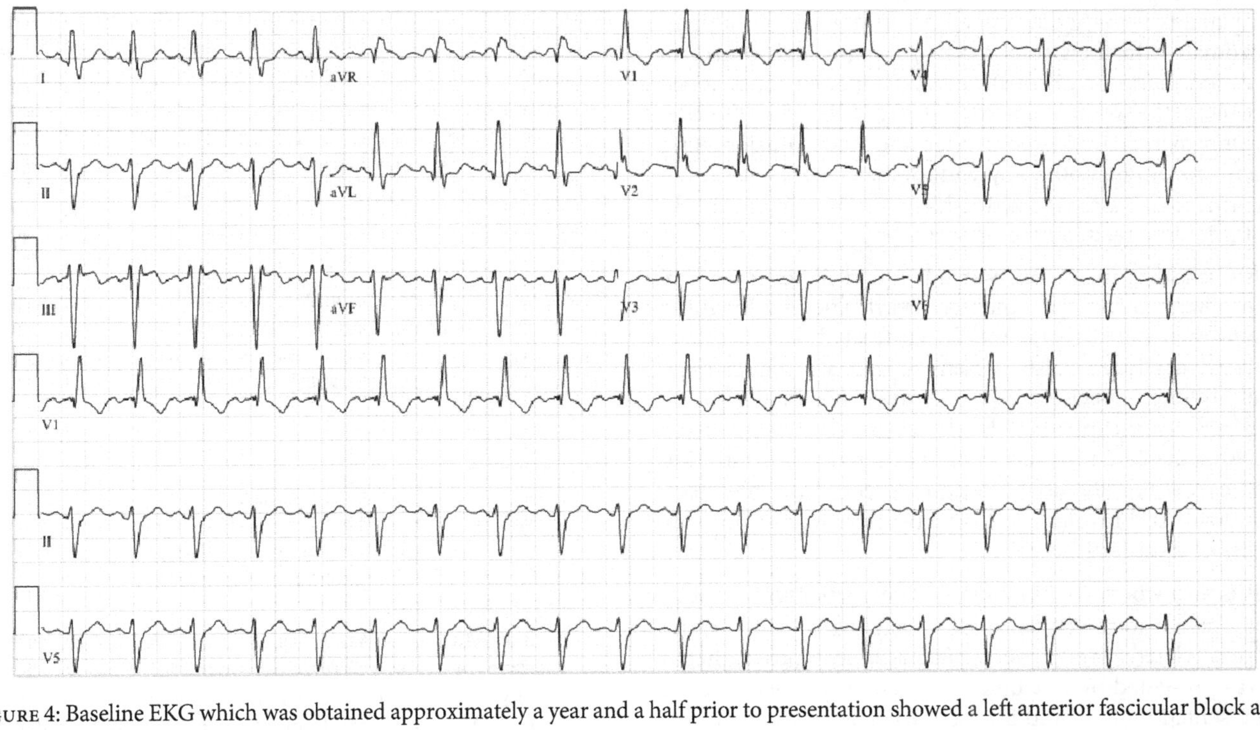

Figure 4: Baseline EKG which was obtained approximately a year and a half prior to presentation showed a left anterior fascicular block and a right bundle branch block.

in order to place the bedpan beneath her, she began to feel lightheaded and her blood pressure dropped to 64/42 mmHg. Repeat EKG at this time showed complete heart block with a ventricular rate of 22 bpm (Figure 2). At this point, she was given a 500 cc bolus and dobutamine drip was initiated. EKG at this time showed complete heart block and idioventricular rhythm with a heart rate of 25 bpm (Figure 3), following which a temporary transvenous pacemaker was emergently placed overnight.

Her labs including a basic metabolic panel and complete metabolic panel were unremarkable. Her magnesium level was 2.2 mg/dL and phosphorus level was 3.2 mg/dL. Troponin T was trended and was negative throughout her admission. Thyroid stimulating hormone level on admission was within normal range at 1.270 mU/mL. Her echocardiogram showed a LVEF of 60-65%. Her baseline EKG obtained approximately a year and a half prior to presentation showed a left anterior fascicular block and a right bundle branch block (Figure 4).

She underwent permanent pacemaker placement the following morning without complication. Prior to discharge, a chest X-ray, electrocardiogram, and device interrogation were performed. She was discharged home in a hemodynamically stable condition.

3. Discussion

Pembrolizumab is commonly associated with immune-related adverse events and is infrequently associated with cardiotoxicities such as myocarditis and heart failure. Conduction disease can be isolated or associated with coexisting myocarditis [8]. However, there are only two case reports in the literature so far in which patients presented with complete heart block. Interestingly, similar to the article by Katsume et al., our patient was receiving pembrolizumab after initial prior treatment with pemetrexed and bevacizumab for NSCLC. Katsume et al.'s patient was also found to have a high PD-L1 expression of >95% and received pembrolizumab at 200 mg 16 days prior to admission [7]. In other words, both patients were highly susceptible to the effects of pembrolizumab with their tumor cells having a high degree of expression (90% or greater), and both patients developed heart block the second time they received the immunotherapy, approximately 3 weeks after the first infusion. Our patient's prior chemotherapy with bevacizumab, a VEGF-A inhibitor, is also a recognized risk factor for immune checkpoint inhibitor-related cardiotoxicity [8].

Moreover, in the second published case of pembrolizumab-induced complete heart block by Jang and Stream, their patient who was being treated for metastatic renal cell carcinoma also presented with worsening exertional dyspnea precisely 3 weeks after his first infusion [9]. His PD-L1 expression level was not documented. Of note, the median interval from the initial administration of other commonly used immune checkpoint inhibitors, ipilimumab and nivolumab, to the development of myocarditis is 17 days [10].

It is also worthwhile to note that the patients in the two other cases were concurrently diagnosed with other immune-related adverse events such as biopsy-proven hepatitis (as presented by Katsume et al.) and myasthenia gravis (as presented by Jang and Stream), whereas our patient was asymptomatic on presentation and her laboratory testing was negative for elevations in troponin, creatine kinase, or liver enzymes. Thus, physicians should be mindful of immune-related adverse events in patients, irrespective of their symptoms and findings on blood work. Since pembrolizumab is administered every three weeks for a variety of indications, increased awareness of possible cardiotoxicity around the time of the second infusion is advised.

There are various proposed mechanisms attempting to explain immune checkpoint inhibitor-mediated arrythmias. Some of these theories include ventricular myocarditis with inflammation and fibrosis or inflammation of the His-Purkinje conduction system, both leading to reentry arrythmias [8]. Atrial or ventricular arrythmias secondary to inflammation without myocarditis, as well as atrial and ventricular arrythmias from functional cardiotoxicity without inflammation, are other possibilities [8]. Interestingly, genetic deletion of PD-1 in mice leads to cardiomyopathy that is caused by autoantibiodies against cardiac troponin I, which may be contributing to the cardiotoxicity caused by immune checkpoint inhibitors [10–12].

Ultimately, we recommend a higher degree of caution among all physicians when dealing with patients on immunotherapy. According to the clinical practice guidelines provided in the American Society of Clinical Oncology Journal for the management of immune-related adverse events in patients treated with immune checkpoint inhibitor therapy, holding checkpoint inhibitor therapy is recommended for all grades of cardiac complications and the appropriateness of rechallenging remains unknown [13]. Discontinuation of the immunotherapy with or without steroid treatment (1 to 2 mg/kg of prednisone) should be considered depending on the grade of toxicity as a therapeutic option [13]. In patients who do not immediately respond to high-dose corticosteroids, methylprednisolone 1 g daily can be attempted [13]. In some cases, further adding mycophenolate, infliximab, or antithymocyte globulin can be considered [13]. Cardiology consultation should always be obtained and transfer to the coronary care unit should be performed in the case of conduction abnormalities or troponemia [13].

Resuming immune checkpoint inhibitor therapy should be considered following multidisciplinary evaluation between cardiology, oncology, and cardiooncology if possible. In the case of our patient, her pembrolizumab was eventually restarted and she has so far tolerated nine additional cycles without any further discernable cardiac toxicities.

References

[1] S. M. Toor, A. S. Syed Khaja, I. Alkurd, and E. Elkord, "In-vitro effect of pembrolizumab on different T regulatory cell subsets," *Clinical and Experimental Immunology*, vol. 191, no. 2, pp. 189–197, 2018.

[2] T. S. K. Mok, Y.-L. Wu, I. Kudaba et al., "Pembrolizumab versus chemotherapy for previously untreated, PD-L1-expressing, locally advanced or metastatic non-small-cell lung cancer (KEYNOTE-042): a randomised, open-label, controlled, phase 3 trial," *The Lancet*, vol. 393, no. 10183, pp. 1819–1830, 2019.

[3] S. S. Mahmood, M. G. Fradley, J. V. Cohen et al., "Myocarditis in patients treated with immune checkpoint inhibitors," *Journal of the American College of Cardiology*, vol. 71, no. 16, pp. 1755–1764, 2018.

[4] G. Varricchi, G. Marone, V. Mercurio, M. R. Galdiero, D. Bonaduce, and C. G. Tocchetti, "Immune checkpoint inhibitors and cardiac toxicity: an emerging issue," *Current Medicinal Chemistry*, vol. 25, no. 11, pp. 1327–1339, 2018.

[5] C.-Y. Hsu, Y.-W. Su, and S.-C. Chen, "Sick sinus syndrome associated with anti-programmed cell death-1," *Journal for ImmunoTherapy of Cancer*, vol. 6, no. 1, p. 72, 2018.

[6] L. Heinzerling, P. A. Ott, F. S. Hodi et al., "Cardiotoxicity associated with CTLA4 and PD1 blocking immunotherapy," *Journal for Immunotherapy of Cancer*, vol. 4, p. 50, 2016.

[7] Y. Katsume, T. Isawa, Y. Toi et al., "Complete atrioventricular block associated with pembrolizumab-induced acute myocarditis: the need for close cardiac monitoring," *Internal Medicine*, vol. 57, no. 21, pp. 3157–3162, 2018.

[8] A. R. Lyon, N. Yousaf, N. M. L. Battisti, J. Moslehi, and J. Larkin, "Immune checkpoint inhibitors and cardiovascular toxicity," *The Lancet Oncology*, vol. 19, no. 9, pp. e447–e458, 2018.

[9] J. Jang and S. Stream, *A Case of Pembrolizumab-induced Complete Heart Block and Myasthenia Gravis*, Hospital Medicine, Orlando, FL, USA, 2018, Abstract 869, https://www.shmabstracts.com/abstract/a-case-of-pembrolizumab-induced-complete-heart-block-and-myasthenia-gravis/.

[10] D. B. Johnson, J. M. Balko, M. L. Compton et al., "Fulminant myocarditis with combination immune checkpoint blockade," *The New England Journal of Medicine*, vol. 375, no. 18, pp. 1749–1755, 2016.

[11] H. Nishimura, T. Okazaki, Y. Tanaka et al., "Autoimmune dilated cardiomyopathy in PD-1 receptor-deficient mice," *Science*, vol. 291, no. 5502, pp. 319–322, 2001.

[12] T. Okazaki, Y. Tanaka, R. Nishio et al., "Autoantibodies against cardiac troponin I are responsible for dilated cardiomyopathy in PD-1-deficient mice," *Nature Medicine*, vol. 9, no. 12, pp. 1477–1483, 2003.

[13] J. R. Brahmer, et al.C. Lacchetti, B. J. Schneider et al., "Management of immune-related adverse events in patients treated with immune checkpoint inhibitor therapy: American Society of Clinical Oncology clinical practice guideline," *Journal of Clinical Oncology*, vol. 36, no. 17, pp. 1714–1768, 2018.

Twiddler Syndrome without Lead Dislodgment Discovered by Remote Monitoring

Catherine Champagne, Nicolas Dognin, Franck Molin, Christian Steinberg, François Philippon, Jean-François Sarrazin, Gilles O'hara, Isabelle Nault, Karine Roy, Benoit Plourde, Louis Blier, and Jean Champagne

Department of Cardiology, Institut Universitaire de Cardiologie et de Pneumologie de Québec, Laval University, Quebec, Canada

Correspondence should be addressed to Jean Champagne; jean.champagne@med.ulaval.ca

Academic Editor: Christopher S. Snyder

Twiddler syndrome is an uncommon yet dangerous phenomenon usually resulting in lead displacement with loss of capture of cardiac implantable electronic devices. In this case report, we present an interesting case of Twiddler syndrome without lead dislodgment which was detected by an alert triggered by an increase in impedance on remote monitoring.

1. Introduction

Twiddler syndrome is a rare complication (0.07-1.1%) following the implantation of cardiac devices and has been observed with different types of cardiac devices [1–4]. Twiddler syndrome is characterized by repeat, patient-initiated manipulation of the pulse generator resulting in rotation of the device and lead twisting that may result in dislodgment of the electrodes and loss of capture. Here, we report a rare case of Twiddler syndrome that was diagnosed with the help of remote monitoring.

2. Case Presentation

A 75-year-old woman with a mixed ischemic/nonischemic cardiomyopathy and depressed left ventricular systolic function (ejection fraction of 25%) underwent the implantation of a single-chamber primary prevention ICD (Boston Scientific Autogen) in January 2017. Her past medical history was significant for multiple other cardiovascular comorbidities including stage III obesity with a body mass index of 41 kg/m^2. She was not known for a history of dementia or impaired cognition.

An active fixation right ventricular (RV) lead (Boston Scientific Reliance 4-Front DF4) was implanted at the RV apex. Six months postimplantation, the RV lead pacing threshold and impedance increased from 0.7 V to 2 V and from 450 ohms to 800 ohms, respectively (Figure 1(a)). It was still considered clinically acceptable and then remained stable for 2 years (Figure 1(b)). No chest X-ray was done during that period. In November 2019, a remote monitoring alert was triggered due to a high pacing impedance. A hospital visit was scheduled to verify the patient's ICD. The patient was asymptomatic and she denied any manipulation of device. The pacing impedance was increased to 1400 ohms, whereas the shock impedance remained stable at 90 ohms (Figure 1(c)). The RV pacing threshold was also increased to 2.9 V at 0.8 msec. Sensing remained unaffected showing a detection of intrinsic R-waves of 10 mV. No noise or inappropriate ventricular arrhythmia therapy had been recorded by the device. A PA/lateral chest X-ray showed typical signs of a Twiddler syndrome (Figure 2), and the ICD lead showed a reduced lead slack with the tip at the RV apex. The patient was admitted for surgical revision. Figure 3 shows the intraoperative device situation after opening of the pocket capsule. The suture sleeve was intact and still tight. The new electrode was placed one centimeter above the old abandoned one. It was impossible to insert a stylet inside the defective ICD lead and an extraction was not performed. The pulse generator was not changed as its longevity was still predicted to last 10 years, but it was fixed to the *pectoralis major* in a new

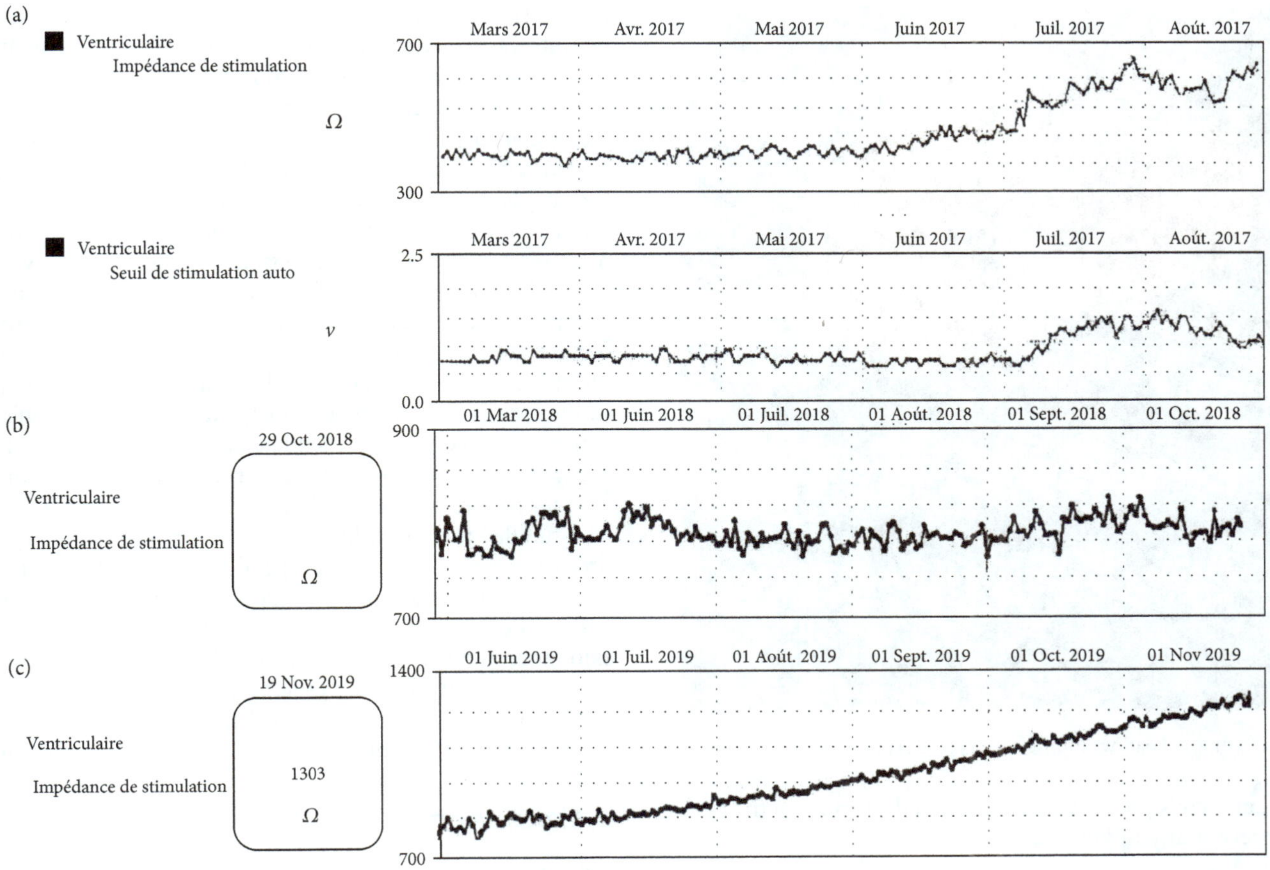

FIGURE 1: Impedance and pacing threshold: (a) simultaneous elevated impedance and threshold six months postimplantation; (b) stabilized impedance and threshold in 2018; (c) remote monitoring of the RV lead showing evidence of an increased impedance.

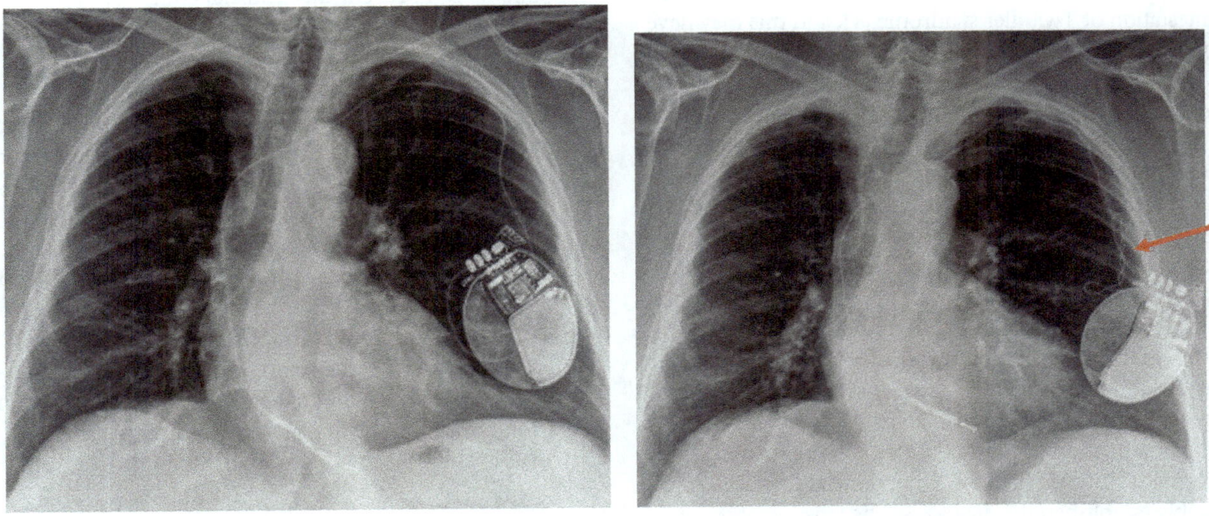

(a) (b)

FIGURE 2: PA chest X-ray one month postimplantation (a) and 3 years postimplantation showing twisting of the lead (b) (red arrow).

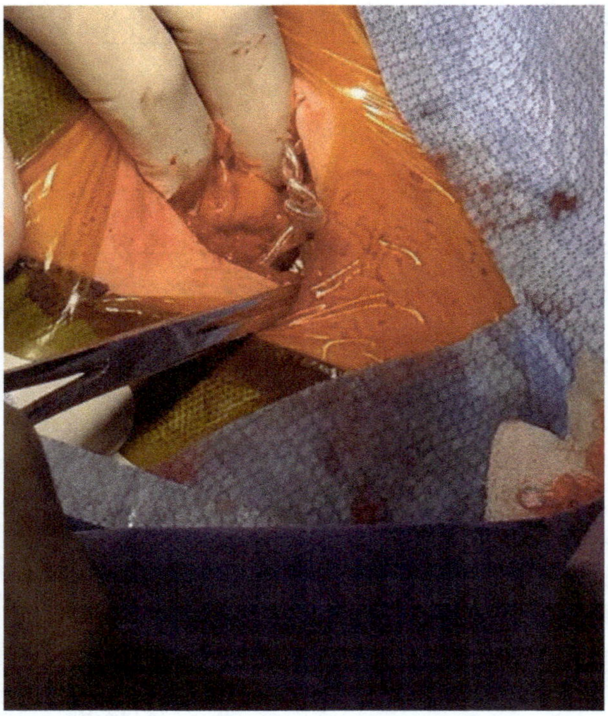

FIGURE 3: Lead wrapping observed during surgical revision.

subcutaneous pocket with a suture in the header of the device to prevent any migration.

3. Discussion

This case report illustrates a Twiddler syndrome without lead dislodgment detected by an impedance lead alert from the remote monitoring system. Failure of the device is often the clinical manifestation of Twiddler syndrome [1], and this may have catastrophic consequences in pacemaker-dependent patients. In patients with ICD, it often presents with the inability of the device to properly shock ventricular arrhythmias and inappropriate ICD therapies and sometimes may lead to sudden cardiac death [5]. The only sign of Twiddler syndrome in this patient was the constant increase in pacing threshold and pacing impedance. Contrarily to most Twiddler syndromes that have been previously reported, the electrode was still tightly attached to the suture sleeve and in contact with the right ventricle. When the voltage threshold increased to 2 V and the impedance went from 450 to 800 ohms, six months postimplantation, Twiddler syndrome was not considered. Since the RV lead threshold and impedance stayed stable after the first elevation six months postimplantation, and pacing was not required, no chest X-ray was performed. However, a chest X-ray done at this time could have possibly established the diagnosis. The twisting of the electrode in the pouch might have damaged the electrode. The inability to place a stylet inside the electrode reveals the loss of integrity of the lead, which probably caused a progressive increase in impedance with conduction resistance.

In a cohort of 1074 patients who underwent cardiac implantable electronic devices, lead macrodislodgment occurred in 19 (1.8%) patients, and the vast majority (89%) of them were detected by a change in lead parameters on remote monitoring [6]. Hence, a remote monitoring system permits the early detection of Twiddler syndrome. Early diagnosis of defibrillation lead dislodgment typically involves a decrease in R-wave amplitude and impedance, with an increase in pacing threshold [7]. Twiddler syndrome should be considered when there is a simultaneous increase in pacing thresholds and lead impedance. Macrodislodgment is usually the manifestation in Twiddler syndrome, but in our patient, microdislodgment should be considered. The chest X-ray confirms a lead traction with loss of the curve. This traction might explain a reduced contact with the right ventricle and threshold elevation. Almost 50% of patients with Twiddler syndromes are asymptomatic or with unrelated symptoms [8]. In the case of lead parameter change detected in the clinic or with remote monitoring, even late after implantation, a chest X-ray should be performed to exclude a Twiddler syndrome.

Our patient was an elderly woman with an increased BMI who fulfilled three well-known risk factors for Twiddler syndrome: increased BMI, female gender, and elderly patient [6, 9]. Obesity limits the physical exam on the pocket site, which makes the assessment of Twiddler syndrome through the skin more difficult. Excessive loose subcutaneous tissue without fixation of the device in the pocket probably contributed to the mobility of the device in the pocket and allowed for rotation of the ICD spontaneously in daily life movements.

4. Conclusion

This case report highlights the utility of remote monitoring for early detection of lead abnormalities or arrhythmia, which can be caused by rare device complications such as Twiddler syndrome. Measures to identify risk factors for Twiddler syndrome and fixation of the device at time of implant in high-risk patients can prevent this unusual complication.

Authors' Contributions

C. Champagne is the first author and was responsible for the research design and data acquisition analysis or interpretation and drafting of the paper. N. Dognin was responsible for the drafting of the paper or revising it critically and approval of the submitted final versions. F. Molin, C. Steinberg, F. Philippon, JF. Sarrazin, G. O'Hara, I. Nault, K. Roy, B. Plourde, and L. Blier were responsible for revising the paper critically and approval of the submitted and final versions. J. Champagne is the senior author and was responsible for the research design and data acquisition analysis or interpretation, drafting the paper or revising it critically, and approval of the submitted and final versions.

References

[1] C. E. Bayliss, D. S. Beanlands, and R. J. Baird, "The pacemaker Twiddler's syndrome: a new complication of implantable transvenous pacemakers," *Canadian Medical Association Journal*, vol. 99, no. 8, pp. 371–373, 1968.

[2] N. G. Boyle, F. Anselme, K. M. Monahan et al., "Twiddler's syndrome variants in ICD patients," *Pacing and Clinical Electrophysiology*, vol. 21, no. 12, pp. 2685–2687, 1998.

[3] M. de Buitleir and C. Canver, "Twiddler's syndrome complicating a transvenous defibrillator lead system," *Chest*, vol. 109, no. 5, pp. 1391–1394, 1996.

[4] P. E. Hill, "Complications of permanent transvenous cardiac pacing: a 14-year review of all transvenous pacemakers inserted at one community hospital," *Pacing and Clinical Electrophysiology*, vol. 10, no. 3, pp. 564–570, 1987.

[5] S. Spencker, A. Poppelbaum, and D. Müller, "An unusual cause of oversensing leading to inappropriate ICD discharges," *International Journal of Cardiology*, vol. 129, no. 1, pp. e24–e26, 2008.

[6] A. S. Tseng, J. N. Shipman, J. Z. Lee et al., "Incidence, patterns, and outcomes after transvenous cardiac device lead macrodislodgment: insights from a population-based study," *Heart Rhythm*, vol. 16, no. 1, pp. 140–147, 2019.

[7] J. A. B. Zaman, K. Chua, A. A. Sovari et al., "Early diagnosis of defibrillation lead dislodgement," *JACC: Clinical Electrophysiology*, vol. 4, no. 8, pp. 1075–1088, 2018.

[8] J. L. Morales, S. Nava, M. F. Márquez et al., "Idiopathic lead Migration," *JACC: Clinical Electrophysiology*, vol. 3, no. 11, pp. 1321–1329, 2017.

[9] H. Kawata, J. Patel, T. McGarry et al., "Obese female patients have higher rates of lead dislodgement after ICD or CRT-D implantation," *International Journal of Cardiology*, vol. 172, no. 3, pp. e522–e524, 2014.

28

Pericardial Effusion-Associated Hyponatremia

Ahmed A. Hanfy, Nicholas T. Manasewitsch, Bryce D. Beutler, Daniel Antwi-Amoabeng, Mohamed Elnaggar, Munadel Awad, and Gurpreet S. Chahal

Department of Internal Medicine, University of Nevada, Reno School of Medicine, Nevada, USA

Correspondence should be addressed to Bryce D. Beutler; brycebeutler@hotmail.com

Academic Editor: Ertugrul Ercan

Pericardial effusion has been identified as a rare cause of hyponatremia. In most patients, pericardiocentesis results in rapid correction. We describe a 67-year-old male who presented with pericardial effusion-associated hyponatremia secondary to cardiac resynchronization therapy-D placement that resolved following evacuation. In addition, we review the literature on pericardial effusion-associated hyponatremia.

1. Introduction

Hyponatremia is defined as a serum sodium concentration below 135 mEq/L. It is most commonly asymptomatic but may manifest with headaches, nausea, seizures, and death due to cerebral edema [1].

Pericardial effusion has been identified as a rare cause of hyponatremia. Interestingly, pericardiocentesis often results in rapid and complete reversal of hyponatremia [2–9]. The mechanism underlying pericardial effusion-related hyponatremia remains to be established. However, it has been hypothesized to result from increased antidiuretic hormone release in the setting of decreased free water excretion [2, 5, 8].

We describe a 67-year-old male with pericardial effusion-associated hyponatremia who experienced rapid and complete normalization of serum sodium following pericardiocentesis.

2. Case Presentation

A 67-year-old male with a history of nonischemic cardiomyopathy, non-insulin–dependent diabetes mellitus, and hypertension presented with progressively worsening dyspnea and cough of three weeks duration. Two months prior to presentation, the patient had undergone cardiac resynchronization therapy-defibrillator (CRT-D) placement for nonischemic cardiomyopathy and left bundle branch block with a left ventricular ejection fraction of less than 35%. No operative complications were reported.

Vital signs were within normal limits (pulse: 84 beats per minute; blood pressure: 132/68 mmHg; temperature: 36.1°C; respiratory rate: 18; oxygen saturation: 94% on room air). Physical examination was significant only for bibasilar rales; no pericardial friction rub or elevated jugular venous pressure were appreciated, and there were no clinical signs or symptoms concerning for tamponade. Laboratory studies demonstrated hyponatremia (sodium: 123 mEq/L; corrected for hyperglycemia: 127 mEq/L), hyperglycemia (glucose: 260 mg/dL), and normocytic anemia (hemoglobin: 11.0 g/dL, mean corpuscular volume: 86.7 fL). N-terminal pro b-type natriuretic peptide (NT-proBNP) was elevated to 239 pg/mL, which was near the patient's baseline. Serum potassium, bicarbonate, blood urea nitrogen, and creatinine were within normal limits. Electrocardiogram (ECG) showed an atrial-paced ventricular rhythm consistent with prior pacemaker placement. Two-view chest radiography revealed an enlarged cardiac silhouette, minimal bibasilar atelectasis, and appropriate placement of the pacemaker leads (Figure 1).

The patient was started on a fluid restriction of 1500 milliliters per day for hyponatremia and suspected heart failure

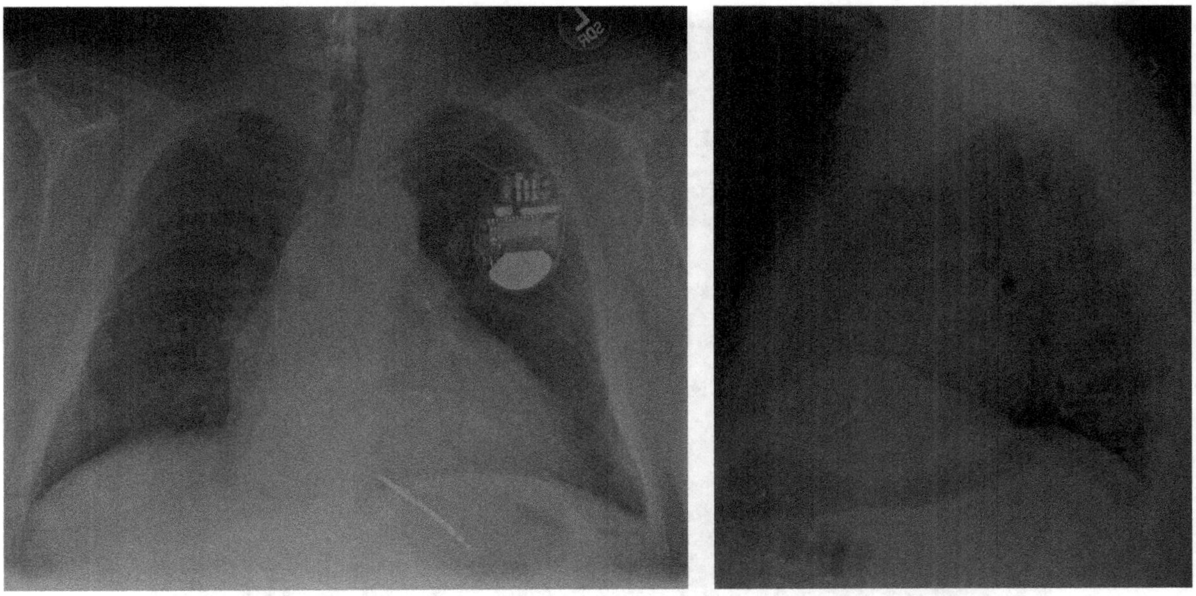

(a) (b)

FIGURE 1: A two-view chest X-ray demonstrating enlarged cardiac silhouette, minimal bibasilar atelectasis, and appropriate placement of pacemaker leads (a, b).

exacerbation. However, subsequent laboratory studies showed significant worsening of the hyponatremia; by the second hospital day, the patient's serum sodium had decreased from 123 to 119 mEq/L (corrected for hyperglycemia: 123 mEq/L). Further investigation revealed serum blood urea nitrogen of 12 mg/dl, serum glucose of 264 mg/dl, calculated serum osmolality of 256 mOsm/kg, urine osmolality of 310 mOsm/kg H2O, and urine sodium of 42 mEq/L. Hypothyroidism was ruled out with a thyroid-stimulating hormone of 2.340 μIU/mL.

An echocardiogram demonstrated a large circumferential pericardial effusion with right atrial collapse (Figure 2). Left ventricular ejection fraction was estimated at 55% with normal diastolic function. Diastolic right ventricular collapse was absent. Echocardiographic features were consistent with early signs of cardiac tamponade. However, there were no clinical signs of tamponade and vital signs remained within normal limits.

An urgent pericardiocentesis was performed with removal of approximately 1200 milliliters of sanguineous fluid. A follow-up echocardiogram was obtained one day after the procedure and demonstrated complete resolution of the effusion (Figure 2(b)). Serum electrolytes were monitored and showed a gradual improvement of the hyponatremia; serum sodium had increased from 120 to 123 mEq/L on the first postoperative day and to 131 mEq within 36 hours of the procedure (Figure 3). Calculated serum osmolality also increased to 278 mOsm/kg. Analysis of the pericardial fluid was negative for malignant cells and pathogens. Our patient's pericardial effusion was presumed to be secondary to his previous CRT-D placement. The patient was discharged home in stable condition on the third postoperative day. Outpatient follow-up four weeks later showed no recurrence of the pericardial effusion.

3. Discussion

Pericardial effusion represents a rare cause of reversible hyponatremia; this has been described in several case reports [2–6, 9] and two retrospective reviews [7, 8]. Our patient presented with progressively worsening hyponatremia in the setting of pericardial effusion with early tamponade and experienced rapid and complete normalization of serum sodium concentration following pericardiocentesis.

Resolution of hyponatremia following pericardiocentesis has been described in case reports by other authors [2–6]. In addition, in a recent review of 31 patients, Jong et al. found that individuals with cardiac tamponade-related hyponatremia demonstrated a statistically significant increase in serum sodium levels within 48 hours of pericardiocentesis [7]. Similar findings were reported in an article by Chang et al. [8]. A review of case reports that demonstrate improvement of hyponatremia following pericardiocentesis is summarized in Table 1.

The underlying cause of cardiac tamponade-related hyponatremia remains to be definitively established. However, a dual mechanism has been proposed: (1) increased cardiac pressure stimulates release of antidiuretic hormone with a consequent decrease in serum sodium from increased free water retention and (2) low cardiac output impairs renal free water excretion [2, 5, 8].

In our patient, malignant and infectious etiologies were ruled out based on pericardial fluid analysis. The pericardial effusion was presumed to be secondary to CRT-D placement two months prior. Postcardiac injury syndrome (PCIS), also called postperiocardiotomy syndrome (PPS), is well-documented following pacemaker placement and is a complication in 10-50% of patients [10, 11]. Pericardial effusion can develop between 5 and 56 days (mean:

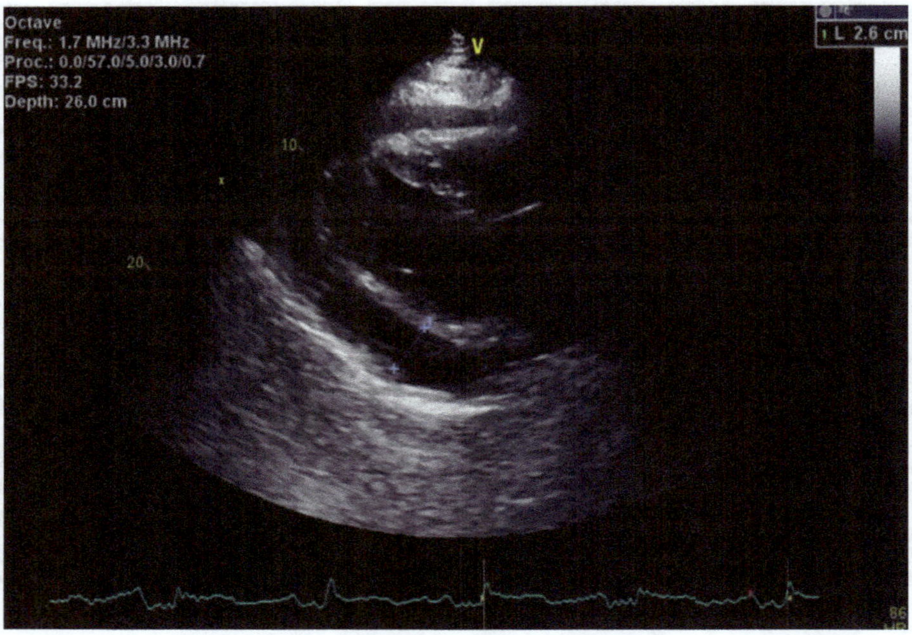

(a)

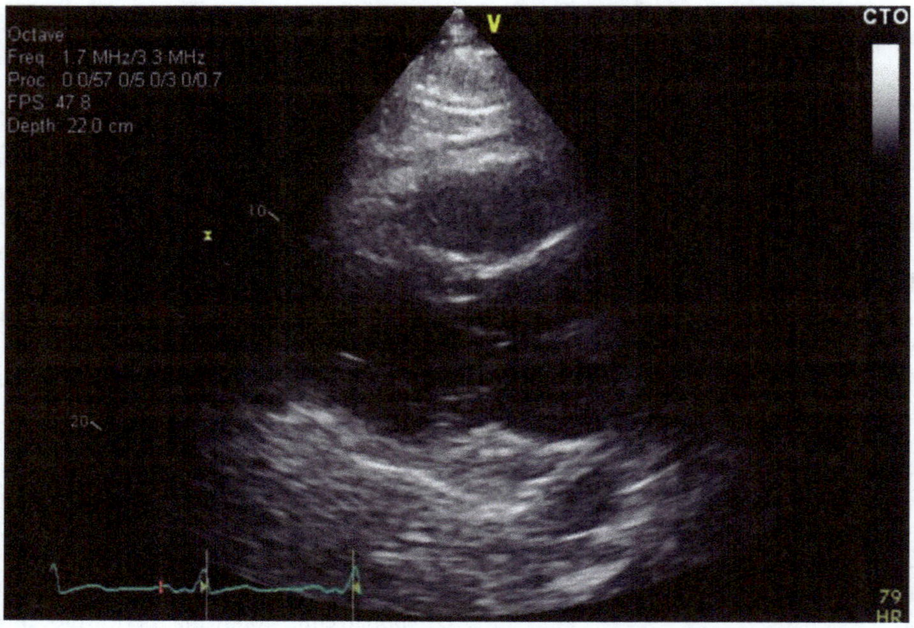

(b)

FIGURE 2: (a) Large circumferential pericardial effusion measuring 2.6 centimeters posteriorly, 1.5 centimeters anteriorly, and 1.8 centimeters at the apex with right atrial collapse and without right ventricular collapse. Significant inflow variation was noted across the mitral and tricuspid valves. Left ventricular ejection fraction was estimated at 55%. Mild concentric left ventricular hypertrophy was present. (b) Echocardiogram obtained the day after pericardial drainage demonstrates resolution of the pericardial effusion.

21.5 days) after pacemaker placement [10]. Cardiac tamponade in PCIS is a rare phenomenon with an incidence of 0.1 to 0.6% [12]. Our patient was discovered to have a pericardial effusion 54 days following his pacemaker placement.

To our knowledge, there are only two reported cases of pericardial effusion-associated hyponatremia in the setting of pacemaker placement [9]. Rakhshan et al. described an 87-year-old woman and an 83-year-old woman in whom pericardial effusion-associated hyponatremia resolved following medical treatment with colchicine. Interestingly, in both of these cases, patients developed pleural effusion in addition to their pericardial effusion. Our case differs in that our patient had echocardiographic evidence of cardiac tamponade. Additionally, our patient was treated with pericardiocentesis rather than with colchicine, suggesting that medical and surgical management may both lead to resolution of hyponatremia.

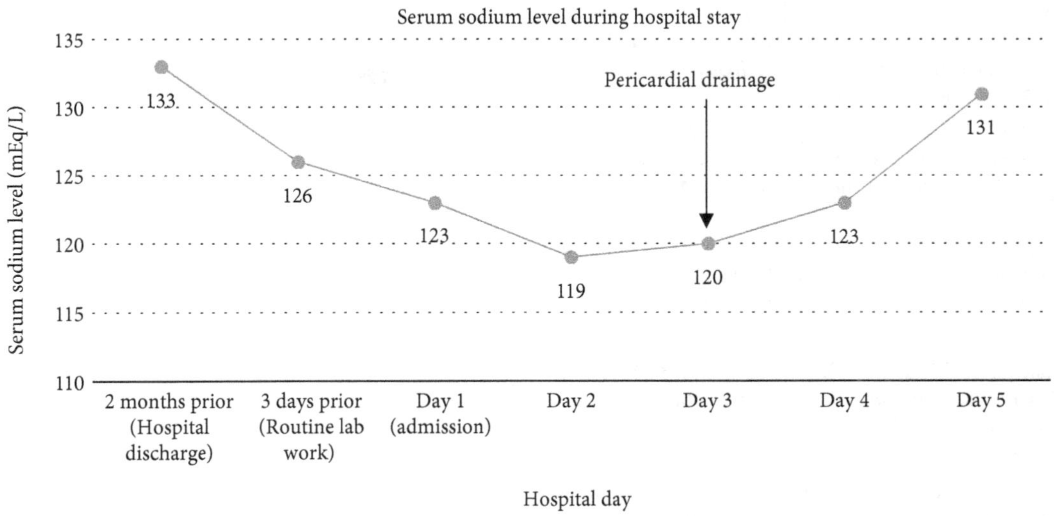

FIGURE 3: Serum sodium level during the hospital stay. Rapid correction of hyponatremia was observed within 36 hours of pericardiocentesis.

TABLE 1: Summary of case reports illustrating resolution of hyponatremia following pericardiocentesis.

Author	Age/gender	Serum sodium level before treatment (mEq/L)	Serum sodium level after treatment (mEq/L)	Pericardiocentesis drainage	Time for resolution of hyponatremia
Present case (2020)	67/M	119	131	1500 mL	36 hours
Dalia et al. [2]	70/F	109	132	750 mL	48 hours
Weekes et al. [3]	49/M	95	134	2200 mL	14 days
Shafique et al. [4]	59/M	105	123	1700 mL	18 hours
Mouallem et al. [5]	58/F	126	139	1500 mL	1 day
Groves et al. [6]	29/M	124	131	1500 mL	36 hours

The documented etiologies of pericardial effusion-associated hyponatremia include uremia [2], malignancy [5, 8], medication [6], and idiopathic [3, 4]. In each of these cases, patients had symptomatic cardiac tamponade with hemodynamic instability. Our case is unique in that our patient lacked clinical signs of tamponade; his only symptoms were cough and dyspnea. In addition, CRT-D placement represents a rare etiology of pericardial effusion.

4. Conclusion

Pericardial effusion-associated hyponatremia has been described in previous case reports [2–6] and retrospective studies [7, 8]. In most patients, hyponatremia resolves following medical management or pericardiocentesis. To the best of our knowledge, this is the first report of resolution of hyponatremia following evacuation of pericardial effusion secondary to CRT-D pacemaker placement. Our case report provides further evidence that treatment of a pericardial effusion rapidly corrects associated hyponatremia.

Additional Points

Take Away Lesson. Hyponatremia is a rare manifestation of pericardial effusion. Serum sodium levels typically normalize following pericardiocentesis. Laboratory studies should be monitored closely in order to reduce the risk of hyponatremia-related complications in patients with an underlying pericardial effusion.

Consent

Informed patient consent was obtained for publication of the case details.

References

[1] Y. H. H. Lien and J. I. Shapiro, "Hyponatremia: clinical diagnosis and management," *The American Journal of Medicine*, vol. 120, no. 8, pp. 653–658, 2007.

[2] T. Dalia, R. Masoomi, K. K. Sahu, and K. Gupta, "Cardiac tamponade causing severe reversible hyponatraemia," *BMJ Case Reports*, vol. 2018, Article ID bcr2017222949, 2018.

[3] M. P. Weekes, B. A. J. Reddi, S. Wharton, and A. Gazis, "Hyponatraemia associated with cardiac tamponade and chronic fluid excess," *BMJ Case Reports*, vol. 2010, no. jul09 1, 2010.

[4] R. Shafique, S. Sarwar, B. M. Wall, and C. R. Cooke, "Reversible hyponatremia related to pericardial tamponade," *American Journal of Kidney Diseases*, vol. 50, no. 2, pp. 336-341, 2007.

[5] M. Mouallem, I. Wolf, G. Mindlin, and Z. Farfel, "Pericardial tamponade-associated hyponatremia," *The American Journal of the Medical Sciences*, vol. 325, no. 1, pp. 51-52, 2003.

[6] P. H. Groves, A. M. Shah, and S. J. Hutchison, "Hyponatraemia secondary to an inappropriately high release of antidiuretic hormone in cardiac tamponade," *British Heart Journal*, vol. 64, no. 3, pp. 206-207, 1990.

[7] B. H. Jong, C. C. Wei, and K. G. Shyu, "Improved hyponatremia after pericardial drainage in patients suffering from cardiac tamponade," *BMC Cardiovascular Disorders*, vol. 16, no. 1, 2016.

[8] F. K. Chang, Y. C. Lee, and C. H. Chiu, "Hyponatremia in patients with symptomatic pericardial effusion," *Journal of the Chinese Medical Association*, vol. 75, no. 10, pp. 509–512, 2012.

[9] E. Rakhshan, S. A. Mirabbasi, B. Khalighi, and K. Khalighi, "Pericarditis-induced hyponatremia after cardiac electronic implantable device (CEID) procedures," *Am J Case Rep.*, vol. 16, pp. 245–249, 2015.

[10] W. C. Tsai, C. T. Liou, C. C. Cheng, K. S. Tsai, S. M. Cheng, and W. S. Lin, "Post-cardiac injury syndrome after permanent pacemaker implantation," *Acta Cardiologica Sinica*, vol. 28, pp. 53–55, 2012.

[11] I. Zeltser, L. A. Rhodes, R. E. Tanel et al., "Postpericardiotomy syndrome after permanent pacemaker implantation in children and young adults," *The Annals of Thoracic Surgery*, vol. 78, no. 5, pp. 1684–1687, 2004.

[12] G. L. Miller, E. B. Coccio, and S. C. Sharma, "Postpericardiotomy syndrome and cardiac tamponade following transvenous pacemaker placement," *Clinical Cardiology*, vol. 19, no. 3, pp. 255-256, 1996.

29

The First Successful Transcatheter Closure of an Inferior Sinus Venosus Defect with Anomalous Drainage of the Right Lower Pulmonary Vein using Bare and Covered Stents

Kritvikrom Durongpisitkul,[1] **Paweena Chungsomprasong**,[1] **Porntip Panjasamanvong**,[2] **and Somrach Thamtorawat**[3]

[1]*Division of Pediatric Cardiology, Department of Pediatrics, Faculty of Medicine Siriraj Hospital, Mahidol University, Bangkok, Thailand*
[2]*Siriraj Piyamaharajkarun Hospital, Mahidol University, Bangkok, Thailand*
[3]*Division of Diagnostic Radiology, Department of Radiology, Faculty of Medicine Siriraj Hospital, Mahidol University, Bangkok, Thailand*

Correspondence should be addressed to Kritvikrom Durongpisitkul; kritvikrom.dur@mahidol.ac.th
Academic Editor: Ertugurul Ercan

Inferior sinus venosus defect (SVD) is less common than a superior one. The lower edge of the defect straddles the orifice of the inferior vena cava, and this makes surgical repair via bicaval cannulation a technical challenge. The orifice of the unroofed right pulmonary vein is caused by the interatrial communication in sinus venosus defects which results in partial anomalous pulmonary vein drainage (PAPVD). Novel transcatheter closure of a superior SVD has recently been described; however, transcatheter closure of an inferior SVD has not yet been reported in the published literature. Here, we report the first successful transcatheter closure of an inferior SVD with bare and covered stents and the rerouting of a PAPVD into the left atrium to avoid occlusion of the hepatic veins. In this single-case report, we carefully describe the planning process, how the procedure was performed, and the steps taken to recapture and reposition a migrated stent. Careful patient selection and intensive assessment of pulmonary and hepatic vein anatomy before and during the procedure were necessary to achieve a successful outcome.

1. Introduction

Ectopic or incomplete resorption of the sinus venosus results in deficiency of the wall that separates the right pulmonary veins from the superior vena cava (SVC), inferior vena cava (IVC), and right atrium resulting in sinus venosus defect (SVD). A defect of this wall leads to abnormal pulmonary venous drainage to the RA which is partial anomalous pulmonary vein drainage (PAPVD) with either the superior and/or middle-right pulmonary vein and less commonly associated with the right lower pulmonary vein (RLPV). Sinus venosus defects are more commonly found at the SVC-RA junction (SVC type) than at the IVC-RA junction (IVC type). Sometimes the defect extends to the right atrium (RA type). Novel techniques of transcatheter closure of superior SVD were reported. The first 5 cases of transcatheter closure of superior SVD were done by Abdullah et al. in 2011 [1] and presented in the conference of CSI-Frankfurt 2013. Later, Garg et al. published the one case report transcatheter closure of an SVD using a stent [2].

Since then, different stents and implantation techniques have been reported [1, 3, 4]. An inferior SVD is less common and is characterized by the lower edge of the defect straddling the orifice of the IVC, and this makes repair via bicaval cannulation a technical challenge. A similar principle was used to describe the transcatheter closure of ASD with absent inferior rim using stent with or without device [5]. To the best of our knowledge, there is only one report of successful transcatheter closure of an inferior SVD, and that closure was achieved using a device [6]. Here, we report the first successful transcatheter closure of an inferior SVD with anomalous drainage of the right lower pulmonary vein using bare and covered stents.

2. Case Report

A 29-year-old Thai female had dyspnea during exertion with past history of surgical atrial septal defect (ASD) closure at another hospital at 8 years old. On cardiac examination, a 2/6 systolic ejection murmur was detected. CXR taken at our hospital showed mild cardiomegaly (Figure 1). Two-dimensional transthoracic echocardiography revealed marked right atrial and right ventricular enlargement with left to right shunt via an inferior SVD with a suspected PAPVD (Figure 2). Cardiac magnetic resonance (CMR) imaging confirmed the diagnosis of an inferior SVD that measured 17.2 mm in length with partial anomalous pulmonary venous drainage (PAPVD) of the RLPV into the IVC (Figures 3(a) and 3(b)). We suspected that diagnosis of secundum ASD previously did not include an inferior PAPVD in this patient; hence, the surgical procedure did not incorporate PAPVD. The patient's right ventricle (RV) was severely dilated with a right ventricular end-diastolic volume index (RVEDVi) of 172 ml/m^2, RV ejection fraction (RVEF) of 59%, a left ventricular end-diastolic volume index (LVEDVi) of 66.2 ml/m^2, and an LVEF of 63%. The QP : QS measurement was 2.17 : 1. It was clear that the shunt was significant and that closure was required. Due to our patient's previous history of open-heart surgery, we decided to opt for transcatheter closure instead of reoperation.

Similar to a superior SVD, a PAPVD in an inferior SVD is caused by a defect in the posterior wall of the IVC and in the anterior wall of the RLPV. We hypothesized that careful placement of one or more covered stents in the IVC could both close the defect and facilitate normal RLPV drainage into the LA. The challenge was where to position the covered stent in the IVC without compromising hepatic venous drainage. Based on three-dimensional (3D) reconstruction of the respiratory-navigated and electrocardiography-(ECG-) gated Dixon CMR sequence, a 3D-printed model (Figure 4(a)) was used to simulate the landing zone for each bare and covered stent deployment, including the preferable angle of angiography. The model was used to evaluate an anterior view of the RA (Figure 4(a)) and by looking into an opening that was artificially cut into the lateral wall of the RA to directly visualize the SVD (Figure 4(b)). An interventional radiologist was invited to our routine heart team meeting. To prevent hepatic vein obstruction, it was decided to anchor bare stent in the IVC just above the left hepatic vein orifice. The 3D model was also used for simulation of balloon sizing to measure the anchoring area diameter of 20.27 mm (Figure 5(a)). The aim of the covered stent was to cover the superior border of the ASD (Figure 5(b)). The length of the stent was decided according to the distance between the features of the IVC just above the entrance of the left hepatic vein and the upper rim of the SVD defect, which was measured to be 60 mm. Since the longest BeGraft ePTFE covered stent (BGA4824_2; Bentley InnoMed GmbH, Hechingen, Germany) is 48 mm in length, we decided to use two overlapping stents, including the aforementioned BeGraft covered stent and one CP8Z45 bare stent (NuMED for Children, Orlando, FL, USA) that is 45 mm in length and that was used as the primary anchoring stent outside of the BeGraft stent.

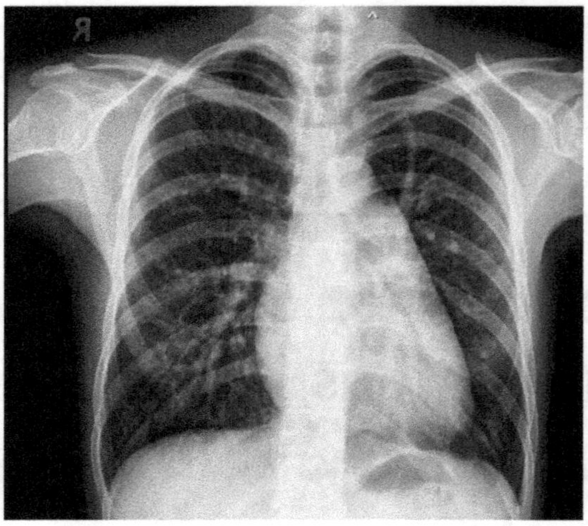

Figure 1: Plain radiograph of the chest showing mild cardiomegaly with left atrialization and slight increase in pulmonary blood flow.

The procedure was performed under general anesthesia in the cardiac catheterization lab. Sheathes were inserted via the right femoral vein and the right femoral artery. Fifty units/kg of unfractionated heparin and ceftriaxone were given intravenously. The activated clotting time (ACT) was monitored and maintained within 200-250 seconds. Angiography was performed in the IVC to visualize hepatic vein entrance into the IVC (Figures 6(a) and 6(b)).

Right pulmonary artery angiography was performed to visualize both the arterial phase (Figure 7(a)) and the levo phase (Figure 7(b)) of RLPV drainage. RLPV venography was performed in the anteroposterior (AP) (Figure 8(a)) and lateral (Figure 8(b)) views to determine the location of the RLPV relative to the posterior wall of the RA. The site of the entrance of the RLPV into the IVC and the lower end of the SVD were also profiled in this angiogram (Figures 7 and 8).

We used the largest available size balloon which is a 30 mm PTS-X balloon (NuMED for Children, Orlando, FL, USA) to generate a 1 atm pressure for sizing. A simultaneous contrast injection was performed at both right (Figures 9(a) and 9(b)) and left (Figures 9(c) and 9(d)) hepatic veins. A higher-pressure balloon will be needed during implantation of the stent. The anchoring CP8Z45 bare stent over a 22 mm × 50 mm Balloon-in-Balloon (BIB) balloon catheter (NuMED for Children, Orlando, FL, USA) was successfully deployed and redilated using a larger 24 mm × 40 mm Z-Med II balloon (NuMED for Children, Orlando, FL, USA) that can expand up to 24 mm in diameter inside the IVC. After stent placement, right hepatic vein flow could freely drain into the stent (Figures 10(a) and 10(b)). The decision

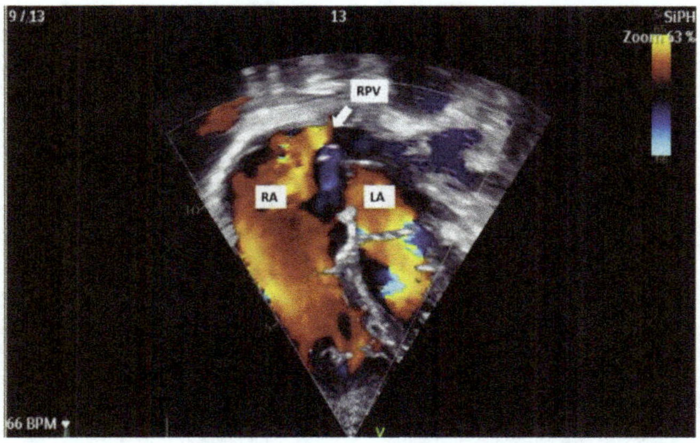

FIGURE 2: Echocardiography showing a four-chamber view with partial anomalous right pulmonary venous drainage with blood flow from the right lower pulmonary vein to inferior vena cava. LA: left atrium; RA: right atrium; RPV: right pulmonary vein.

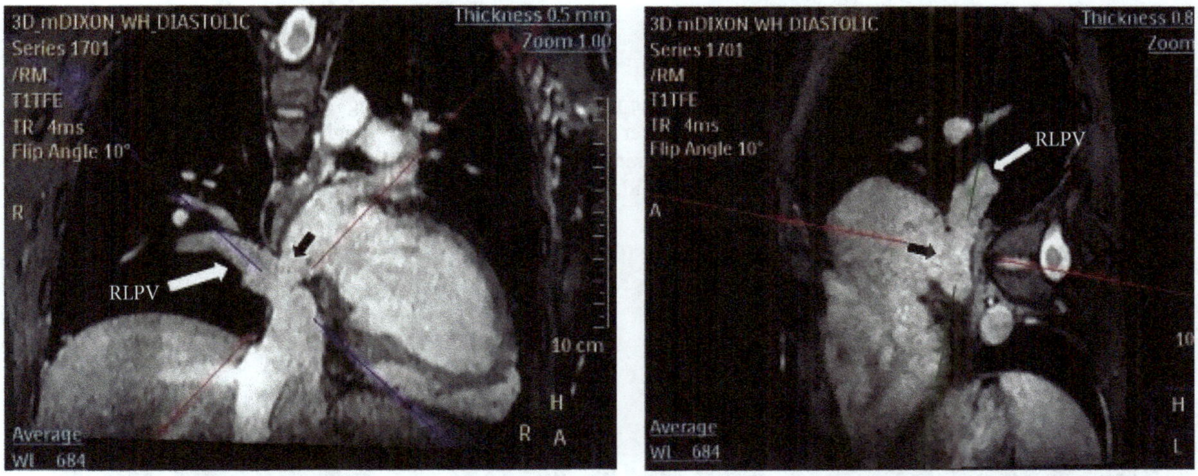

FIGURE 3: Cardiac magnetic resonance imaging shows a residual sinus venosus defect (black arrow) between the right lower pulmonary vein (RLPV) and inferior vena cava. (a) Coronal view and (b) sagittal view from the left side. Anomalous right lower pulmonary vein drainage can also be observed.

was made to place the lower end of the covered stent above the entrance of the hepatic veins, but the bare stent had been positioned lower down than proper position making the overlapping segment shorter than 50% as shown in Figure 10 as angiogram is more practical and informative during the procedure than CMR, cardiac CT, or 3D printing. Placement of the planned subsequent covered stent using a 24 mm × 48 mm BeGraft ePTFE Covered Stent (AccuPath Medical Technologies Co., Ltd., Shanghai, China) was positioned at the superior aspect of the primary anchoring stent at just above the left hepatic vein drainage. We estimated that this positioning would allow enough distance above the openings of both the right and left hepatic veins (Figure 10). However, this reduced the overlap between stents, which compromised the stability of the covered stent. Nonetheless, the covered stent was finally deployed at the intended position (Figures 11(a) and 11(b)).

The covered stent then unexpectedly migrated into the RA shortly after it was deployed (Figure 12). The first attempt to reposition the covered stent using a balloon inflated inside the stent to try to pull it backwards and back into position was unsuccessful. We then deployed a second 24 mm × 40 mm Z-Med II balloon in an attempt to use an external force to squeeze or push the migrated covered stent to a smaller diameter to be able to pull back inside first stent, squeeze; however, this attempt was also unsuccessful due to the strong radial force of the covered stent (Figures 13(a) and 13(b)).

We then deployed a 35 mm Amplatz Gooseneck Snare (Medtronic, Minneapolis, MN, USA) via a delivery catheter in an attempt to grasp distal wire position of from the left femoral vein and was used to snuggle the distal part of the migrated covered stent (Figures 14(a) and 14(b)). The deployed snare was used to squeeze the middle part of the stent with simultaneous inflation of the distal balloon to pull the dislodged stent back into the anchoring bare stent. However, this led to the angulation of the covered stent. We then attempted to snare the stent without balloon inflation, but this strategy was also not successful. We then decided to

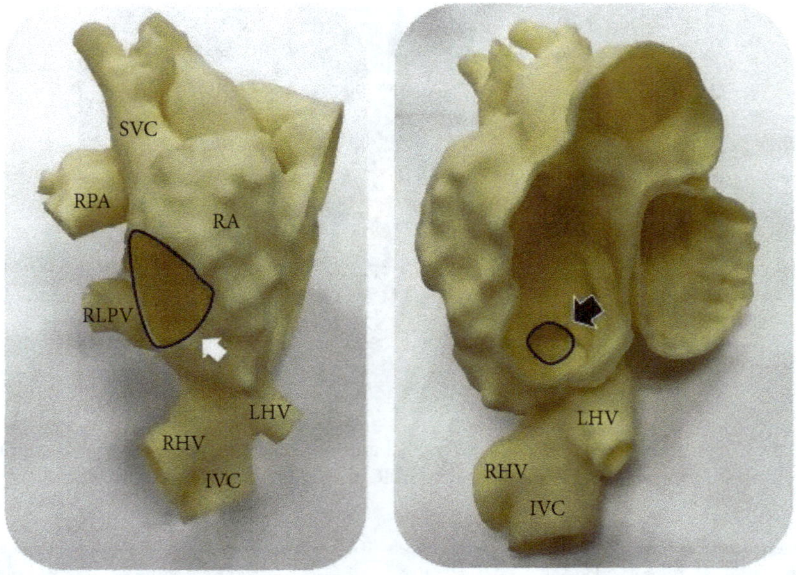

(a) (b)

FIGURE 4: Anterior aspect of a 3-dimensional model from cardiac magnetic resonance imaging. (a) The superior vena cava- (SVC-) right atrium (RA) junction, right pulmonary artery (RPA), right lower pulmonary vein (RLPV), right hepatic vein (RHV), left hepatic vein (LHV), and inferior vena cava (IVC) can be observed. An opening was artificially created (white arrow) to facilitate a simulated view into the lateral aspect of the RA. (b) A sinus venosus defect was identified at the IVC-RA junction (black arrow).

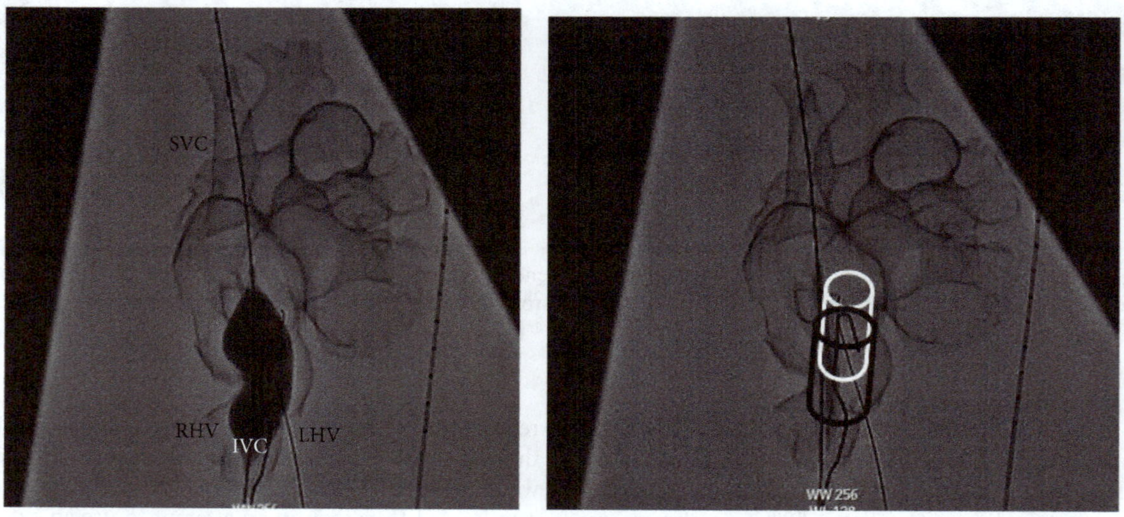

(a) (b)

FIGURE 5: A 3-dimensional model was created to simulate balloon sizing in the inferior vena cava (IVC) (a). The critical point at the IVC-right atrium junction was 20.3 mm. A decision was made to position a 24 mm anchored bare stent (black outlined stent) at this location (b). A long wire was placed in the superior vena cava (SVC), and a short wire was placed in both the left hepatic vein (LHV) and the IVC. The aim of the placement of the bare stent (black outlined stent) and the subsequently positioned covered stent (white outlined stent) was to cover the sinus venosus defect and to ensure no obstruction of blood flow in the LHV and the right hepatic vein (RHV).

snare the stent with simultaneous inflation of the distal part of the stent to make it coaxial/telescopic to the anchored bare stent, and this strategy successfully released the migrated stent and allowed us to pull it back into position within the bare stent (Figures 14(c)–14(f)). However, once back inside the bare stent, the snare could not be released from the covered stent. The balloon, covered stent, and snare were then pushed back out of the bare stent. The snare was then repositioned to the distal part of the stent to facilitate successful release of the snare once the covered stent was repositioned within the bare stent (Figures 14(g) and 14(h)). This strategy resulted in the successful repositioning of the covered stent and the successful release of the snare (Figures 15(a) and 15(b)).

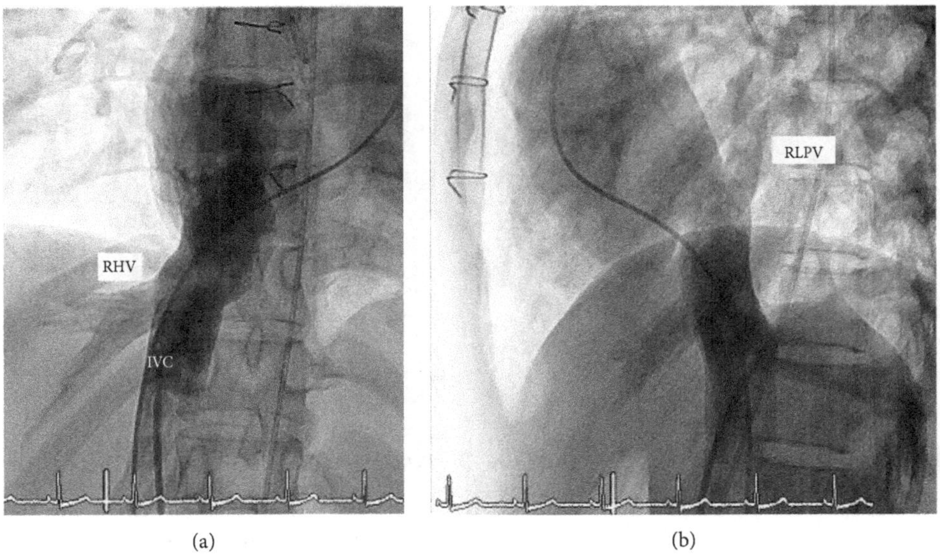

FIGURE 6: Angiography was performed in the inferior vena cava (IVC). The (a) anterior and (b) lateral views show the connection between the right lower pulmonary vein (RLPV) and the right atrium. The decision was made to place the lower end of the covered stent above the entrance of the left and right hepatic veins (RHV).

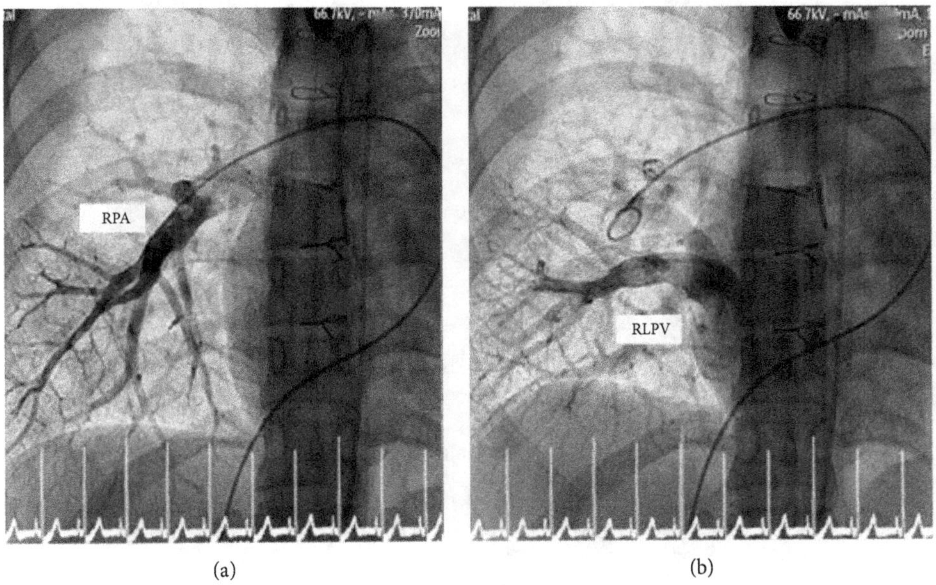

FIGURE 7: The (a) arterial phase and (b) levo phase of right pulmonary artery (RPA) angiography shows drainage of the right lower pulmonary vein (RLPV) into the right atrium.

A second CP8Z45 bare stent that was mounted on a 22 mm × 5 cm BIB-balloon catheter was then applied over the overlapping section of the first bare stent and the covered stent in order to stabilize both the structure of the combination stent and the patency of the affected vasculature (Figures 16(a) and 16(b)). Postprocedural angiogram showed the second bare stent in place with good blood flow in the hepatic veins and no residual RLPV drainage to the RA (Figures 16(c) and 16(d)). The overall procedure time was 193 minutes, and the fluoroscopy time was 56 minutes. The laboratory results showed normal liver function test. The patient was discharged the following day and aspirin was prescribed. Cardiac CT angiogram (CTA) showed normal RLPV drainage to the LA with a small residual SVD at the superior border of the ASD shunt due to the angulation of the IVC into the interatrial septum (Figure 17). On CTA, both the left and right hepatic veins were patent with no evidence of venous obstruction. A thrombus was suspected in the lower part of the IVC, so oral anticoagulant drug was given. At the 1-month follow-up, duplex ultrasound of the IVC showed complete resolution of the suspected thrombus.

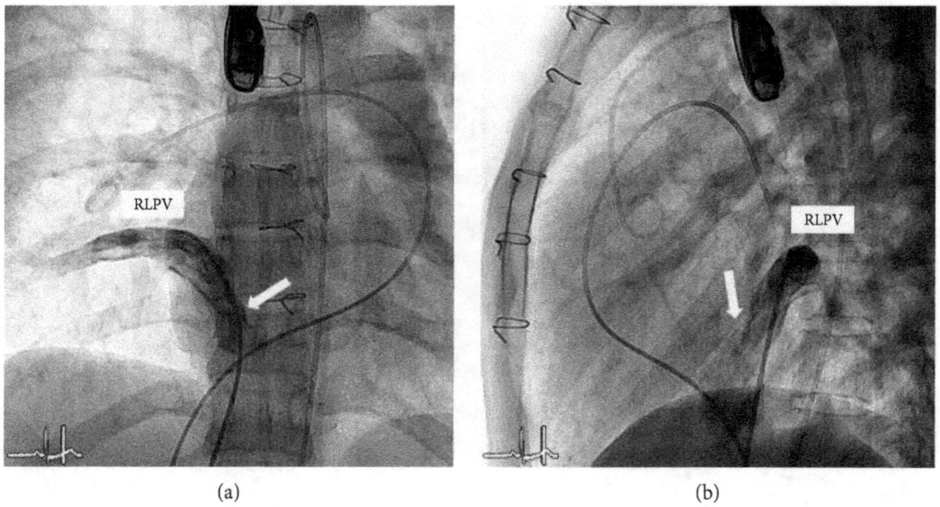

FIGURE 8: Right lower pulmonary vein (RLPV) angiography was performed simultaneous both (a) anterior view and (b) lateral view of the right atrium. The drainage of the RLPV into the right atrium (white arrow) was also shown in both views. (a) The decision was made to place the upper part of the covered stent and anterior and above the entrance of this RLPV (white arrow) to direct the pulmonary venous blood return to the left atrium.

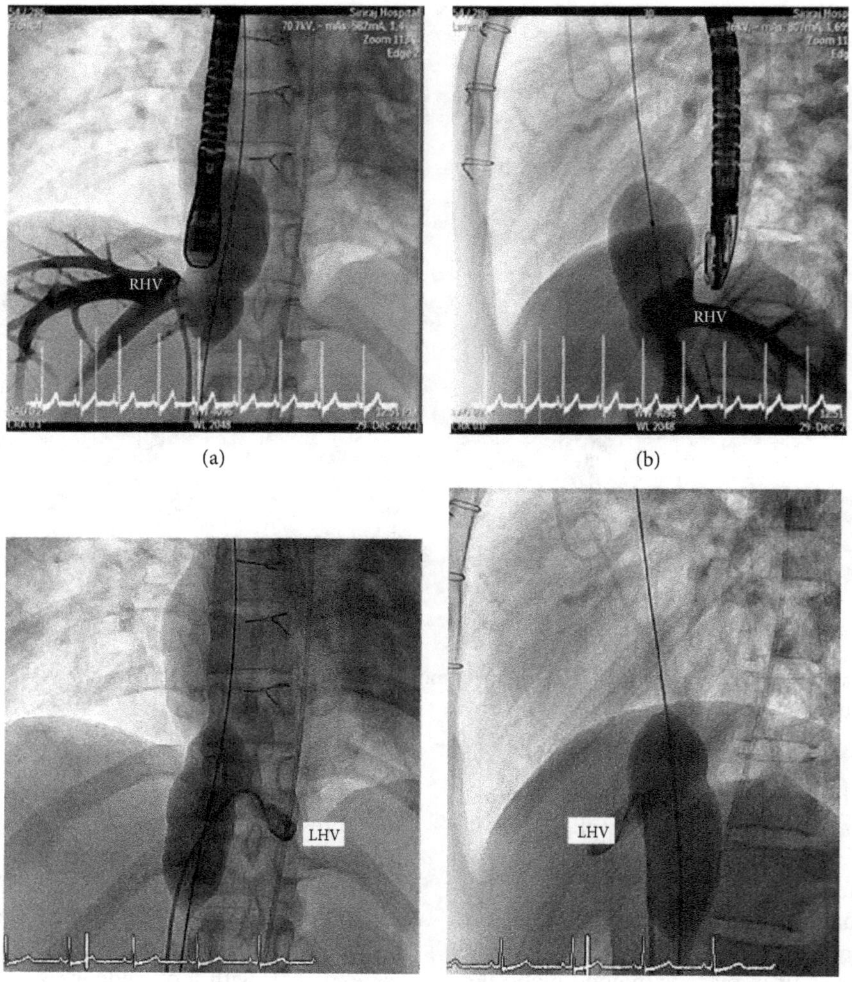

FIGURE 9: Balloon sizing of the sinus venosus defect that was performed at the inferior vena cava (IVC)-right atrium junction ((a) anterior and (b) lateral views on angiography) showed the right hepatic vein (RHV) to be occluded by the balloon. During the same occlusion, we placed a catheter in the left hepatic vein (LHV) and simultaneously injected contrast showing the LHV connection ((c) anterior and (d) lateral views).

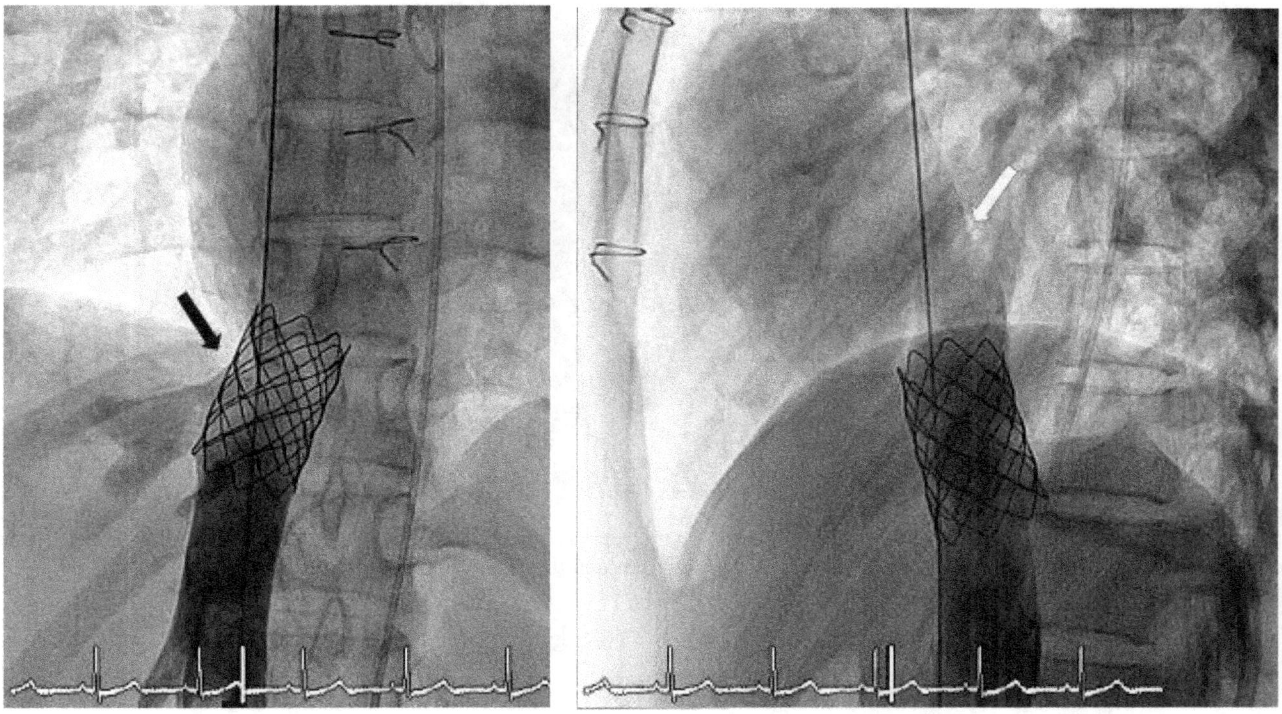

(a) (b)

FIGURE 10: The bare stent, which was placed first, was positioned at the inferior vena cava-right atrium junction ((a) anteroposterior and (b) lateral views on angiography). The decision was then made to position the lower end of the planned covered stent, which will be placed later, above the entrances of the right and also left hepatic veins (black arrow), and that the covered stent would overlap with the bare stent approximately 50%. It was also noted that the distal part of this covered stents should position just above the entrance of the right lower pulmonary vein (white arrow).

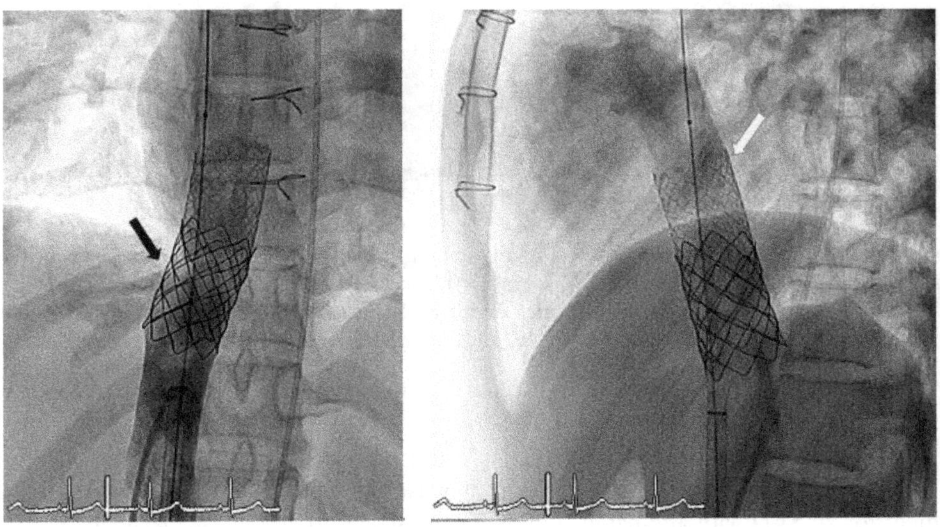

(a) (b)

FIGURE 11: The covered stent (white arrow), which was placed second, is positioned superior to the anchored bare stent (black arrow) in the inferior vena cava ((a) anteroposterior and (b) lateral views on angiography). The placement of covered stent was supposed to be above the entrance of the right lower pulmonary vein (RLPV) but at the expense of overlapping segment because the bare stent was placed lower enough into the IVC. This can be compared with final position of the covered stent after repositioning almost covering the entrance of RLPV but lower than the first position (Figure 15). The stitch can be used as a guide line.

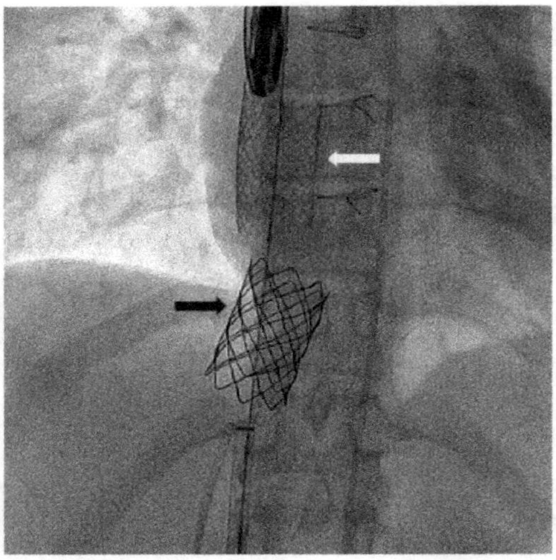

FIGURE 12: The covered stent unexpectedly embolized into the right atrium as visualized on anterior view angiography of the right atrium. The black arrow and white arrow indicate the position of the bare stent and the covered stent, respectively.

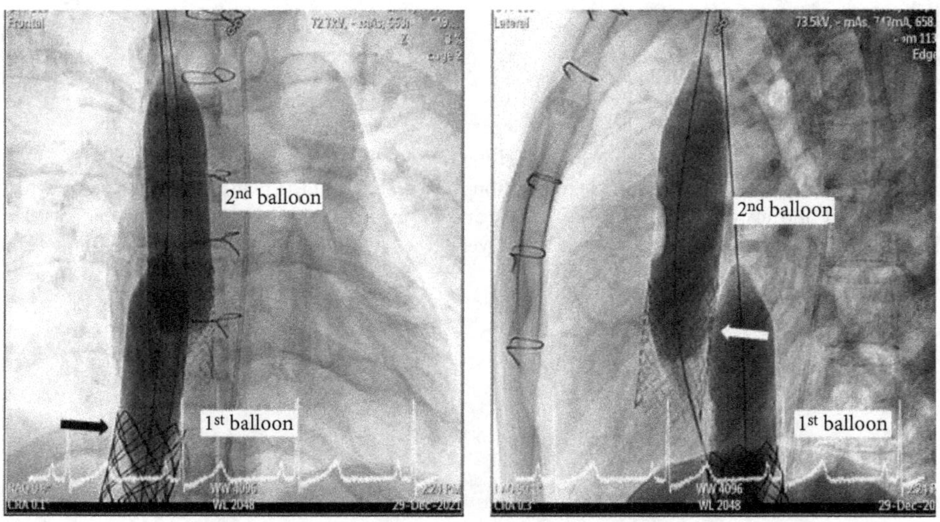

(a) (b)

FIGURE 13: The balloon inside the covered stent was inflated in an attempt to pull down and reposition the embolized covered stent, but that attempt was unsuccessful. We then deployed another 24 mm × 40 mm Z-Med balloon in an attempt to use an external force to squeeze or pushing the embolized covered stent to a smaller diameter to be able to pull back inside first stent, but that was also unsuccessful due to the strong radial force of the covered graft (a, b). The black arrow and white arrow indicate the position of the bare stent and the covered stent, respectively.

3. Discussion

The standard treatment for an SVD with anomalous drainage of pulmonary veins is surgical closure. This surgical procedure yields an excellent complete closure rate; however, some patients develop stenosis of the SVC that requires reoperation. Transcatheter closure of an SVD with PAPVD is a currently available alternative treatment due to its ability to stent the SVC to prevent subsequent stenosis. Several studies reported the success of this procedure using covered stents or device closure in patients having the appropriate anatomy [2–4, 7]. The use of 3-dimensional- (3D-) printed heart models enhances the feasibility of transcatheter closure and promotes improved understanding of the relationship between the structure and surrounding vessels. A 3D-printed heart model can facilitate a simulation of stent or device deployment and can demonstrate successful occlusion of the SVD with redirection of the pulmonary vein to the left atrium [8–10]. The majority of these procedures have been performed in superior SVDs. The first case report of transcatheter closure of an inferior SVD was reported by Kim et al. [6]. Later, He et al. reported a case series of transcatheter closure of inferior SVDs using a device [9]. The challenge of device closure of an inferior SVD is navigating the rim of the atrial septum. In the case series from He et al. [9], all included patients had to have at least two defects,

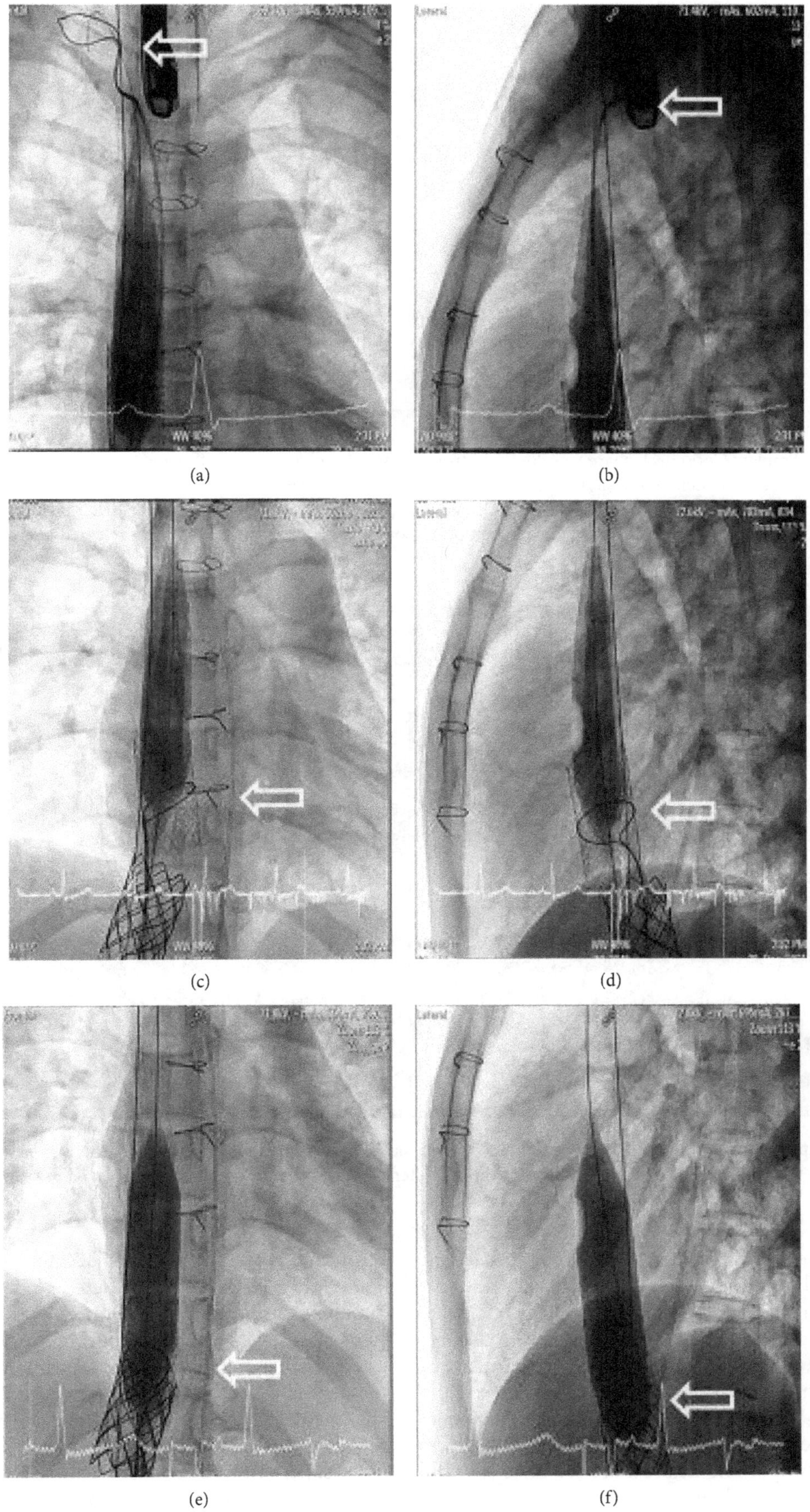

(a) (b) (c) (d) (e) (f)

FIGURE 14: Continued.

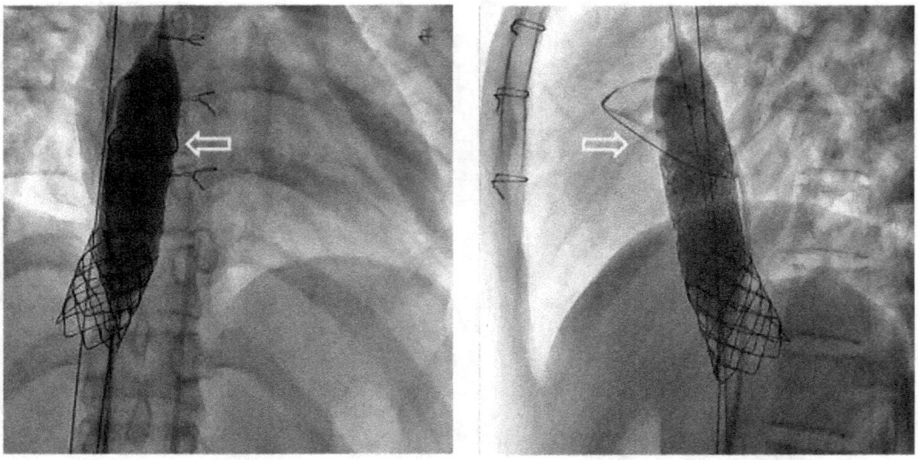

(g) (h)

Figure 14: A 35 mm Amplatz Gooseneck snare was deployed from a distal Amplatz Super Stiff wire (a, b). The snare was used to grasp the middle of the embolized covered stent and to pull it back inside the anchored bare stent (c, d); however, we were not able to release the snare once the covered stent was back inside the bare stent (e, f). We then redeployed the snare at a more distal position and then pulled the embolized stent with balloon inflated in the more distal position to coaxial both stents and eventually released snare (g, h).

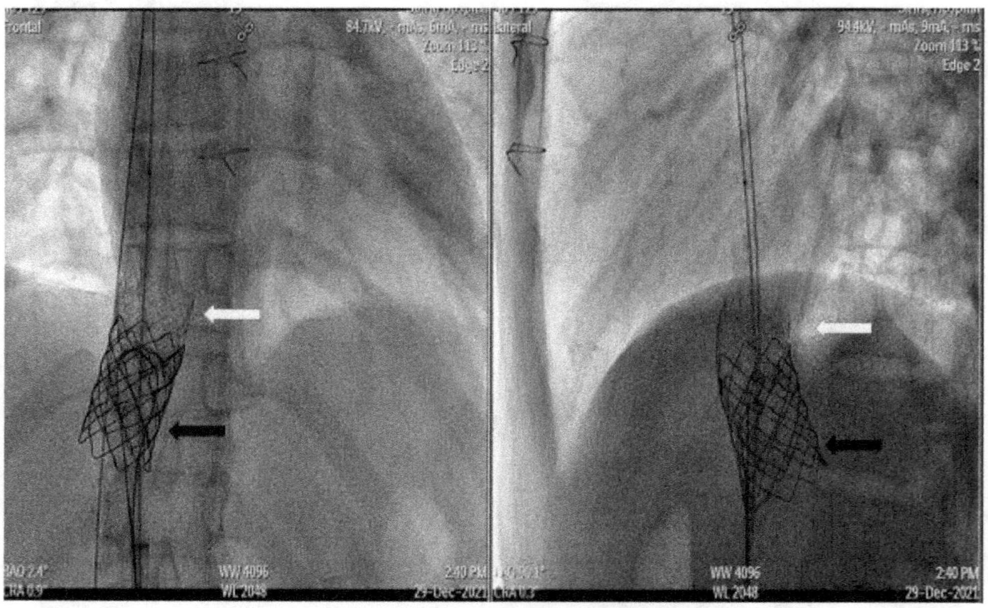

Figure 15: Angiography showing the previously embolized covered stent successfully pulled back inside the primary anchored bare stent. The black arrow and white arrow indicate the position of the bare stent and the covered stent, respectively.

including an inferior SVD. In contrast, the patient profiled in this case report had only one ASD, so device closure was not considered to be an appropriate treatment strategy.

Here, we report the first successful transcatheter closure of an inferior SVD using bare and covered stents. Similar to transcatheter closure of a superior SVD, transcatheter closure of an inferior SVD involves closure of the pulmonary vein defect to redirect pulmonary vein flow to the LA. However, there are four important factors that need to be considered when considering or planning for transcatheter closure of an inferior SVD. First, the position of the hepatic veins needs to be carefully assessed by MRI, CT, or 3D printing before the procedure so that placement of the anchor stent will avoid occlusion of the left and right hepatic veins. Simultaneous venography to ensure that the position of the stent was not too far down during the procedure was also extremely helpful. Second, the angulation of the IVC which pointed more directly to interatrial septum will prevent well alignment of the covered stent than in the SVC showed in the postprocedural CT here that there was a small leakage at the superior rim of the ASD. Third, the effects and severity of intraprocedural complications, such as the stent migration observed in our patient, can be mitigated via intensive preprocedural preparation and a comprehensive inventory

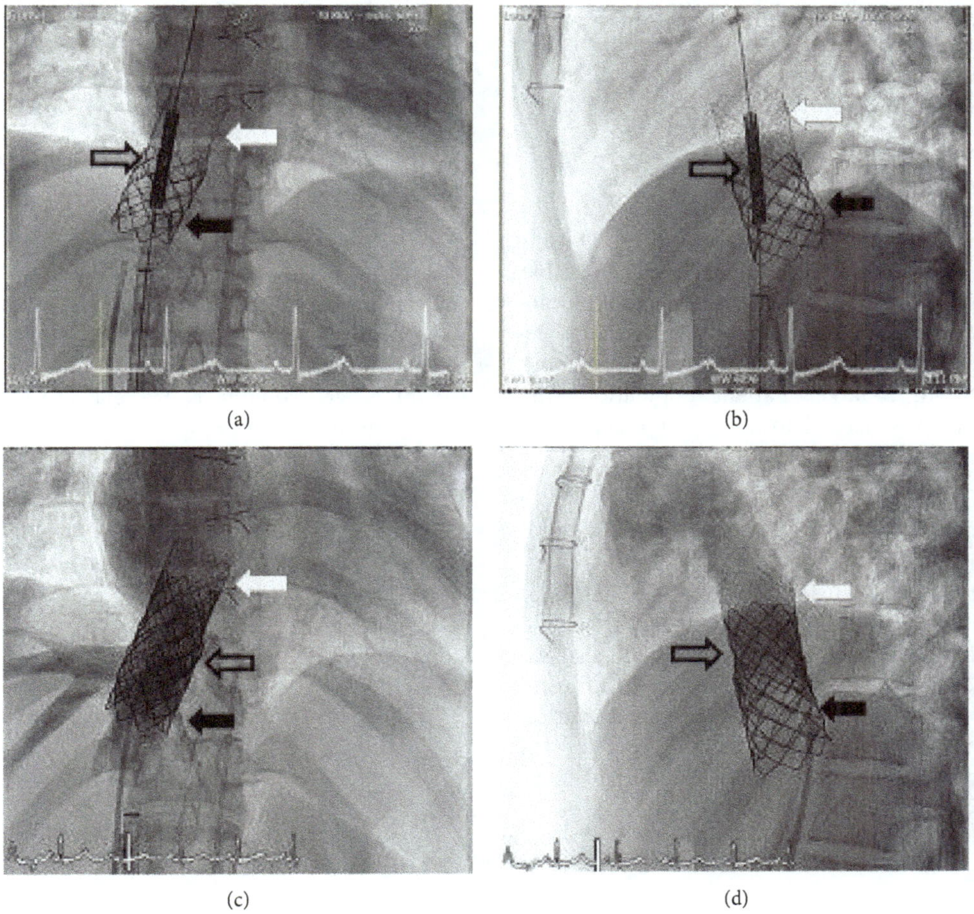

FIGURE 16: A second bare stent was then applied over the overlapping section of the first bare stent and the covered stent in order to stabilize both the structure of the combination stent and the patency of the affected vasculature ((a) anterior and (b) lateral views on angiography). Postprocedural angiogram showed the second bare stent in place with good blood flow in the hepatic veins ((c) anterior and (d) lateral views on angiography). No contrast was observed filling in the pulmonary vein. The black arrow, white arrow, and black outline arrow indicate the position of the first bare stent, the covered stent, and the second bare stent, respectively.

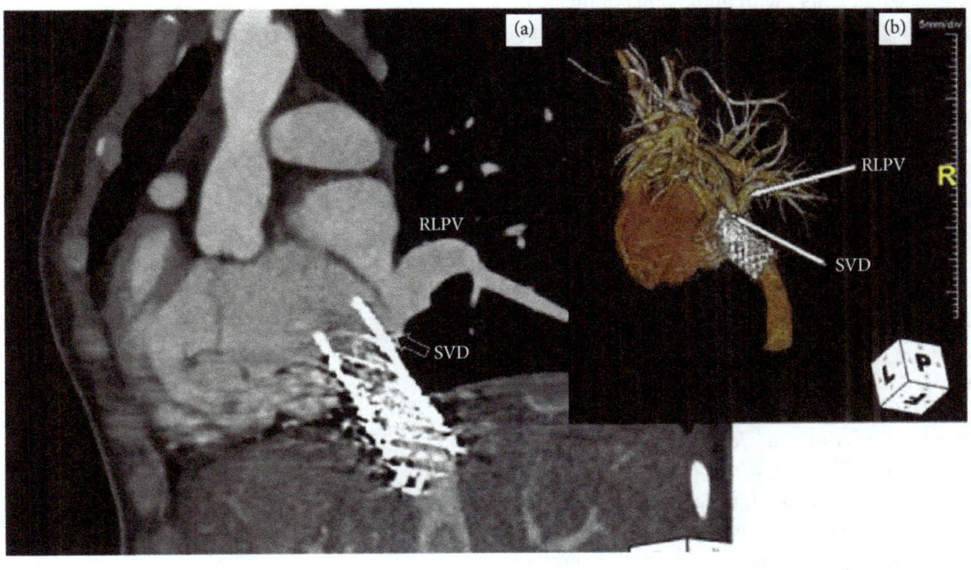

FIGURE 17: Postprocedural computed tomography angiogram showing (a) a sagittal image and (b) a rendered image of a patent 3-stent structure in the inferior vena cava. The stent structure covers the sinus venosus defect (SVD) with the upper end almost opposed to the interatrial septum causing a small residual opening (black arrow) and unobstructed blood flow from the right lower pulmonary vein (RLPV) to the left atrium (a). The superior segment of the covered stent should be flared by balloon to prevent residual shunt.

of medicines, equipment, and techniques in the cardiac catheterization laboratory. Forth and last, double anti-platelet should be administered to avoid thrombosis of the stents deployed in IVC with slow venous flow.

4. Conclusion

Transcatheter closure of an inferior SVD with PAPVD using bare and covered stents in the IVC was shown to be feasible. Careful patient selection and intensive assessment of pulmonary and hepatic vein anatomy before and during the procedure were necessary to achieve a successful outcome. However, a study in a larger patient population with longer-term follow-up is needed to assess the efficacy and safety of this technique.

Acknowledgments

The authors gratefully acknowledge the patient described in this report for granting us permission to report details and images specific to her case. The authors would also like to thank Dr. Prakul Chanthong, Dr. Pornrawee Plearntummakun, and the staff members of the cardiac catheterization laboratory at Her Majesty Cardiac Center of the Faculty of Medicine Siriraj Hospital, Mahidol University, for their assistance.

References

[1] H. A. M. Abdullah, H. A. Alsalkhi, and K. A. Khalid, "Transcatheter closure of sinus venosus atrial septal defect with anomalous pulmonary venous drainage: innovative technique with long-term follow-up," *Catheterization and Cardiovascular Interventions*, vol. 95, no. 4, pp. 743–747, 2020.

[2] G. Garg, H. Tyagi, and A. S. Radha, "Transcatheter closure of sinus venosus atrial septal defect with anomalous drainage of right upper pulmonary vein into superior vena cava–an innovative technique," *Catheterization and Cardiovascular Interventions*, vol. 84, no. 3, pp. 473–477, 2014.

[3] M. Riahi, M. N. Velasco Forte, N. Byrne et al., "Early experience of transcatheter correction of superior sinus venosus atrial septal defect with partial anomalous pulmonary venous drainage," *EuroIntervention*, vol. 14, no. 8, pp. 868–876, 2018.

[4] E. Rosenthal, S. A. Qureshi, M. Jones et al., "Correction of sinus venosus atrial septal defects with the 10 zig covered Cheatham-platinum stent – an international registry," *Catheterization and Cardiovascular Interventions*, vol. 98, no. 1, pp. 128–136, 2021.

[5] H. Abdulwahab, M. R. Husain, and K. A. Khalid, "Feasibility of transcatheter closure of large secundum atrial septal defect with absent superior or inferior rim," *Journal of Interventional Cardiology*, vol. 2022, pp. 2764296–2764298, 2022.

[6] H. D. Kim, M. S. Kim, K. J. Yun, S. M. Bae, S. H. Her, and J. H. Lee, "Successful transcatheter closure of an inferior sinus venosus atrial septal defect," *The Korean Journal of Internal Medicine*, vol. 31, no. 1, pp. 176–178, 2016.

[7] A. E. Baruteau, M. I. Jones, G. Butera, S. A. Qureshi, and E. Rosenthal, "Correction percutanee d'une communication interatriale (CIA) sinus venosus avec retour veineux pulmonaire anormal partiel: la procedure de choix chez des patients selectionnes ?," *Archives of Cardiovascular Diseases*, vol. 113, no. 2, pp. 92–95, 2020.

[8] A. N. Thakkar, P. Chinnadurai, J. P. Breinholt, and C. H. Lin, "Transcatheter closure of a sinus venosus atrial septal defect using 3D printing and image fusion guidance," *Catheterization and Cardiovascular Diagnosis*, vol. 92, no. 2, pp. 353–357, 2018.

[9] L. He, G. S. Cheng, Y. J. Du, and Y. S. Zhang, "Feasibility of device closure for multiple atrial septal defects with an inferior sinus venosus defect: procedural planning using three-dimensional printed models," *Heart, Lung & Circulation*, vol. 29, no. 6, pp. 914–920, 2020.

[10] M. N. Velasco Forte, N. Byrne, I. Valverde et al., "Interventional correction of sinus venosus atrial septal defect and partial anomalous pulmonary venous drainage: procedural planning using 3D printed models," *JACC: Cardiovascular Imaging*, vol. 11, no. 2, pp. 275–278, 2018.

30

Acute Inflammatory Pericarditis following First Dose of COVID-19 Vaccine (AstraZeneca)

Mohammed Alshaikh,[1] Abdullah Muharib ,[1] Radhi Alshehri,[1] Abdulaziz Alshoaibi,[1] Mohammed Qattea,[2] and Shahad AlOtaiby[3]

[1]*Medical Imaging, King Fahad Medical City, Central Second Health Cluster, Ministry of Health, Riyadh, Saudi Arabia*
[2]*King Salman Heart Center, King Fahad Medical City, Central Second Health Cluster, Ministry of Health, Riyadh, Saudi Arabia*
[3]*Research Center, King Fahad Medical City, Central Second Health Cluster, Ministry of Health, Riyadh, Saudi Arabia*

Correspondence should be addressed to Abdullah Muharib; amuharib@kfmc.med.sa

Academic Editor: Christopher Snyder

Background. Clinical trials of the COVID-19 vaccine reported the safety and efficacy of mRNA vaccines (AstraZeneca) to help control the disease. Few previous reports have shown various side effects associated with COVID-19 vaccines that vary in severity. The possibility of pericarditis and myocarditis has been observed in people who have received an mRNA COVID-19 vaccine which we are reporting. Acute inflammatory pericarditis can be a rare presentation after receiving the first dose of this vaccine, and it is enriching to share such rare presentations in the era of COVID-19 for better management and outcomes after vaccination. *Case Presentation.* This is a case of acute inflammatory pericarditis with a small pericardial effusion after receiving the first dose of AstraZeneca COVID-19 vaccine in a healthy adult patient who had no other symptoms suggestive of other viral illness in addition to the negative COVID-19 PCR. A 48-year-old healthy male presented nine days after receiving the first dose of COVID-19 AstraZeneca vaccine. The symptoms started three days after the vaccine, when he complained of progressive retrosternal chest pain with low-grade fever and generalized fatigue, followed by exertional dyspnea after a few days. The diagnosis of acute inflammatory pericarditis with small pericardial effusion was established, and the patient was accordingly treated. One week later, the patient showed significant clinical improvement with the resolution of his pericardial effusion. After 39 days, there was a significant radiological resolution of signs of acute pericarditis. *Conclusion.* The ongoing COVID-19 outbreak is still under investigation, and guidelines are regularly modified since we are continuously learning about this novel disease, although multiple vaccines have been shown to be effective against COVID-19. However, we report a case of unique clinical manifestation that has not been reported widely in the literature, after receiving the first dose of AstraZeneca COVID-19 vaccine, and that it may help raise awareness of the possible diagnosis and the possibility of inflammatory pericarditis after COVID-19 vaccination.

1. Introduction

The viral respiratory infection associated with the novel coronavirus disease (COVID-19) that firstly emerged in Wuhan in China in December 2019 has spread out rapidly among people worldwide [1]. This disease caused a global health crisis, and it has been confirmed as a pandemic and as a Public Health Emergency of International Concern (PHEIC) by the World Health Organization (WHO) [2]. A vaccination campaign against the SARS-CoV-2 virus is the only efficacious intervention to control the outbreak nationally and worldwide [3, 4]. The AstraZeneca vaccine is made up of the adenovirus- (Ad-) vectored AZD1222 (Covishield or Vaxzevria, ChAdOx1-S, Oxford-AstraZeneca) that has been reported to carry active immunization to prevent COVID-19 caused by SARS-CoV-2, in individuals ≥ 18 years old [5]. It has reported a rare side effect such as myocarditis/pericarditis after mRNA COVID-19 vaccines in adults, in several countries including the USA, Israel, UK, Canada, and Italy [6–8]. In this case, we are documenting a rare complication of Oxford-AstraZeneca vaccine which is acute pericarditis that occurs due to inflammation of the pericardium. Pericarditis can be attributed to several factors, including viral, bacterial, or fungal, or it can happen as an isolated condition or as part of a systemic disease [9]. Other possible causes of pericarditis include heart attack, cardiac surgical intervention, and other medical conditions related to injuries and medications. The complications of pericarditis include a spectrum of conditions that varies from mild symptoms like tachycardia to severe symptoms such as cardiac tamponade from the accumulated pericardial effusion [10].

2. Case Presentation

A 48-year-old male with an unremarkable medical history presented with retrosternal chest pain aggravated by lying supine and relieved in a sitting position. Also, he had a low-grade fever, fatigue, and exertional dyspnea. The low-grade fever was mildly improving when the patient took paracetamol. The chest pain started three days after he had received the first dose of the COVID-19 vaccine AstraZeneca. A written consent form was obtained from the patient before collecting any information about his medical condition.

Vital signs and physical examination were within normal limits. Initial laboratory workup including complete blood count, cardiac enzymes, liver function test, and renal function test was within normal limits including a negative COVID-19 PCR. However, the C-reactive protein and the erythrocyte sedimentation rate were elevated reaching 75 mg/L and 77 mm/h, respectively. In addition, the D-dimer test showed a high result reaching 1.44 mg/L. The patient's chest X-ray (Figure 1) showed faint left lower lung zone opacity. Further examination was done on the patient (CT pulmonary angiogram) to rule out pulmonary embolism. CT scan (Figure 2) shows pericardial thickening with surrounding fat stranding and small pericardial and left pleural effusions. After that, an echocardiogram was done (Figures 3 and 4) which showed a small pericardial effusion and pericardial thickening around the apex of the left and right ventricles. No echocardiographic signs of constriction were noted and no echocardiographic evidence of cardiac tamponade. An electrocardiogram (Figure 5) showed sinus rhythm and PR segment elevation in lead aVR. The patient's diagnosis of pericarditis was established due to the patient's symptoms and the relevant data. The initiated treatment plan included ibuprofen of 400 milligrams three times a day for 2 weeks and colchicine of 0.5 milligrams twice a day for 3 months.

3. Outcome and Follow-Up

The patient was seen after one week in the cardiology clinic where he showed significant clinical improvement, with the resolution of the chest pain and fever, with minor exertional dyspnea. A timely follow-up with the patient was set after 39 days of the treatment, where he showed total resolution of his symptoms except for mild dyspnea. An enhanced CT scan of the chest (Figure 6) showed marked interval improvement of the pericardial thickening with interval resolution of the pericardial and left pleural effusions. Also, an echocardiogram was done (Figure 7) showing interval improvement of the pericardial thickening with interval resolution of the pericardial effusion, and the C-reactive protein turned to the normal limit.

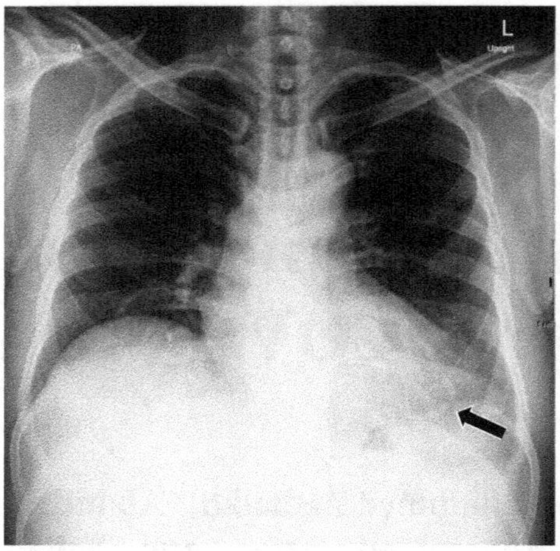

Figure 1: Upright PA chest X-ray showing faint opacity in the lower zone of the left lung.

4. Discussion

About 58 vaccines against severe acute respiratory syndrome coronavirus 2 (SARS-CoV-2) have been developed, and in clinical trials, one of them is the AstraZeneca vaccine. [11]. Once the vaccine was approved and put into use, vaccine safety was continuously monitored to identify any serious adverse events. The early safety monitoring of the AstraZeneca vaccine detected multiple postvaccination complications that include anaphylaxis, allergic reactions, thrombotic and embolic events, and immunothrombocytopenia [12, 13]. COVID-19 vaccine AstraZeneca has been studied and approved for its safety and efficacy in preventing severe disease and hospitalization IN 100% as well as preventing symptomatic COVID-19 in 76% and reaching 85% in people aged 65 years and older. The most common side effects of the vaccine are mild to moderate severity while the most serious ones are very rare making the benefits of the vaccine outweigh its risks [12].

The occurrence of pericarditis after immunization is extremely rare, and the number of cases of pericarditis reported after immunization to other vaccines such as influenza and hepatitis B virus is low [14]. On the other, hand when a patient presents with symptoms of acute chest pain to the hospital after receiving the AstraZeneca COVID-19 vaccine, this raises concern for the possibility of pericarditis. This can be further confirmed clinically by typical symptoms of acute pericarditis and reflected by elevation of C-reactive protein, erythrocyte sedimentation rate, D-Dimer, and ECG changes and may be complicated by pericardial effusion. A recent review shows COVID-19 vaccine-related

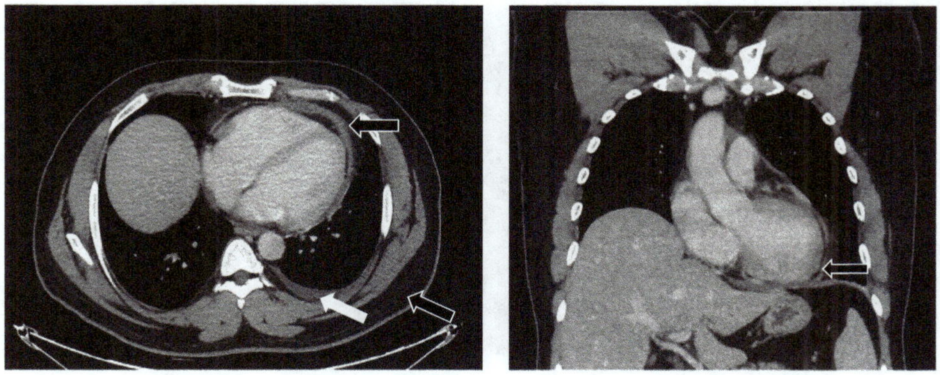

(a) (b)

FIGURE 2: (a) The axial image and (b) the coronal image of the CT scan of the chest post administration of IV contrast showing diffuse pericardial thickening and pericardial fat stranding (black arrow) with small left pleural effusion (white arrow).

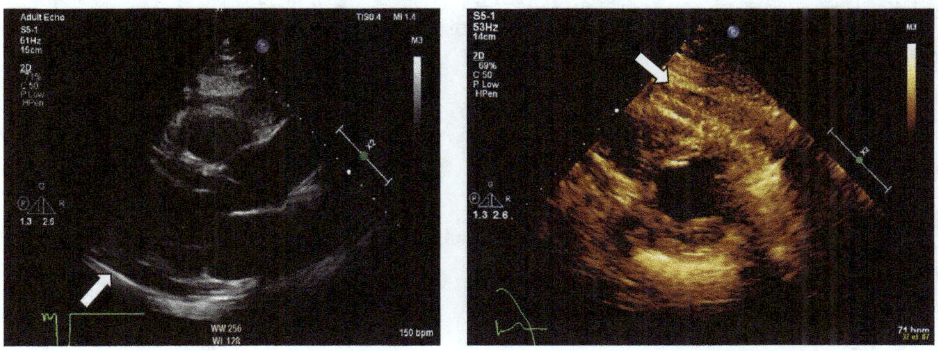

(a) (b)

FIGURE 3: Transthoracic echocardiogram in the long parasternal axis view (a) and short axis view (b).

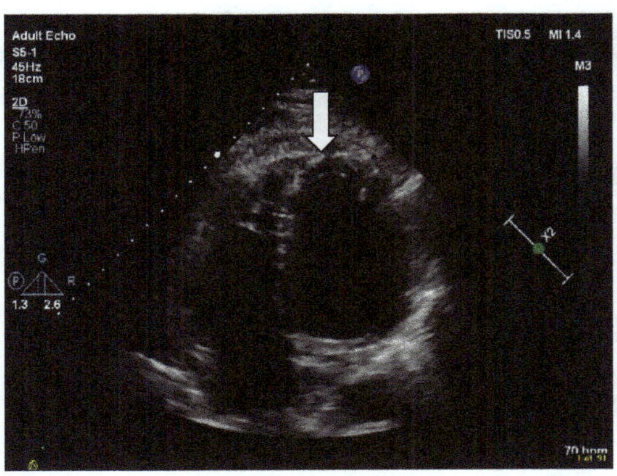

FIGURE 4: Apical 4 chamber views show pericardial thickening around the apex of left and right ventricles. White arrows; in addition to small pericardial effusion.

myocardial injury usually presents in young Caucasian males with a median age of 36 years, at 3–10 days postinjection [15]. In our case, symptoms occurred 3 days postvaccination, and the 48-year-old male who complained of continuous chest pain did not need to be hospitalized compared to a similar case in Taiwan [16].

The most common cause of pericarditis is a viral infection which could be direct or secondary immune-mediated. It has been suggested that vaccination may trigger an autoimmune response due to antigenic mimicry as well as due activation of quiescent autoreactive T and B cells [17]. Our case shows the importance of having an index with suspicion of pericarditis during the clinical assessment in any patient who presents with continuous chest pain, fever, and dyspnea a few days postvaccination. COVID-19 itself is associated with a substantially higher risk of myocarditis and other cardiac complications compared with vaccination, and primary infection should be ruled out as the first step before claiming the vaccine as a cause of the acute inflammatory condition. The negative PCR result of the COVID-19 virus and a dramatic improvement in ibuprofen and colchicine were enough to totally exclude COVID-19 infection and consider this acute pericarditis as a side effect of the vaccine, not a complication from COVID-19 infection.

It is difficult to confirm a definitive link between pericarditis and the COVID-19 vaccine; however, a link may exist which is supported by the fact that the patient is a previously healthy male without a previous history of the same symptoms. Additionally, several case reports suggest that COVID-19 infection, COVID-19 vaccine, and other vaccines may trigger an autoimmune reaction [18]. The

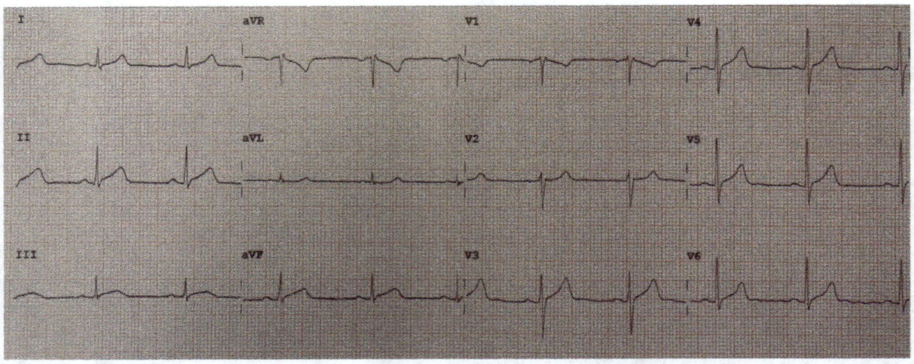

Figure 5: The patient's electrocardiogram showed sinus rhythm, with PR segment elevation in lead aVR (12 lead).

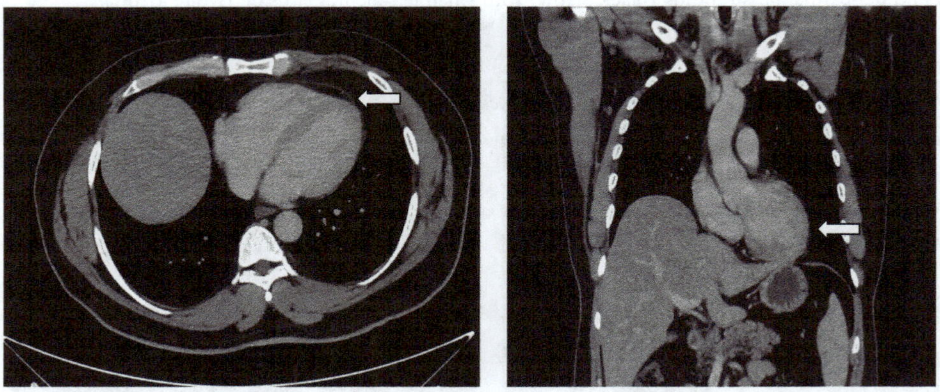

(a) (b)

Figure 6: Enhanced CT scan of the chest after a complete course of colchicine and ibuprofen showing improvement of the pericarditis evident by significant improvement of the pericardial thickening and resolution of the pericardial and left pleural effusions.

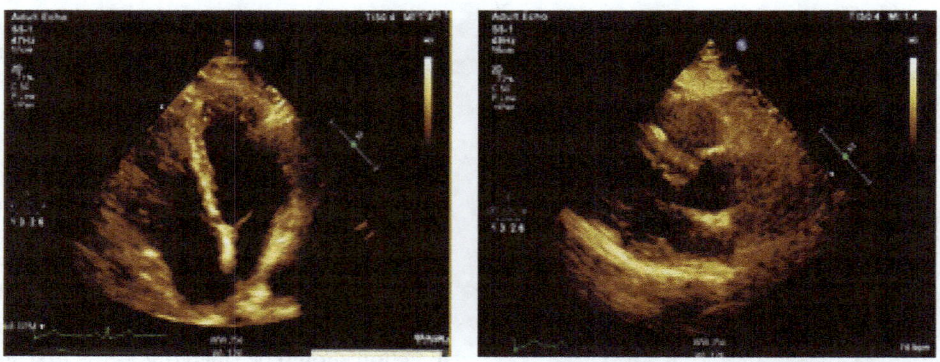

(a) (b)

Figure 7: (a) Selected image of transthoracic echocardiogram in apical 4 chamber view and (b) a parasternal long axis view showing marked interval improvement of the pericardial thickening with resolution of the pericardial effusion.

diagnosis can be established by history and physical examination in addition to the imaging features of pericarditis and pericardial effusion seen in the echocardiography and computed tomography. The appropriate management of this condition can be achieved by the standard treatment of noninfectious pericarditis utilizing Colchicine and nonsteroidal anti-inflammatory drugs. The symptoms are expected to be resolved within two weeks.

5. Conclusions

Although pericarditis is emerging as a potential rare adverse effect after COVID-19 vaccination (AstraZeneca), it is rare and the majority of cases of myocarditis/pericarditis reported after mRNA COVID-19 vaccines have occurred within 1-5 days (median 2 days) following the second dose. However, every effort should be made to diagnose early any crucial cardiac complication followed by the COVID-19 vaccination. Although the overall benefit-risk of the COVID-19 AstraZeneca vaccine remains positive, yet the healthcare provider needs to maintain a high index of cardiac symptoms to prevent further consequences.

Acknowledgments

The authors would like to thank the Research Centre, King Fahad Medical City, Riyadh, Saudi Arabia, for providing support in preparing this manuscript.

References

[1] World Health Organization (WHO), "Coronavirus," 2021, <https://www.who.int/health-topics/coronavirus#tab=tab_1>2.

[2] World Health Organization (WHO), "Coronavirus Disease (COVID-19) Situation Reports," 2021, https://www.who.int/emergencies/diseases/novel-coronavirus-2019/situation-reports.

[3] R. M. Magadmi and F. O. Kamel, "Beliefs and barriers associated with COVID-19 vaccination among the general population in Saudi Arabia," *BMC Public Health 21*, vol. 1438, no. 1, pp. 1–8, 2021.

[4] K. B. Megha, S. A. Nayar, and P. V. Mohanan, "Vaccine and vaccination as a part of human life: in view of COVID-19," *Biotechnology Journal*, vol. 17, article 2100188, 2021.

[5] European Medicines Agency, *AstraZeneca's COVID-19 vaccine: EMA finds possible link to very rare cases of unusual blood clots with low blood platelets*, 2021.

[6] J. Montgomery, M. Ryan, R. Engler et al., "Myocarditis following immunization with mRNA COVID-19 vaccines in members of the US military," *JAMA Cardiology*, vol. 6, no. 10, pp. 1202–1206, 2021.

[7] H. W. Kim, E. R. Jenista, D. C. Wendell et al., "Patients with acute myocarditis following mRNA COVID-19 vaccination," *JAMA Cardiology*, vol. 6, no. 10, pp. 1196–1201, 2021.

[8] C. M. Rosner, L. Genovese, B. N. Tehrani et al., "Myocarditis temporally associated with COVID-19 vaccination," *Circulation*, vol. 144, no. 6, pp. 502–505.

[9] J. G. Chiabrando, A. Bonaventura, A. Vecchié et al., "Management of acute and recurrent pericarditis:," *Journal of the American College of Cardiology*, vol. 75, no. 1, pp. 76–92, 2020.

[10] M. Noutsias, S. Pankuweit, and B. Maisch, "Chapter 56 Myocarditis, cardiac tamponade, and pericarditis," *The ESC Textbook of Intensive and Acute Cardiac Care*, 2011.

[11] M. D. Knoll and C. Wonodi, "Oxford-AstraZeneca COVID-19 vaccine efficacy," *The Lancet*, vol. 397, no. 10269, pp. 72–74, 2021.

[12] National Institutes of Health (NIH), "Phase III double-blind, placebo-controlled study of AZD1222 for the prevention of COVID-19 in adults," 2020, https://clinicaltrials.gov/ct2/show/study/NCT04516746.

[13] N. Barda, N. Dagan, Y. Ben-Shlomo et al., "Safety of the BNT162b2 mRNA Covid-19COVID-19 vaccine in a nationwide setting," *The New England Journal of Medicine*, vol. 385, no. 12, pp. 1078–1090, 2021.

[14] R. Mei, E. Raschi, E. Forcesi, I. Diemberger, F. De Ponti, and E. Poluzzi, "Myocarditis and pericarditis after immunization: gaining insights through the vVaccine adverse event reporting system," *International Journal of Cardiology*, vol. 273, pp. 183–186, 2018.

[15] G. A. Diaz, G. T. Parsons, S. K. Gering, A. R. Meier, I. V. Hutchinson, and A. Robicsek, "Myocarditis and pericarditis after vaccination for COVID-19," *JAMA*, vol. 326, no. 12, pp. 1210–1212, 2021.

[16] Y. P. Hung and K. S. Sun, "A case of myopericarditis with pleuritis following AstraZeneca COVID-19 vaccination," *QJM: An International Journal of Medicine*, vol. 114, no. 12, p. 879, 2021.

[17] D. C. Wraith, M. Goldman, and P. H. Lambert, "Vaccination and autoimmune disease: what is the evidence?," *The Lancet*, vol. 362, no. 9396, pp. 1659–1666, 2003.

[18] M. Radwi and S. Farsi, "A case report of acquired hemophilia following COVID-19 vaccine," *Journal of Thrombosis and Haemostasis*, vol. 19, no. 6, pp. 1515–1518, 2021.

31

Aortic Root Abscess with Aorta to Right Atrium Fistula due to Vancomycin-Intermediate Staphylococcus aureus (VISA)

Stephen J. Hankinson, Elliot A. Sultanik, and Gautam V. Ramani

Department of Medicine, Division of Cardiovascular Medicine, University of Maryland School of Medicine, Baltimore, Maryland 21201, USA

Correspondence should be addressed to Stephen J. Hankinson; shankinson@som.umaryland.edu

Academic Editor: Antonio de Padua Mansur

We present a case of root abscess with aorta to right atrium fistula due to vancomycin-intermediate Staphylococcus aureus (VISA) after limb amputation and cardiac surgery. Patient underwent redo aortic valve replacement, patch repair of aorta to right atrial fistula, and tricuspid valve repair with a ring. Fistula formation is a rare complication of prosthetic valve endocarditis (PVE). This is the first case to discuss aortocavitary fistula (ACF) formation due to VISA. Transesophageal echocardiogram (TEE) is the preferred imaging modality to diagnose ACF.

1. Introduction

The emergence of multidrug-resistant (MDR) organisms makes the medical management of endocarditis increasingly difficult. TEE is the preferred imaging modality to diagnose ACF. Surgical repair continues to be the definitive treatment option for ACF.

2. Case Presentation

Our patient is a 74-year-old man with a history of rheumatoid arthritis (on prednisone), left below the knee amputation (BKA), coronary artery bypass graft (CABG) with a saphenous vein graft to the right coronary artery (SVG to RCA), aortic valve replacement (AVR) with a bioprosthetic valve, and mitral valve replacement (MVR) with a bioprosthetic valve who presented with fever, chills, and generalized weakness after a prolonged course of vancomycin for methicillin-resistant Staphylococcus aureus (MRSA) bacteremia.

The patient was previously admitted for left foot MRSA osteomyelitis. During that hospitalization, the patient had a myocardial infarction. Source control obtained with BKA of the left leg and five days later subsequently underwent CABG (SVG to RCA), AVR for severe aortic stenosis (AS), and MVR for severe mitral regurgitation (MR). The patient was discharged with a six-week course of vancomycin; however, vancomycin course was extended due to BKA wound that required skin graft surgery. Eighty-eight days after cardiac surgery, the patient was readmitted for MRSA bacteremia attributed to cellulitis of the BKA stump vs. endocarditis. Transthoracic echocardiogram (TTE) at that time was negative for PVE. Patient was treated with a six-week course of vancomycin, and BKA stump cellulitis subsequently resolved. Five days after completing antibiotics, the patient presented with MRSA bacteremia, which progressed to VISA bacteremia with a vancomycin minimum inhibitory concentration (MIC) of 4 μg/mL (Table 1). The patient was started on daptomycin, ceftaroline, and rifampin for VISA bacteremia. TEE showed aortic root thickening suggestive of abscess with associated structural defect, a mobile 2.4 cm × 1.9 cm echodensity projecting into the right atrium (RA) (Figure 1(a)), and left to right shunting (Figure 1(b)).

The patient subsequently underwent cardiac surgery for redo AVR with a bovine pericardial tissue valve, patch repair of aorta to right atrial fistula with a bovine pericardial patching material from both the left ventricular side and right atrial side, and tricuspid valve repair with a ring. Postsurgery TTE demonstrated a normal left ventricle size and systolic

Table 1: Culture data during protracted use of vancomycin.

Type of culture	Date	Organism	Vancomycin MIC (μg/mL)
Left foot wound	11/10/2017	MRSA	≤0.5
Blood	2/27/2018	MRSA	1
Blood	4/16/2018	MRSA	2
Blood	4/26/2018	MRSA	4

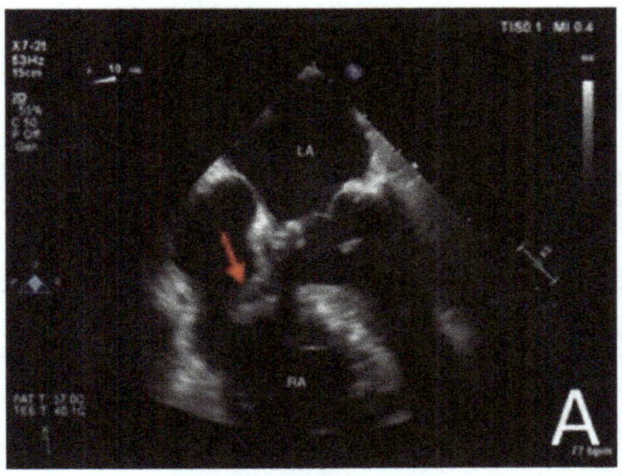

(a)

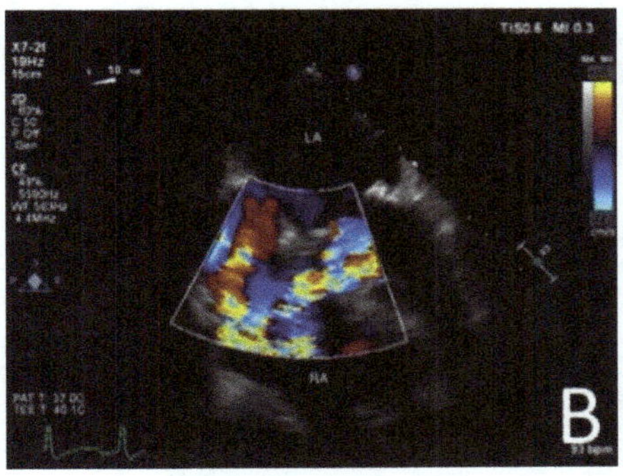

(b)

Figure 1: TEE demonstrates mobile echodensity (red arrow) measuring 2.4 cm × 1.9 cm in the RA associated with the wall of the atrium at the site of the suspected defect (a). TEE demonstrates atrioventricular defect and a systolic left to right shunt suggestive of aortic root abscess and erosion into the RA (b).

function, a normal right ventricle size and function, a bioprosthetic valve in aortic position (mean gradient 20 mmHg and peak gradient 45 mmHg) and no aortic regurgitation, and an annuloplasty ring indicative of tricuspid valve repair.

3. Discussion

This case discusses ACF formation as a complication of cardiac surgery shortly after limb amputation. PVE is a devastating complication of valve replacement with the prevalence being 4.1% at 4 years after primary valve replacement with the greatest risk occurring 1 to 2 months after surgery [1].

ACF is a rare condition caused by congenital abnormalities, aortic dissection, valve replacement, and infective endocarditis (IE) [2]. The pathogenesis of ACF related to infection is caused by extension and infiltration of abscesses related to endocarditis. Annular infection affects contiguous tissue leading to pyogenesis and tissue necrosis, which causes formation of an abscess cavity. As a result, the weakened necrotic myocardium may expand and rupture which may create intracardiac fistulous communications or even pericardial shunts [3]. Echocardiography can be used to identify the location of the lesion while angiography is often used to demonstrate the course of the lesion and define the surgical approach. Anguera et al. demonstrated that the detection of ACF for TTE and TEE is 53% and 97%, respectively [4]. TEE is the superior imaging technique because the flow across the fistula is highly turbulent and Doppler mapping can easily detect pressure differences between the aorta and cardiac chambers even when the fistulous orifice is small; therefore, TEE allows for the detection of almost all fistulas and allows the optimal characterization of each fistula tract. Additionally, TEE is superior to TTE in assessing valve function and morphology as well as delineating intracardiac pathology such as complications of endocarditis, namely, root abscess and fistulas. Furthermore, TEE has a better signal to the noise ratio and proximity of the transducer to the heart leading to higher quality images with lesser attenuation [5].

Our case is unique because it is the first case of ACF due to VISA. Our patient had extensive comorbidities prior to BKA including cardiac issues, sepsis, and steroid use, all of which have been shown to be predictors of increased mortality and postoperative complications within 30 days after BKA [6]. Given these comorbidities, perhaps a longer time course should have elapsed between the BKA in order to further optimize the patient prior to cardiac surgery. Overall, these comorbidities lead to a prolonged course of vancomycin, which resulted in the development of a MDR organism.

VISA and vancomycin-resistant S. aureus (VRSA) are relatively rare infections that occur in the setting of heavy prior use of glycopeptide antibiotics [7]. The Clinical Laboratory Standards Institute (CLSI) defines VISA as a vancomycin MIC of 4-8 μg/mL and VRSA as a vancomycin MIC of ≥16 μg/mL [8]. Vancomycin MIC ≥ 4 μg/mL is associated with vancomycin treatment failures in MRSA IE, which is a novel concept for this cohort [9]. MRSA resistance to vancomycin occurs through a variety of mechanisms including cell wall thickening, decreased autolysis, reduced production of cell surface protein A, increased capsule expressions, increased D-alanylation of teichoic acids, and reduced *agr* activity [8]. Given the prolonged course of vancomycin prior to the discovery of the ACF, it is difficult to identify whether the valve annulus was seeded during implantation of the valve or BKA stump cellulitis lead to hematogenous seeding of the valve.

4. Conclusion

Presented above was a case of a patient with an ACF due to VISA. This case demonstrated that protracted use of vancomycin resulted in VISA IE. Clinicians should exercise caution in patients with high bacterial load infections after prolonged antibiotic use. Infectious disease specialist consultation, change in antibiotic regimen, and aggressive surgical management are appropriate for the management of VISA IE.

References

[1] J. F. Sabik, B. W. Lytle, E. H. Blackstone, A. G. M. Marullo, G. B. Pettersson, and D. M. Cosgrove, "Aortic root replacement with cryopreserved allograft for prosthetic valve endocarditis," *The Annals of Thoracic Surgery*, vol. 74, no. 3, pp. 650–659, 2002, discussion 659.

[2] E. A. Fierro, R. R. Sikachi, A. Agrawal, I. Verma, M. Ojrzanowski, and S. Sahni, "Aorto-atrial fistulas: a contemporary review," *Cardiology in Review*, vol. 26, no. 3, pp. 137–144, 2018.

[3] N. Kang, S. Wan, C. S. Ng, and M. J. Underwood, "Periannular extension of infective endocarditis," *Annals of thoracic and cardiovascular surgery: official journal of the Association of Thoracic and Cardiovascular Surgeons of Asia*, vol. 15, no. 2, pp. 74–81, 2009.

[4] I. Anguera, J. M. Miro, I. Vilacosta et al., "Aorto-cavitary fistulous tract formation in infective endocarditis: clinical and echocardiographic features of 76 cases and risk factors for mortality," *European Heart Journal*, vol. 26, no. 3, pp. 288–297, 2005.

[5] K. Ananthasubramaniam, "Clinical and echocardiographic features of aorto-atrial fistulas," *Cardiovascular Ultrasound*, vol. 3, no. 1, 2005.

[6] P. J. Belmont Jr., S. Davey, J. D. Orr, L. M. Ochoa, J. O. Bader, and A. J. Schoenfeld, "Risk factors for 30-day postoperative complications and mortality after below-knee amputation: a study of 2,911 patients from the national surgical quality improvement program," *Journal of the American College of Surgeons*, vol. 213, no. 3, pp. 370–378, 2011.

[7] G. Chesi, A. Colli, C. A. Mestres, G. Gambarati, F. Boni, and T. Gherli, "Multiresistant-MRSA tricuspid valve infective endocarditis with ancient osteomyelitis locus," *BMC Infectious Diseases*, vol. 6, no. 1, 2006.

[8] B. P. Howden, J. K. Davies, P. D. Johnson, T. P. Stinear, and M. L. Grayson, "Reduced vancomycin susceptibility in Staphylococcus aureus, including vancomycin-intermediate and heterogeneous vancomycin-intermediate strains: resistance mechanisms, laboratory detection, and clinical implications," *Clinical Microbiology Reviews*, vol. 23, no. 1, pp. 99–139, 2010.

[9] A. M. Casapao, S. L. Davis, J. P. McRoberts et al., "Evaluation of vancomycin population susceptibility analysis profile as a predictor of outcomes for patients with infective endocarditis due to methicillin-resistant Staphylococcus aureus," *Antimicrobial Agents and Chemotherapy*, vol. 58, no. 8, pp. 4636–4641, 2014.

32

Idiopathic Chylopericardium in a Young Adult: Diagnosis and Management

João Pedro E. Sant'Ana,[1] **Amanda O. Vicente**,[1] **Amanda S. Pereira**,[1] **Pedro V. Bertozzi**,[1] **and Rodrigo A. S. Sardenberg**[2]

[1]*Advanced Research Center in Medicine, School of Medicine, União das Faculdades dos Grandes Lagos (UNILAGO), São José do Rio Preto SP, Brazil*
[2]*Thoracic Surgeon Hospital Alemão Oswaldo Cruz, Thoracic Surgery Departament, São Paulo (SP), Brazil*

Correspondence should be addressed to João Pedro E. Sant'Ana; joaosantana1199@gmail.com

Academic Editor: Antonio de Padua Mansur

Primary idiopathic chylopericardium (PIC) is an uncommon cardiologic disorder; it is defined as accumulation of lymph in the pericardial sac without any know precipitating factor. A 25-year-old presented with dyspnea and chest pain for over two months. The patient underwent a chest X-ray, which revealed an enlargement of cardiac silhouette and signs of cardiac tamponade. Chest CT was performed, revealing large pericardial effusion and small pleural effusion on the right hemithorax. The patient was referred to the ICU and underwent a pericardial window through VATS, which revealed 500 ml of a milky fluid.

1. Introduction

Primary idiopathic chylopericardium (PIC) is an uncommon cardiologic disorder, first reported by Hasebroek et al. in 1888 [1]. The term PIC was initially used by Groves and Effler in 1954, with a case of isolated lymph accumulation in the pericardium without any other evident cause [2]. Other secondary causes may occur, such as complications due to trauma, mediastinal tumors, lymphoma, cardiothoracic surgery, mediastinal tuberculosis, radiotherapy, and subclavian vein thrombosis [3]. Congenital lymphangiomatosis or lymphangiectasia may also be a cause of chylopericardium. There are relatively few published reports of PIC, and its pathogenesis remains unknown.

The present study reports a case of PIC in a 25-year-old female patient, who remained symptomatic for two months. Because of cardiac tamponade, she was treated successfully by surgical approach.

2. Case Report

A 25-year-old female patient was admitted to the emergency room complaining of dyspnea and chest pain, which persisted for the last two months. Upon physical examination on admission, the blood pressure was 120/80 mmHg and the pulse was at 100 bpm. The patient was alert, and there was no elevated jugular venous pressure, but she had muffled heart sounds and the lungs were clear on auscultation. Chest radiography presented enlargement of the cardiac silhouette (Figure 1), and electrocardiography showed low-voltage complexes. Transthoracic echocardiography demonstrated a large pericardial effusion and signs consistent with cardiac tamponade. Chest TC was performed, showing large pericardial effusion and small pleural effusion on the right hemithorax (Figure 2).

The patient was referred to the ICU and underwent a pericardial window through a right video-assisted

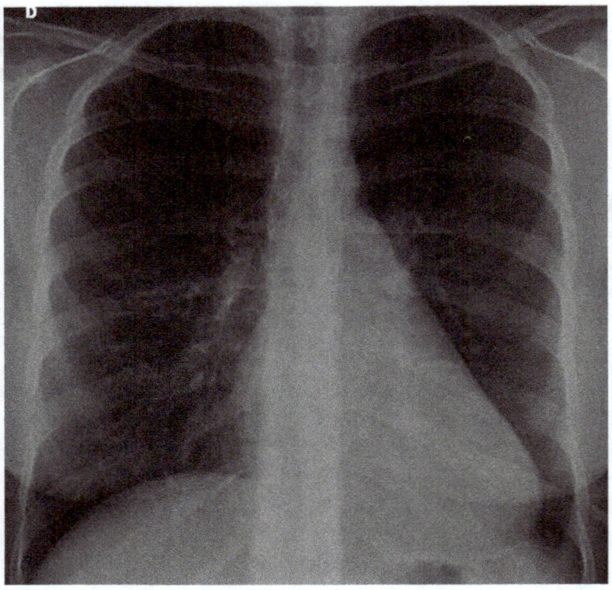

Figure 1: Chest X-ray showing enlargement of cardiac silhouette.

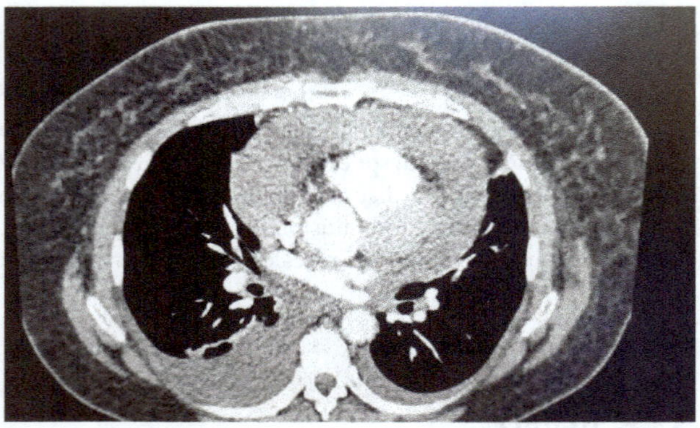

Figure 2: Chest TC showing pericardial effusion and pleural effusion on the right hemithorax.

thoracoscopy surgery (VATS) (Figure 3). Pericardial window showed 500 ml of a milky fluid. There were no pleural remarkable findings.

During hospital stay, lymphangioscintigraphy showed no abnormal findings. Pericardial fluid examination revealed a triglyceride level of 2050 mg/dl, total protein 5.6 g/l and glucose 154 mg/dl, all values consistent with chylopericardium. The postoperative course was uneventful; the chest tube was removed on day three, and the patient was discharged on day five. After one-year follow-up, the patient was in good condition and presented no signs of recurrence.

3. Discussion

Chylopericardium is defined as accumulation of lymph in the pericardial sac, a condition that occurs most frequently after cardiothoracic surgery and trauma or in association with tumors. The condition is defined as an idiopathic chylopericardium when it happens without any known precipitating factor [1, 2]. The pathogenesis might be explained by damage to the thoracic duct valves and increased permeability in the lymphatic vessels associated with elevated pressure in the thoracic duct or communication between the thoracic duct and pericardial lymphatics [2]. Besides the unclear pathophysiology, recent reports identified lymphatic leakage and communication with the pericardial sac, as explanations for the etiology of the disease [2, 3]. Until 2017, 104 cases were found in the literature and among these cases, approximately, 56% were idiopathic [4].

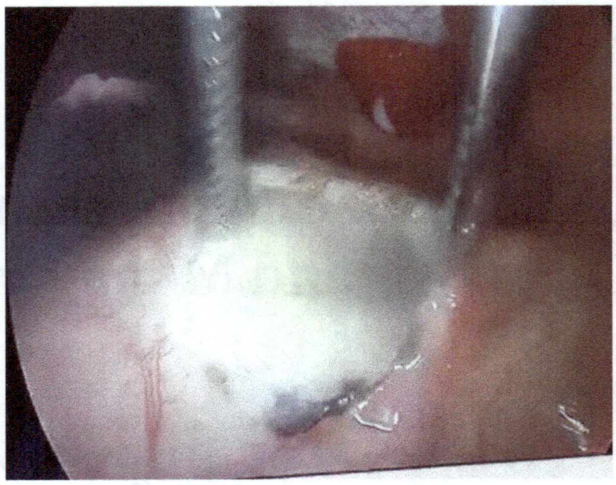

Figure 3: Pericardial window through VATS showing the presence of a milky fluid in the pericardium.

A normal pericardial space contains 25-30 ml of fluid [4]. In patients with chylopericardium, the fluid has a milky yellowish appearance, a cholesterol/triglyceride ratio < 1.0, triglycerides > 500 mg/dL, lymphocyte dominant fluid cell count, and negative fluid cultures [3]. Its suspect diagnosis is made mainly by imaging exams such as echocardiography, radiography, and chest CT, in addition to noninvasive techniques, such as scintigraphy with sestamibi-99mTc, a radiopharmaceutical with high cardiac absorption [3, 5]. It can also be confirmed by ingesting triglycerides or fatty acids radiologically labeled with 131I-triolein, glycerol, which acts on the lipid absorption mechanism [3, 6].

The disorder takes place in all ages and shows no sex-related variation [2, 3]. Clinical manifestations vary from asymptomatic patients, dyspnea, cough, and fatigue [2]. A recent review about the theme collected all reported cases in literature, and the most common symptoms were dyspnea (53.9%), cough (10.8%), and palpitation (9.62%). The second major part of the patients was asymptomatic (39.42%), and the most uncommon sign was edema (1.92%). On physical examination, 22.12% of the patients presented jugular venous distention and 32.69% presented muffled heart sound [3].

The ideal treatment for PIC is still uncertain; management options include diet therapy with medium-chain triglycerides, ligation of the thoracic duct, pericardiocentesis, and pericardial window. The surgical treatment should be prioritized, even in asymptomatic patients, to prevent the progression and exacerbation of the patient's clinical condition. Conservative treatment is usually not satisfactory and presents high failure rates; therefore, it should be considered when surgery is not a possibility [2].

4. Conclusion

Even though PIC is a rare condition, clinicians should keep in mind its possibility as a differential diagnosis. This condition requires a rapid evaluation to prevent complications and pericardial window, which, even when presenting risk of recurrence, is an effective and safe treatment option. In case of relapse of such condition, surgical ligation of thoracic duct should be considered.

References

[1] M. Itkin, N. M. Swe, S. E. Shapiro, and J. B. Shrager, "Spontaneous chylopericardium: delineation of the underlying anatomic pathology by CT lymphangiography," *The Annals of Thoracic Surgery*, vol. 87, no. 5, pp. 1595–1597, 2009.

[2] Z. Han, S. Li, H. Jing, and H. Liu, "Primary idiopathic chylopericardium: a retrospective case series," *BMC Surgery*, vol. 15, no. 1, p. 61, 2015.

[3] J. B. Kwon, S. Y. Choi, C. K. Kim, and C. B. Park, "Primary idiopathic silent chylopericardium," *Journal of Cardiothoracic Surgery*, vol. 8, no. 1, p. 28, 2013.

[4] X. Yu, N. Jia, S. Ye, M. Zhou, and D. Liu, "Primary chylopericardium: a case report and literature review," *Experimental and Therapeutic Medicine*, vol. 15, no. 1, pp. 419–425, 2017.

[5] P. C. M. Oliveira and A. M. Rocha, "Utilização de radiofármacos marcados com tecnécio 99m como potenciais marcadores na obtenção de imagens de perfusão miocárdica," *Arquivos de Ciências da Saúde da UNIPAR*, vol. 23, no. 3, pp. 221–226, 2019.

[6] T. Nakamoto, "Standard methods of 131I-triolein test and 131I-oleic acid test for lipid absorption study, and their clinical investigation," *Journal of the Japanese Society of Gastroenterology*, vol. 65, pp. 363–382, 2007.

33

Torsades de Pointes due to Excessive Marijuana Use in a Susceptible Patient

Vivek D. Shah[1] **Adeba Mohammad**[1] **Shuktika Nandkeolyar**[2] **Liset Stoletniy**[2] **and Tahmeed Contractor**[2]

[1]*Department of Internal Medicine, Loma Linda University Medical Center, CA, USA*
[2]*Department of Internal Medicine, Division of Cardiology, Loma Linda University Medical Center, CA, USA*

Correspondence should be addressed to Tahmeed Contractor; tcontractor@llu.edu

Academic Editor: Tong Liu

There are several recent reports of tetrahydrocannabinol vaping-related sudden cardiac arrest, and the mechanisms are unclear. We report a unique case of a 19-year-old female who suffered documented prolonged QTc leading to Torsades de pointes and cardiac arrest in the setting of frequent marijuana wax vaping. While she demonstrated normal baseline QTc measurements years earlier, she was found to have a genetic predisposition to QTc prolongation (genetic mutation, family history of prolonged QTc), suggesting that specific patient populations are at higher risk of these adverse events. The patient was acutely managed with isoproterenol to increase the heart rate and was discharged on nadolol after placement of an implantable cardioverter-defibrillator. Marijuana wax vaping and dabbing may cause fatal Torsades de pointes in susceptible patients, and further research is required to identify these patients a priori.

1. Introduction

In 2018, 3.9% of the global population from 15-64 years of age, or 192 million individuals, used tetrahydrocannabinol (THC), making it the most commonly used recreational drug [1]. This use has consistently increased since 2007 in young adults aged 18-25 with the advent of synthetic forms of cannabis [1]. These synthetic sources are up to 10 times more potent especially when consumed via wax vaping (dabbing), which involves the use of butane hash oil—made by extracting solely the hydrophobic components of marijuana plants. This form of cannabis is highly concentrated in THC (50%+) compared to the medicinal plant, which has a concentration of 4-8% [2]. With these shifts in the use and forms of THC come increasing evidence of associated adverse cardiac events including cardiac arrest, which may be related to prolongation of the QTc interval [3]. In this report, we discuss the case of a 19-year-old female who frequently used marijuana and suffered QTc prolongation-related ventricular fibrillation (VF) arrest at home followed by recurrent Torsades de pointes (Tdp) during hospitalization. Unique to her case is a normal QTc interval in the past, genetic mutation for long QT syndrome type 2 (LQTS2), and family history of sudden cardiac arrest as well as QTc prolongation. This case highlights the fact that certain individuals may be at risk of fatal arrhythmias with the use of recreational marijuana that is otherwise considered safe and legal in many states in the USA.

2. Case Presentation

2.1. Patient Information. A 19-year-old female with a family history of prolonged QTc and social history of frequent use of marijuana through dabbing had a witnessed episode of loss of consciousness. The family performed cardiopulmonary resuscitation for 20 minutes until emergency medical services arrived. The initial rhythm was VF (Figure 1(a)), and she was defibrillated with return of spontaneous circulation. She was intubated at the scene and transferred to our hospital. A detailed assessment of her family history revealed

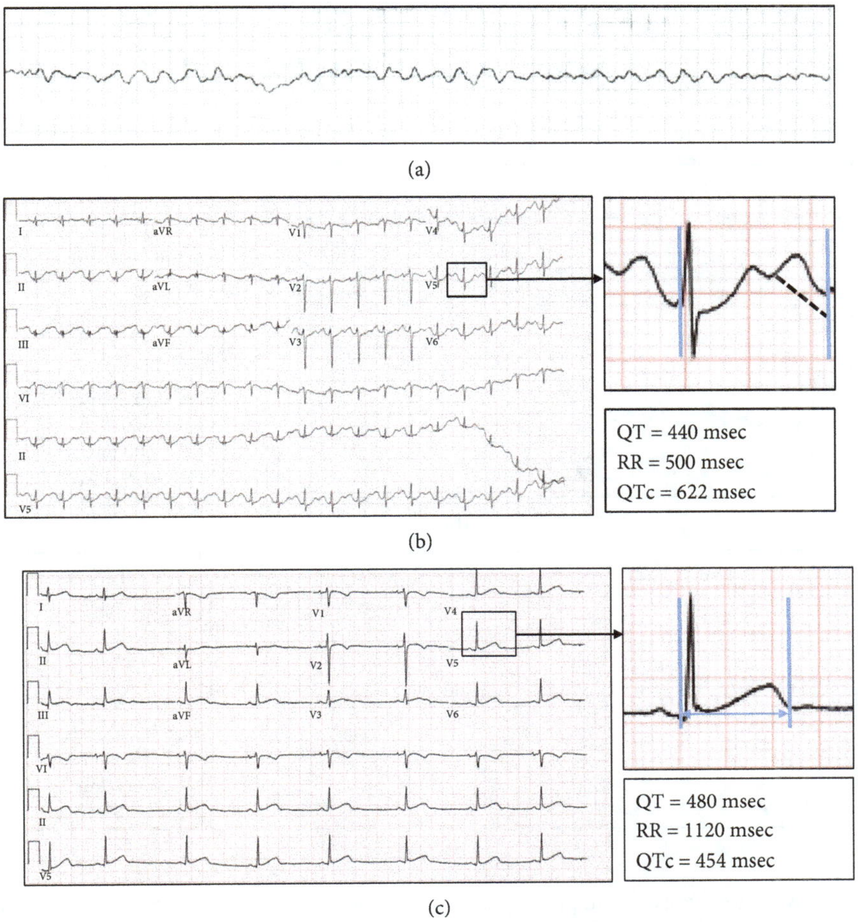

FIGURE 1: (a) Ventricular fibrillation detected by emergency medical services requiring defibrillation; (b) QTc measured in ECG obtained after correction of electrolyte abnormalities (measured by U-wave avoidance technique and calculated by the Bazett Formula: $QTc = QT/\sqrt{RR}$); (c) measurement of QTc from baseline ECG done several years prior.

sudden cardiac arrest in a 28-year-old maternal cousin. A maternal aunt died of cardiac arrest at age 65 years. The patient's mother and sister both had a history of prolonged QTc diagnosed on electrocardiogram (ECG) by each of their primary care physicians with no further work-up performed.

2.2. Clinical Findings. Upon arrival to the hospital, the initial physical exam was notable for a respiratory rate of 24 and heart rate of 114. She had mechanical breath sounds bilaterally.

2.3. Diagnostic Assessment. Our differential diagnosis for Tdp-related cardiac arrest included QTc prolongation (either from inherited arrhythmia syndromes or secondary causes such as drug ingestion and electrolyte derangements), Brugada syndrome, catecholaminergic polymorphic ventricular tachycardia (CPVT), and structural heart diseases such as arrhythmogenic right ventricular dysplasia (ARVD) or hypertrophic cardiomyopathy.

Initial labs demonstrated metabolic acidosis with pH 7.28; all electrolytes were within normal limits with a magnesium level of 1.2 (reference 0.7-1.1 mmol/L) and a potassium level of 3.7 (reference 3.5-5.0 mmol/L). Cardiac enzymes were obtained, revealing mildly elevated troponin T levels at 0.04 ng/mL (normal ≤ 0.03 ng/mL), which increased to a maximum of 0.96 ng/mL and then normalized. Toxicology work-up was negative for acetaminophen, salicylate, and prescription drug toxicity. Urine drug screen revealed cannabinoid use. ECG was obtained after correction of electrolyte abnormalities and showed prolonged QTc of 622 msec (Figure 1(b)). Notably, previous ECG on record from 5 years prior was normal with a QTc of 454 msec (Figure 1(c)). Initial echocardiogram revealed left ventricular ejection fraction (LVEF) of 25-30%.

2.4. Therapeutic Intervention. Hypothermia protocol was initiated, and the patient was admitted to the intensive care unit. Initial management included (1) intravenous calcium gluconate and magnesium for prolonged QTc, (2) propofol for sedation, and (3) amiodarone drip for prevention of recurrent ventricular arrhythmias.

We provided calcium carbonate and magnesium as treatments for this patient's arrhythmia before initial labs were available to ensure stabilization of the cardiac membranes and since hypocalcemia and hypomagnesemia are known risk factors for prolonged QTc and TdP [4, 5].

After admission, she had two episodes of Tdp, requiring cardioversion. Telemetry demonstrated persistently prolonged

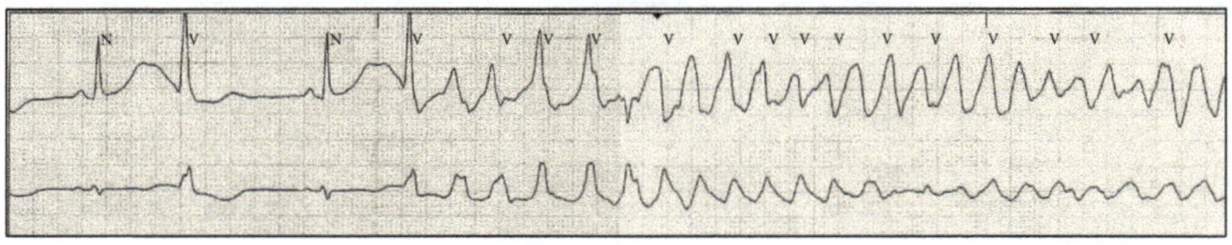

(a)

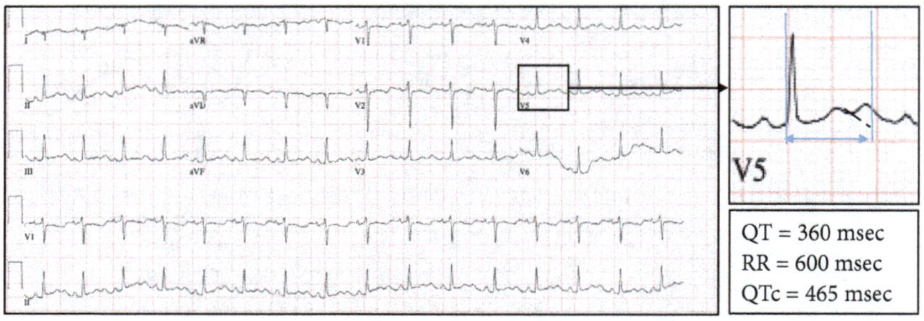

(b)

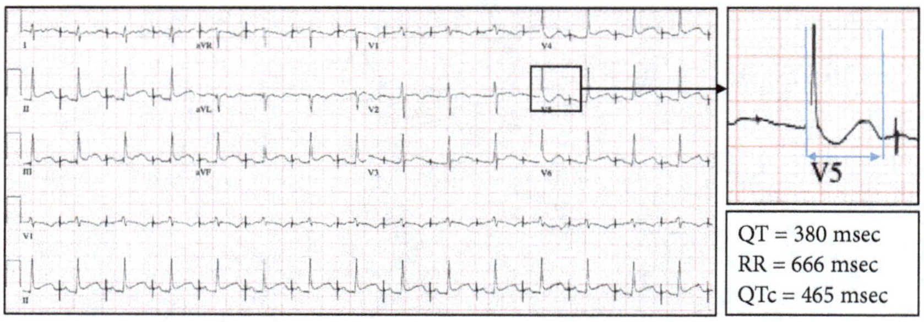

(c)

FIGURE 2: (a) Telemetry strip showing bradycardia with prolonged QTc and R-on-T premature ventricular contraction initiating Torsades de pointes; (b) ECG after starting isoproterenol drip with QTc reduction to 465 msec. (c) ECG showing atrial pacing after placement of dual-chamber ICD, with QTc of 465 msec, prior to starting nadolol.

QTc intervals and bradycardia with a subsequent R-on-T premature ventricular complex initiating these episodes (Figure 2(a)). Amiodarone drip was thus discontinued, and the patient was started on an isoproterenol drip with a decrease in QTc to 465 msec and resolution of ventricular arrhythmias (Figure 2(b)), and the patient was extubated in three days.

Cardiac magnetic resonance imaging (MRI) with delayed gadolinium was performed, which did not demonstrate any scar but did demonstrate a normalized LVEF, indicating that the initial echocardiographic changes were likely related to the cardiac arrest. While the prolonged QTc and the resultant TdP could have been "reversible" from marijuana use, the propensity of the patient to develop future episodes with other QTc-prolonging medications/triggers, especially with significant family history, was discussed. In a shared decision-making process with the patient and her family, it was decided to proceed with dual-chamber implantable cardioverter-defibrillator (ICD). At the time of discharge, she was atrially paced at 90 BPM (Figure 2(c)) and started on nadolol 40 mg twice daily.

The patient underwent genetic testing for long QT syndromes, which revealed a variant of unknown significance in KCNH2 (exon 10 c.2407_2409del (p.Asp803del)). Gene KCNH2 (also known as hERG) has been implicated in LQTS2; however, the specific variant seen in this patient has yet to be reported as associated with risk for LQTS. She was also noted to have mutations in PKP2, which is associated with ARVD, and TRDN, which is associated with CPVT. The normal MRI and QTc prolongation-related VF episodes did not support a clinical diagnosis of ARVD or CPVT.

2.5. Follow-Up and Outcomes. At the three-month follow-up, the patient had no further episodes of Tdp, and interrogation of ICD revealed no recurrence of ventricular arrhythmias. Her atrial pacing rate was dropped to 70 beats per minute, with QTc found at 463 msec. Echocardiogram performed at the three-month follow-up reveals an ejection fraction of 65%.

3. Discussion

THC has been associated with different types of ventricular arrhythmias, including VF from QTc prolongation or Brugada syndrome and monomorphic VT attributed to ischemia [3, 6, 7]. This case highlights the importance of pharmacogenomics in the pathophysiology of arrhythmia associated with the relatively common practice of THC dabbing. In this patient with a normal QTc interval as a child,

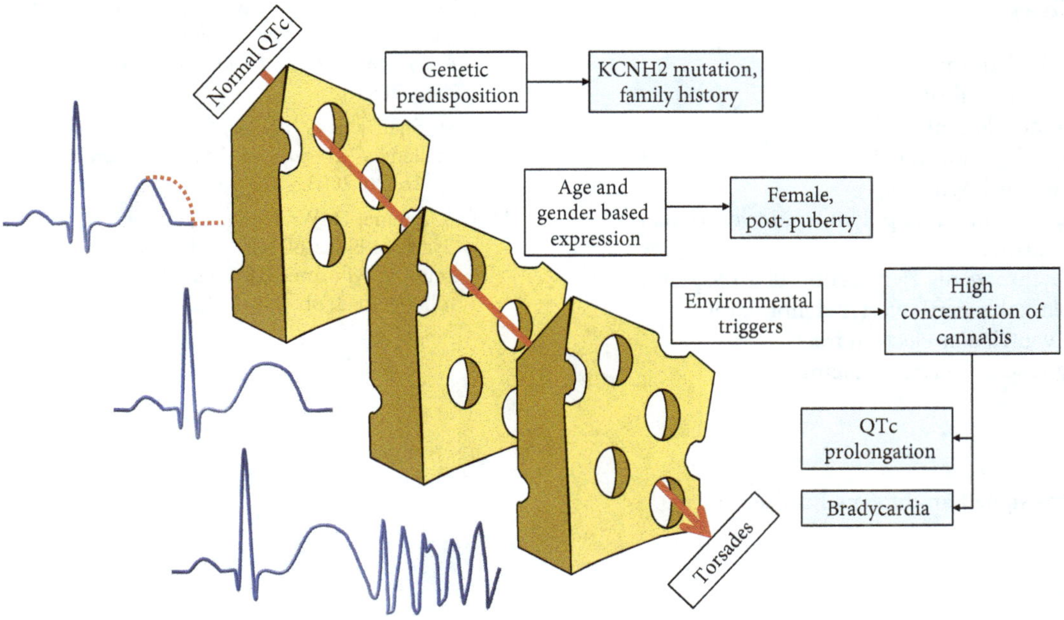

FIGURE 3: Representation of "the perfect storm" that led up to Tdp and cardiac arrest. Normal QTc several years ago was likely secondary to lack of age/gender-based expression. However, when postpubertal and in the presence of a potent environmental trigger, she developed QTc prolongation and bradycardia resulting in Tdp and cardiac arrest.

the combination of (1) genetic predisposition (family history, genetic mutation), (2) being a postpubertal female, and (3) consumption of high-concentration THC products provided the "perfect storm" for Tdp [8] (Figure 3). THC can cause Tdp via 2 mechanisms: (1) chronic THC results in increased parasympathetic and reduced sympathetic activity, with resultant bradycardia that predisposes to further prolongation of QTc and early after depolarizations [9], and (2) use of marijuana has been associated with long QTc via inhibition of the delayed rectifier potassium channel (coded for by hERG gene) [10, 11], through a mechanism similar to LQTS2 [12]. Genetic testing in this patient revealed a mutation in genes coding the same ion channels associated with THC-induced QTc prolongation.

The management of THC vaping or dabbing-related Tdp remains unclear. As in other cases of prolonged QTc-mediated TdP, increasing the heart rate with isoproterenol may provide a temporary solution. As a nonspecific β_1/β_2-adrenoceptor agonist, isoproterenol increases the heart rate, thus shortening the QTc interval and refractory period [5]. Long-term management requires a shared process of decision-making regarding consideration of ICD, in conjunction with pharmacologic therapies. Beta blockers, such as nadolol, may reduce recurrence of ventricular arrhythmias, with the postulated mechanism being a combination of reduction in dispersion of repolarization across the myocardium, decrease in after depolarizations, and in some cases a shortened QTc [13]. In addition, nadolol blocks late Na-currents (i.e., I_{Na} that continue to flow during the action potential plateau) that then shortens the repolarization phase [14]. In the absence of any other obvious triggers, we also recommend such patients abstain from further use of marijuana products and any other potential QTc-prolonging products including certain medications.

4. Conclusions

There are an increasing number of cases reporting sudden cardiac arrest related to THC use, and the mechanisms are unclear (3). In the setting of genetic propensity for QTc prolongation, THC dabbing, which results in high concentrations of the compound, may be a potent trigger of TdP due to a combination of sympathetic suppression by a high concentration of THC, and QTc prolongation, even in the setting of a baseline normal QTc interval. Genetic testing may assist in identifying patients at the highest risk of arrhythmia, initially screened with appropriate family history. Acute treatment involves temporary shortening of QTc interval through nonspecific beta agonists such as isoproterenol. Long-term management may involve the use of nonspecific beta blockers, shared decision-making to determine appropriateness of ICD, and avoidance of QTc-prolonging triggers.

5. Patient Perspective

The patient had limited recollection of her hospitalization course; however, she has expressed her gratitude regarding her hospital and postdischarge care. She reports that after her experience, she has stopped using cannabis and has made drastic changes to her lifestyle including exercise and diet changes. As a result of her hospitalization, her sister has stopped using cannabis and has inspired her peers to also refrain from using it. Her mother and sister visited their primary care physicians and were found to have prolonged QTc on screening ECGs. They were instructed to avoid QT-prolonging drugs but have not performed genetic testing yet.

Abbreviations

THC: Tetrahydrocannabinol
VF: Ventricular fibrillation
Tdp: Torsades de pointes
LQTS2: Long QT syndrome 2
ECG: Electrocardiogram
CPVT: Catecholaminergic polymorphic ventricular tachycardia
ARVD: Arrhythmogenic right ventricular dysplasia
ICD: Implantable cardioverter-defibrillator
LVEF: Left ventricular ejection fraction
MRI: Magnetic resonance imaging.

Consent

The patient has signed an informed consent form.

References

[1] UNODC, "World Drug Report Drug Use and Health Consequences," 2020, http://www.unodc.org/wdr2020.

[2] I. Al-Zouabi, J. M. Stogner, B. L. Miller, and E. S. Lane, "Butane hash oil and dabbing: insights into use, amateur production techniques, and potential harm mitigation," *Substance Abuse and Rehabilitation*, vol. Volume 9, pp. 91–101, 2018.

[3] T. Ahmed, A. Khan, V. Y. See, and S. Robinson, "Cardiac arrest associated with synthetic cannabinoid use and acquired prolonged QTc interval: a case report and review of literature," *HeartRhythm Case Reports*, vol. 6, no. 5, pp. 283–286, 2020.

[4] N. K. Eryol, R. Çolak, Özdoğru et al., "Effects of calcium treatment on QT interval and QT dispersion in hypocalcemia," *The American Journal of Cardiology*, vol. 91, no. 6, pp. 750–752, 2003.

[5] S. H. Thomas and E. R. Behr, "Pharmacological treatment of acquired QT prolongation and torsades de pointes," *British Journal of Clinical Pharmacology*, vol. 81, no. 3, pp. 420–427, 2016.

[6] P. J. Sampat, S. Riaz, M. Bisen, and R. Carhart, "An Unusual Case of Ventricular Tachycardia in a Young Patient Associated with Cannabis Use," *Case reports in Cardiology*, vol. 2020, 4 pages, 2020.

[7] P. Kariyanna, P. Wengrofsky, A. Jayarangaiah et al., "Marijuana and cardiac arrhythmias: a scoping study," *International journal of clinical research & trials*, vol. 4, no. 1, p. 132, 2019.

[8] T. Sedlak, C. Shufelt, C. Iribarren, and M. CNB, "Sex hormones and the QT interval: a review," *Journal of Women's Health*, vol. 21, no. 9, pp. 933–941, 2012.

[9] H. Goyal, H. H. Awad, and J. K. Ghali, "Role of cannabis in cardiovascular disorders," *Journal of Thoracic Disease*, vol. 9, no. 7, pp. 2079–2092, 2017.

[10] K. Ramphul and J. Joynauth, "Cardiac arrhythmias among teenagers using Cannabis in the United States," *The American Journal of Cardiology*, vol. 124, no. 12, p. 1966, 2019.

[11] J. Yun, K. S. Yoon, T. H. Lee et al., "Synthetic cannabinoid, JWH-030, induces QT prolongation through hERG channel inhibition," *Toxicology Research*, vol. 5, no. 6, pp. 1663–1671, 2016.

[12] W. Shimizu, A. J. Moss, A. A. Wilde et al., "Genotype-phenotype aspects of type 2 long QT syndrome," *Journal of the American College of Cardiology*, vol. 54, no. 22, pp. 2052–2062, 2009.

[13] M. Shah and C. Carter, "Long QT syndrome: a therapeutic challenge," *Annals of Pediatric Cardiology*, vol. 1, no. 1, pp. 18–26, 2008.

[14] A. Besana, D. W. Wang, A. L. George Jr., and P. J. Schwartz, "Nadolol block of Nav1.5 does not explain its efficacy in the long QT syndrome," *Journal of Cardiovascular Pharmacology*, vol. 59, no. 3, pp. 249–253, 2012.

A Case of Severe Tricuspid Regurgitation Related to Traumatic Papillary Muscle Rupture

Ruchika Meel,[1] Bongane Ngutshane,[2] Ricardo Gonçalves,[3] and Shungu Mogaladi[2]

[1]*Department of Internal Medicine, Division of Cardiology, Chris Hani Baragwanath Hospital, University of the Witwatersrand, Johannesburg, South Africa*
[2]*Department of General Surgery, Division of Cardio-Thoracic Surgery, Charlotte Maxeke Hospital, University of the Witwatersrand, Johannesburg, South Africa*
[3]*Olivedale Hospital, Johannesburg, South Africa*

Correspondence should be addressed to Ruchika Meel; ruchikameel@gmail.com

Academic Editor: Man-Hong Jim

A 25-year-old male presented after a motor vehicle accident with tricuspid valve (TV) regurgitation, due to a flail TV secondary to papillary muscle rupture. We highlight the importance of three-dimensional echocardiographic imaging of the tricuspid valve and its utility in aiding a successful surgical repair.

1. Introduction

The majority of injuries to the tricuspid valve (TV) apparatus are related to blunt chest trauma [1]. Motor vehicle accidents (MVA) are a common cause of blunt trauma to the heart. It is unusual for the TV to be involved in isolation [2–4]. The aortic valve is most commonly involved, followed by the mitral valve and finally the TV. The postulated mechanism of injury to the TV in these cases tends to be a rapid deceleration force combined with an increase in intracardiac right chamber pressures [5]. In a vast number of cases of MVA, cardiac injury tends to be overlooked due to other overt injuries [6]. Injury to the TV can be silent depending on the severity of structural damage [7]. Therefore, some authors have advocated routine and timeous use of echocardiography in patients sustaining blunt trauma to the chest [6]. The advent of newer echocardiographic techniques such as three-dimensional (3D) imaging acts as a supplementary tool in characterising the precise location of injury to the TV [8].

2. Case Presentation

A 25-year-old healthy male presented to a peripheral hospital in Johannesburg, South Africa, after an MVA. He was an unrestrained passenger who hit the car dashboard after sudden deceleration from high speed. He sustained multiple injuries including bilateral hemopneumothoraxes. An admission transthoracic echocardiogram (TTE) revealed severe TR of unclear mechanism.

He was referred 2 weeks after the index admission to a tertiary hospital. On arrival, he was asymptomatic and haemodynamically stable. He had abrasion marks on the chest (Figure 1). Cardiovascular examination revealed prominent internal jugular vein c-v waves and a soft grade 2/6 pansystolic murmur at the left lower parasternal border. He was not in heart failure. Sinus tachycardia and an early repolarisation pattern were noted on the 12-lead electrocardiogram. He had normal laboratory blood parameters. On TTE, a moderately enlarged right ventricle (RV) and right atrium, with preserved RV systolic function, was noted. There was a flail TV leaflet and an oscillating mass in the right atrium (Figure 2(a)). Avulsion of the anterior papillary muscle from the RV wall was suspected. The colour flow Doppler revealed severe TR with an early peaking triangular jet velocity of 2.16 m/sec (Figures 2(b) and 3(a)). There was systolic flow reversal in the hepatic veins (Figure 3(b)). A 3D transoesophageal echocardiogram (TEE) was performed which confirmed a flail anterior TV leaflet due to rupture of the

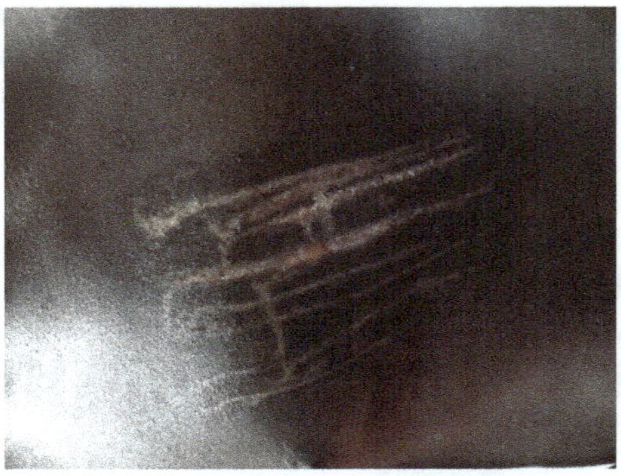

FIGURE 1: Abrasion marks on the anterior chest wall secondary to blunt chest trauma.

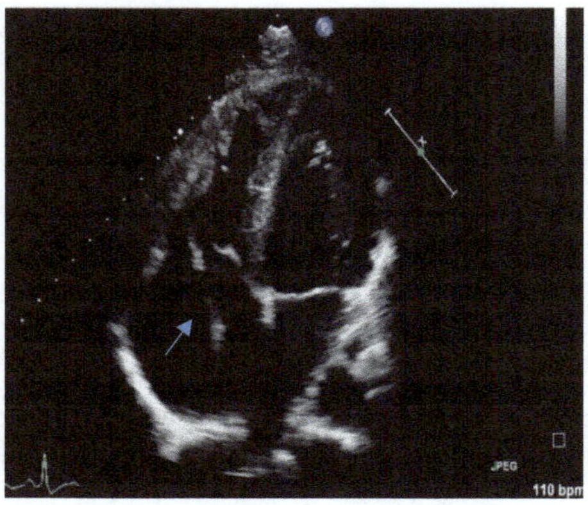

(a)

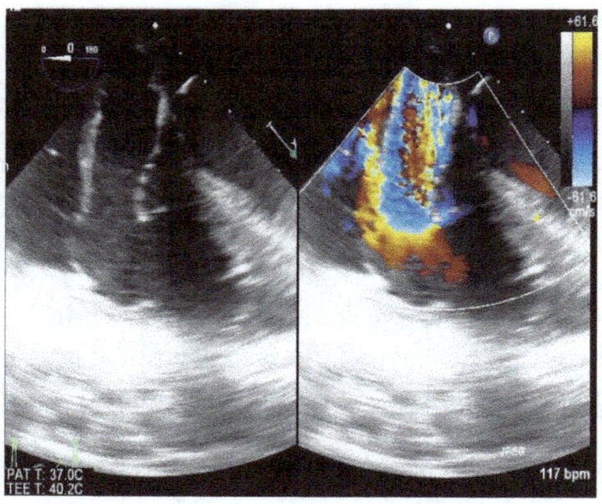

(b)

FIGURE 2: (a) Transthoracic apical 4-chamber echocardiographic view showing flail anterior tricuspid valve leaflet (arrow) and (b) transoesophageal right ventricle long axis views depicting severe tricuspid valve regurgitation.

anterior papillary muscle (Figures 4(a), 5(a), and 5(b)). On 3D colour flow, the TR was severe, with the jet filling greater than 50% of the right atrium (Figure 4(b)).

The patient underwent a successful surgical repair of the TV (Figure 6). A flail anterior TV leaflet due to anterior papillary muscle rupture was identified with a residual papillary muscle stump on the RV. The anterior papillary muscle was reattached to the stump with pledgeted 4-0 polypropylene sutures. Additionally, a modified De Vega annuloplasty was done. Finally, the valve competency was tested by saline

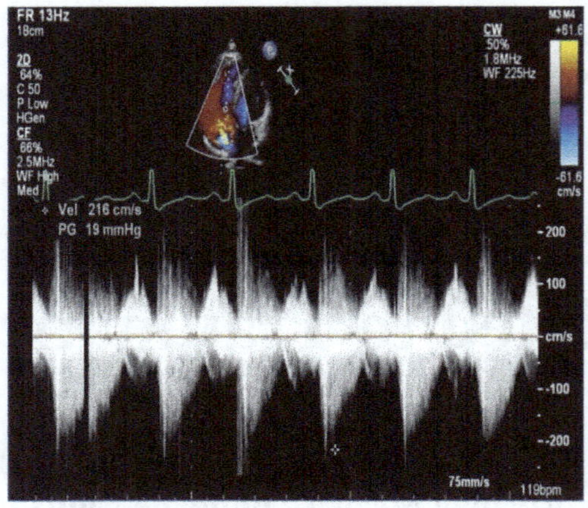

(a)

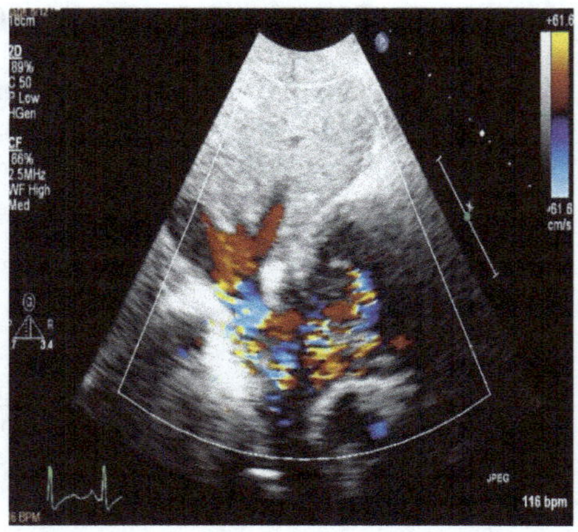

(b)

FIGURE 3: (a) Continuous wave Doppler through the tricuspid valve in 4-chamber view showing an early peaking triangular tricuspid regurgitation velocity. (b) A subcostal view showing hepatic vein systolic flow reversal due to severe tricuspid valve regurgitation on colour flow imaging.

injection into the RV and confirmed by TEE after coming off cardiopulmonary bypass. Trivial TR was noted. The patient had an uneventful postoperative course.

3. Discussion

Our case brings attention to the following pertinent aspects related to traumatic tricuspid valve insufficiency: (1) underreporting of TV injury in Africa and the importance of meticulous screening for TV injury in patients with history of blunt chest trauma; (2) the value of three-dimensional imaging of the TV prior to surgical referral; and (3) early referral for surgery of patients with severe TR due to TV injury.

Motor vehicle accidents are an important cause of TV injury [9, 10]. South Africa has one of the highest motor vehicle accident-related fatalities [11, 12]. Yet, there is a paucity of data regarding TV trauma related to MVA. This is possibly due to TV injuries being missed in a polytrauma patient, lack of resources in terms of imaging in low- and middle-income countries, or underutilisation of existing imaging modalities due to a lack of expertise. Additionally, the true prevalence of TV regurgitation due

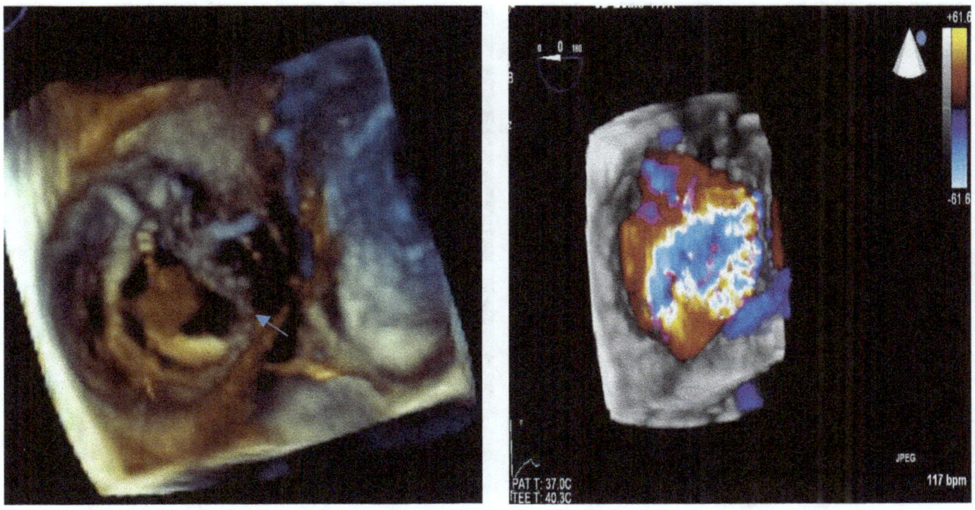

(a) (b)

FIGURE 4: (a) Three-dimensional view of the tricuspid valve from the right atrial aspect showing flail anterior tricuspid valve leaflet and ruptured papillary muscle (arrow) and (b) three-dimensional colour imaging showing severe tricuspid regurgitation into the right atrium.

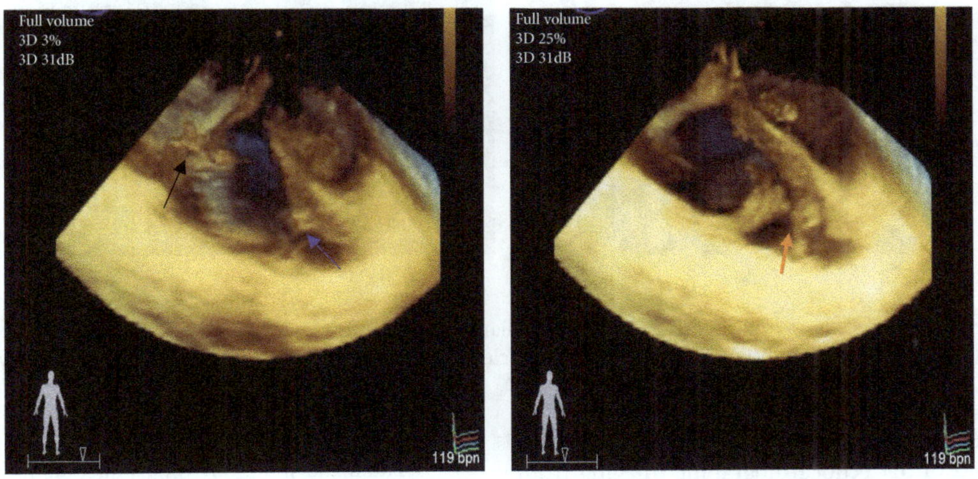

(a) (b)

FIGURE 5: Three-dimensional transoesophageal views of the right ventricle showing the attachment point of the anterior papillary muscle ((a) blue and (b) orange arrows) and flail anterior tricuspid leaflet with ruptured papillary muscle ((a) black arrow).

to trauma is underreported as patients experience minimal or no symptoms for a prolonged period of time [13]. TTE is a useful bedside tool for assessing cardiac structure and function in a trauma patient [14]. It is freely available at most institutions, noninvasive, inexpensive, and radiation- and contrast-free [15]. It has been validated as a useful tool for right heart, TV, and subvalvular apparatus assessment. Transoesophageal echocardiography (TEE) can be utilised in cases where TTE provides insufficient information for decision making[14]. However, TEE is not widely available and needs specialized expertise.

Recently, more attention has been focused on 3-dimensional imaging of the TV [16]. It allows "enface" views of the valve and thus easy discrimination of the 3 TV leaflets. Accurate anatomical information aided in planning this TV repair by identifying the exact site anterior papillary muscle rupture. The literature suggests a lower success rate for surgical repair when the mechanism for TV regurgitation is not papillary muscle rupture [13]. In the current era of 3D imaging, successful TV repair for TR due to papillary muscle rupture has been reported [17].

A surgeon with sufficient skill and experience in repairing tricuspid valves is crucial, and all imaging is complementary to direct anatomical inspection. Early referral of patients with severe TR is advised to prevent right ventricular dysfunction from chronic volume overload [13]. It has been noted that if the operation is delayed, valve repair becomes more challenging due to the development of fibrosis of the valve and subvalvular apparatus [18]. For these reasons, early surgical referral was preferred and led to a successful outcome. Follow-up of the patient is important as TR may recur.

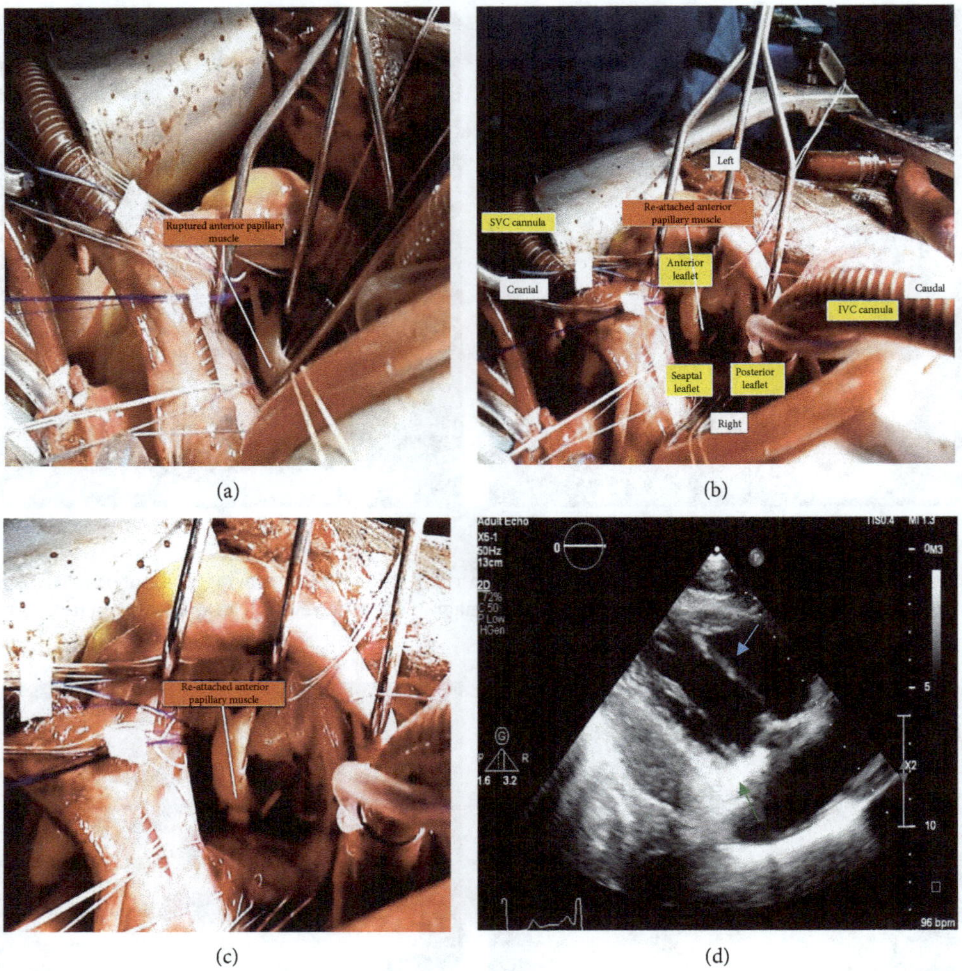

FIGURE 6: (a–c) Intraoperative images of ruptured anterior papillary muscle and its repair and (d) transthoracic postoperative right ventricular inflow view showing the repaired anterior papillary muscle (blue arrow) and annuloplasty ring (orange arrow).

In conclusion, we have presented a case of successful TV repair with the aid of 3D echocardiographic imaging from Africa. We hope that this case will stimulate readers to actively search for and report on TV-related injury in a patient with a history of chest trauma.

Acknowledgments

The first author is the recipient of postdoctoral Carnegie fellowship award.

References

[1] G. Avegliano, M. Corneli, D. Conde, and R. Ronderos, "Traumatic rupture of the tricuspid valve and multi-modality imaging," *Cardiovascular diagnosis and therapy*, vol. 4, no. 5, pp. 401–405, 2014.

[2] L. F. Parmley, W. C. Manion, and T. W. Mattingly, "Nonpenetrating traumatic injury of the heart," *Circulation*, vol. 18, no. 3, pp. 371–396, 1958.

[3] A. Cordovil, C. H. Fischer, A. C. T. Rodrigues et al., "Papillary muscle rupture after blunt chest trauma," *Journal of the American Society of Echocardiography*, vol. 19, no. 4, pp. 469.e1–469.e3, 2006.

[4] M. Pasquier, C. Sierro, B. Yersin, D. Delay, and P. N. Carron, "Traumatic mitral valve injury after blunt chest trauma: a case report and review of the literature," *The Journal of Trauma*, vol. 68, no. 1, pp. 243–246, 2010.

[5] S. Sbar and E. E. Harrison, *Chronic tricuspid insufficiency due to trauma. The Heart: Update III*, McGraw-Hill, New York, 1980.

[6] S. Khurana, R. Puri, D. Wong et al., "Latent tricuspid valve rupture after motor vehicle accident and routine echocardiography in all chest-wall traumas," *Texas Heart Institute Journal*, vol. 36, no. 6, pp. 615–617, 2009.

[7] B. Stoica, S. Paun, I. Tanase, I. Negoi, A. Runcanu, and M. Beuran, "Traumatic Tricuspid Valve Rupture after Blunt Chest Trauma - A case Report and Review of the Literature," *Chirurgia*, vol. 110, no. 5, pp. 467–470, 2015.

[8] I. Stankovic, A. M. Daraban, R. Jasaityte, A. N. Neskovic, P. Claus, and J. U. Voigt, "Incremental value of the en face view of the tricuspid valve by two-dimensional and three-dimensional echocardiography for accurate identification of tricuspid valve leaflets," *Journal of the American Society of Echocardiography*, vol. 27, no. 4, pp. 376–384, 2014.

[9] G. Dounis, E. Matsakas, J. Poularas, K. Papakonstantinou, A. Kalogeromitros, and A. Karabinis, "Traumatic tricuspid insufficiency: a case report with a review of the literature,"

European Journal of Emergency Medicine, vol. 9, no. 3, pp. 258–261, 2002.

[10] C. L. Jiang, T. X. Gu, Z. W. Zhang, and Z. Y. Xiu, "Diagnosis and treatment of traumatic tricuspid valve insufficiency," *Chinese Journal of Traumatology*, vol. 6, no. 6, pp. 379–381, 2003.

[11] N. B. Moodley, C. Aldous, and D. L. Clarke, "An audit of trauma-related mortality in a provincial capital in South Africa," *South African Journal of Surgery*, vol. 52, no. 4, pp. 101–104, 2014.

[12] "Accident crash statistics - arrive alive," February 2019, https://www.arrivealive.mobi/accident-crash-statistics.

[13] F. Maisano et al., "Valve repair for traumatic tricuspid regurgitation," *European Journal of Cardio-Thoracic Surgery*, vol. 10, no. 10, pp. 867–873, 1996.

[14] S. J. Co, C. J. Yong-Hing, S. Galea-Soler et al., "Role of imaging in penetrating and blunt traumatic injury to the heart," *Radiographics*, vol. 31, no. 4, pp. E101–E115, 2011.

[15] A. Kossaify, "Echocardiographic assessment of the right ventricle, from the conventional approach to speckle tracking and three-dimensional imaging, and insights into the "right way" to explore the forgotten chamber," *Clinical Medicine Insights: Cardiology*, vol. 9, pp. 65–75, 2015.

[16] D. Muraru, R. T. Hahn, O. I. Soliman, F. F. Faletra, C. Basso, and L. P. Badano, "3-dimensional echocardiography in imaging the tricuspid valve," *JACC: Cardiovascular Imaging*, vol. 12, no. 3, pp. 500–515, 2019.

[17] K. Nishimura, H. Okayama, K. Inoue et al., "Visualization of traumatic tricuspid insufficiency by three-dimensional echocardiography," *Journal of Cardiology*, vol. 55, no. 1, pp. 143–146, 2010.

[18] J. A. M. van Son, G. K. Danielson, H. V. Schaff, and F. A. Miller Jr., "Traumatic tricuspid valve insufficiency: Experience in thirteen patients," *The Journal of Thoracic and Cardiovascular Surgery*, vol. 108, no. 5, pp. 893–898, 1994.

35

Infectious Aortitis with Abdominal Aortic Aneurysm in a 47-Year-Old Female with Systemic Lupus Erythematosus

Valerie R. Ramiro ,[1] Carmegie C. Saliba,[2] John Anthony D. Tindoc,[3] Marinette R. Jambaro,[4] Enrique M. Chua III,[5] Donna Ricca M. Hornilla,[1] and Maria Teresa B. Abola[1]

[1]*Section of Cardiology, University of the Philippines–Philippine General Hospital, Manila, Philippines*
[2]*Department of Medicine, University of the Philippines–Philippine General Hospital, Manila, Philippines*
[3]*Department of Pathology, University of the Philippines–Philippine General Hospital, Manila, Philippines*
[4]*Section of Rheumatology, University of the Philippines–Philippine General Hospital, Manila, Philippines*
[5]*Section of Thoracic Cardiovascular Surgery, University of the Philippines–Philippine General Hospital, Manila, Philippines*

Correspondence should be addressed to Valerie R. Ramiro; vrramiro@yahoo.com

Academic Editor: Hajime Kataoka

Aortic aneurysms are not commonly reported among patients with systemic lupus erythematosus (SLE). We report a case of a 47-year-old Filipino female diagnosed with SLE 17 years ago maintained on prolonged oral steroids, azathioprine, and hydroxychloroquine. She also had lupus nephritis, secondary hypertension, and dyslipidemia. She initially presented with a week-long watery nonbloody diarrhea with associated diffuse crampy abdominal pain and generalized weakness. She was admitted for a week at a provincial hospital and was given an unrecalled antibiotic with resolution of symptoms. Upon discharge, however, she experienced two weeks of severe right lower quadrant pain radiating to the back and left lower quadrant, with no history of diarrhea, vomiting, dysuria, and fever. Complete blood count showed slight leukocytosis and elevated C-reactive protein. Abdominal imaging revealed a saccular infrarenal aneurysm with dissection. An atherosclerotic mechanism was primarily considered, but a vasculitic process was likewise considered due to elevated acute phase reactants. The initial plan was Endovascular Aneurysm Repair (EVAR) but due to financial limitations, an exploratory laparotomy with infrarenal endoaneurysmorrhaphy was eventually performed. Intraoperative findings were a saccular infrarenal aneurysm with dissection up to the proximal right common iliac artery and an abscess compartment within the false lumen in the anterior aortic wall. Abscess culture yielded high growth of *Salmonella* group B. Micrographs of the aortic wall biopsy showed fibrin deposition necrosis and calcification with peripheral viable cellular infiltrates consisting of neutrophils and foamy macrophages. Inadvertently placing an endovascular graft in an infected aortic aneurysm would have led to graft infection and catastrophic morbidity. We highlight the significance of having a high index of suspicion for infectious causes of aortitis among immunocompromised patients presenting with aneurysm prior to pursuing an endovascular versus an open approach for repair.

1. Introduction

Systemic lupus erythematosus (SLE) is an autoimmune disease with a multifaceted pathophysiology and multiorgan involvement. Cardiovascular disease is a major cause of morbidity and mortality complicating SLE [1]. However, diseases of the aorta, particularly aneurysms and dissections, among SLE patients are uncommonly reported [2].

2. Case

We report a case of a 47-year-old Filipino female diagnosed with SLE 17 years ago maintained on prolonged oral prednisone 10 mg/day, azathioprine, and hydroxychloroquine. She also had chronic kidney disease from lupus nephritis, secondary hypertension, and dyslipidemia. She was a nonsmoker.

She initially presented with a week-long watery nonbloody diarrhea with associated diffuse crampy abdominal pain and generalized weakness. There was no fever nor vomiting. She was admitted for a week at a provincial hospital and was given an unrecalled antibiotic with resolution of symptoms. Upon discharge, however, she experienced severe right lower quadrant pain radiating to the back and left lower quadrant for two weeks, with no history of diarrhea, vomiting, dysuria, and fever. She was readmitted at the provincial hospital where diagnostics revealed anemia and urinary tract infection, for which she was transfused with packed red blood cell units and given unrecalled intravenous antibiotics, respectively. Blood cultures were initially negative. Abdominal imaging revealed bilateral renal parenchymal disease and an infrarenal aortic aneurysm. Appendicitis was ruled out by symptomatology and imaging. She was then transferred to our institution for surgical repair of the aneurysm.

During her admission at the surgical ward, antihypertensive medications were titrated to keep her blood pressures less than 120/80. Prednisone was given at 1 mg/kg/day. Hydroxychloroquine 200 mg OD, mycophenolate mofetil 500 mg BID, and atorvastatin 40 mg OD were continued. She continued to have intermittent abdominal pain. There was no fever, overt bleeding, dysuria, or recurrence of diarrhea. Complete blood count showed slight leukocytosis, and the C-reactive protein was elevated. A computed tomography (CT) aortogram revealed an infrarenal aneurysm with signs of dissection and retroperitoneal hematoma formation, indicative of leakage (see Figures 1–3). Given the absence of fever and no signs of ongoing infection, antibiotics were not yet started. An atherosclerotic mechanism was primarily considered, but a vasculitic process was likewise considered due to elevated acute phase reactants.

The initial plan was Endovascular Aneurysm Repair (EVAR) but due to financial limitations, an exploratory laparotomy with infrarenal endoaneurysmorrhaphy was eventually performed. Intraoperative findings were a saccular infrarenal aneurysm with dissection up to the proximal right common iliac artery and an abscess compartment, with an aspirated volume of approximately 5 mL, within the false lumen in the anterior aortic wall. The entire infected aneurysmal segment was resected, and piperacillin-tazobactam was immediately started. Abscess culture yielded a high growth of *Salmonella* group B. Guided by the sensitivity pattern, the antibiotic was shifted to Ceftriaxone. This was continued after discharge as outpatient parenteral antibiotic therapy to complete 6 weeks then a lifetime of chronic suppressive therapy with trimethoprim-sulfamethoxazole (TMP-SMX) 160/800 mg OD. Syphilis and HIV screening were both negative. Micrographs of the aortic wall biopsy showed fibrin deposition necrosis and calcification with

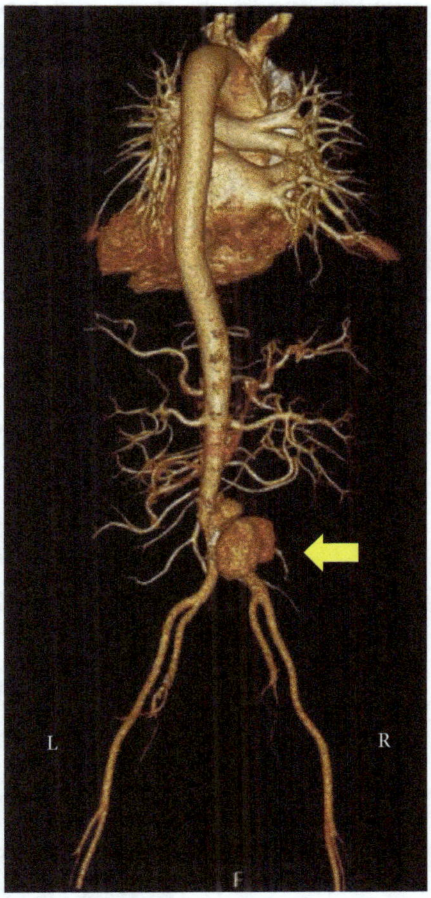

FIGURE 1: This is a 3-dimensional reconstruction of the CT aortogram, with the arrow indicating the saccular component of the aneurysm.

peripheral viable cellular infiltrates consisting of neutrophils and foamy macrophages consistent with an atherosclerotic process (see Figures 4–6). Given the histopathologic findings that favored aortitis rather than vasculitis, steroids were tapered down gradually. Aspirin was started postoperatively. Atorvastatin and antihypertensive medications were continued. She was discharged after 2 weeks and followed up regularly at the outpatient clinic.

3. Discussion

The etiology of SLE remains unknown but is likely multifactorial from genetic, immunologic, and environmental mechanisms. It occurs more commonly among women of reproductive age. The prevalence rate in the United States is around 20 to 150 per 100,000 women [3]. Among Asian countries, the prevalence rate falls within 30-50/100,000 people [4]. Aortic involvement has been found among many rheumatologic conditions and may present with a plethora of clinical manifestations [5]. Aortic diseases in SLE are not commonly reported. However, a case-control study found that SLE patients have a higher proportion of aortic aneurysms compared with age- and sex-matched controls, with an odds ratio of 4.5 [6].

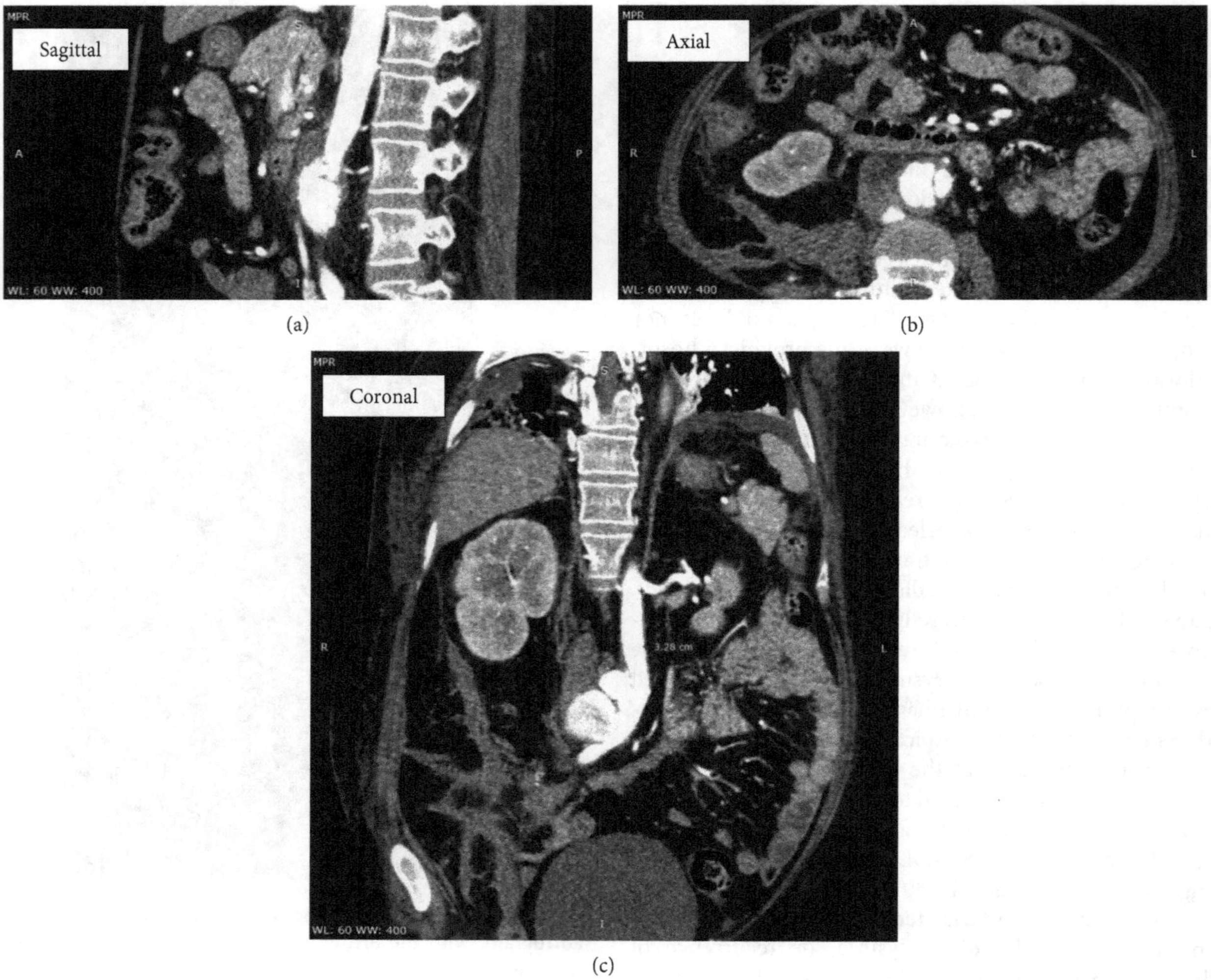

FIGURE 2: Multiplanar images demonstrating the infrarenal abdominal aorta. The dissection is seen arising 3.3 cm distal to the take-off of the left renal artery and extending to the iliac bifurcation, with an involved length of 7 cm.

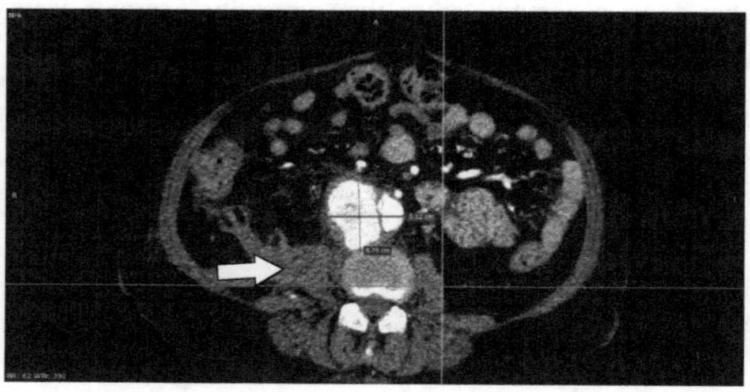

FIGURE 3: This is an axial view at the level of L4, demonstrating the saccular aneurysm at its maximal caliber of 5.1 × 4.8 cm (W × AP). An intimal flap is seen along the right lateral aspect of this dilatation. The saccular component of the aneurysm arises from the false lumen and is oriented anterolaterally to the right. No definite perivascular contrast extravasation is appreciated indicating that the point of rupture has likely been walled off. A heterogenous, predominantly hypodense fluid collection exhibiting minimal peripheral enhancement is appreciated at the right retroperitoneum, probably subacute hematoma (arrow).

Several pathophysiologic hypotheses have been purported to explain the occurrence of aortic aneurysms in SLE. Popular theories include an autoimmune process, such as vasculitis with associated medial degeneration, or an atherosclerotic process due to longstanding steroid use, hypertension, and dyslipidemia [2, 7]. Transforming growth factor $\beta 1$ (TGF-$\beta 1$) is a suppressor of vascular wall inflammation as well as inhibitor of smooth muscle proliferation; type I interferon is associated with impaired endothelial function. Downregulation of TGF-$\beta 1$ and activation of interferons in SLE have been suggested as immunologic mechanisms contributing to arterial wall dysfunction [6]. A meta-analysis conducted by Kurata and colleagues in 2011 examined the pathophysiological relationship of certain clinical and histopathologic findings to the formation of aortic aneurysms in SLE. They included 35 cases reported over the past 40 years of SLE with aortic aneurysms, including those complicated by dissection. The study found that aortic involvement in SLE affected relatively younger individuals, with an average age of 44.5 years, and that the thoracic aorta was more commonly involved. This is contrary to aneurysms found in the general population which are usually discovered in the sixth decade of life and more commonly affecting the

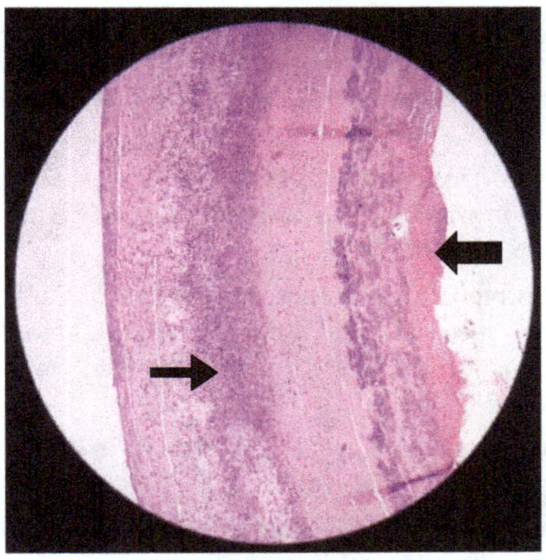

FIGURE 4: This is a section of the vascular wall adjacent to the main thrombus. Neutrophilic infiltrates (thin arrow) can be appreciated within the layers of the wall. At the intimal side, there is fibrin deposition (thick arrow) indicating an endothelial state favorable towards coagulation.

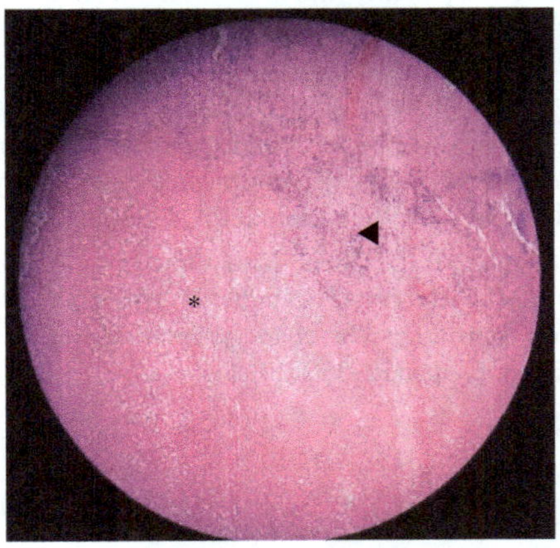

FIGURE 5: This is a section taken from the main thrombus showing heavy deposition of eosinophilic fibrin material (∗) with entrapped erythrocytes and inflammatory cells (◀).

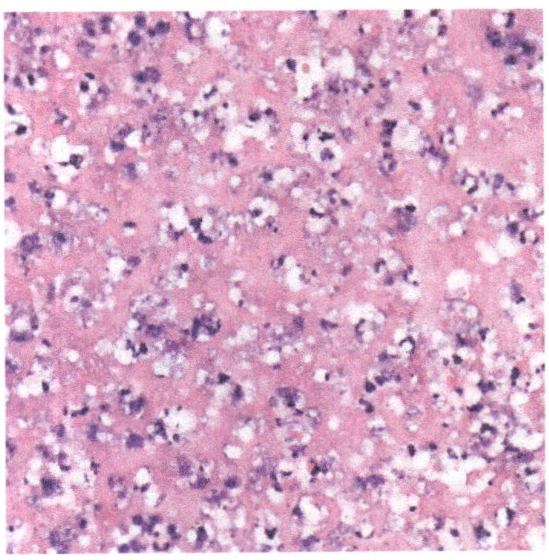

FIGURE 6: At the periphery of the thrombus with viable cellular material, clusters of foamy macrophages or foam cells can be seen.

abdominal rather than the thoracic segments. Correlation analysis led the authors to outline two distinct pathways of aortic aneurysm formation in SLE. Thoracic aortic aneurysms were not linked with atherosclerosis but were positively correlated with vasculitis, cystic medial degeneration, dissection, and higher mortality rate. Abdominal aortic aneurysms on the other hand showed positive correlation with atherosclerosis associated with prolonged steroid treatment and with better prognosis [2].

Aortitis, the pathologic term for inflammation of the aorta, is broadly subdivided into noninfectious and infectious aortitis. The majority of aortitis cases are noninfectious and include large-vessel vasculitides and other rheumatologic conditions. Infectious aortitis are less common [8]. A normal aorta is normally not prone to infection. However, damage to the aortic wall, such as in cases of atherosclerotic disease, aneurysm, cystic medial degeneration, endothelial damage from diabetes, medical devices, or surgery, makes it weak and vulnerable to infection. Microorganisms can seed hematogenously via the vasa vasorum, contiguously from the adjacent infected tissues, or by traumatic or iatrogenic means. Commonly implicated pathogens include *Salmonella*, *Staphylococcal*, and *Streptococcus* species. Tuberculous aortitis is infrequent in the developed countries [7, 8]. However, due to the high prevalence of tuberculous infections in our country, it is still relevant to include a tuberculous etiology in the differentials. According to a cross-sectional study in 2012, *Staphylococcus aureus* and *Salmonella* species are the most common pathogens (40%), with *Salmonella* as the most prevalent in abdominal aortitis, native aorta, and mycotic aneurysms [9]. Majority of adult cases inflicted with nontyphoid salmonellosis are group B (38%), then followed by group D (30%) and group C (23%) [10]. The known risk factors for invasive *Salmonella* infections are achlorhydria (i.e., intake of proton pump inhibitors) and immunosuppression (i.e., chronic steroids, immunocompromised host, and HIV infection). A minimum of three weeks post source control up to 6-12 weeks is recommended for endovascular infection. And chronic suppressive therapy is advised for patients with infected prosthetic materials, biliary tract abnormalities, and people living with HIV with nontyphoidal bacteremia, low CD4 counts, or those poorly responding to antiretroviral therapy. TMP-SMX 160/800 mg OD, levofloxacin 500 mg OD, or ciprofloxacin 500-750 mg OD can be given indefinitely [11].

In our patient's case, evidence of inflammation was demonstrated in the histopathologic sections of the excised aorta. The infiltrates were predominantly neutrophilic with foam cells thereby favoring an atherosclerotic over a vasculitic pathophysiology of the aneurysm. This is in contrast with the primarily lymphocytic inflammatory pattern of SLE vasculitis [12]. We can therefore surmise that our patient's chronic SLE, coupled with the long-term steroid use, contributed to accelerated atherosclerosis and eventual aneurysm formation. This became a nidus for bacterial infiltration and proliferation, which in turn, may have further perpetuated aneurysmal growth and dissection. We hypothesize that the initial diarrhea of our patient may be due to inadequately treated *Salmonella*, with bacterial seeding on the abdominal aneurysm causing aortitis and the abscess formation. SLE patients have increased susceptibility to *Salmonella* presumably due to defective lymphocyte function, impaired effector cells (e.g., macrophage, monocytes, and granulocytes), and depletion of C3 opsonizing activity [13]. Our patient did not present with classic signs and symptoms of infection because she has been chronically maintained on multiple immunosuppressive agents to control SLE activity. The open repair allowed for gross inspection and discovery of the small pocket of abscess which was missed on the CT aortogram. It also allowed us to obtain biopsies and better understand the underlying disease process of aneurysm formation.

4. Conclusion

Aortic complications are uncommon manifestations of SLE. These can be caused by vasculitis, atherosclerosis, infection, or a combination of these mechanisms. We highlight the significance of having a high index of suspicion for infectious causes of aortitis among immunocompromised patients presenting with aneurysm prior to pursuing an endovascular versus an open approach for repair. Inadvertently placing an endovascular graft in an infected aortic aneurysm would have led to graft infection and catastrophic morbidity.

Disclosure

This case report has been presented in the following conferences: first place, oral presentation, Case Report Category, Philippine Heart Association 49th Annual Convention, May 2018; oral presentation, Case Report Category, Korean Society of Cardiology 62nd Annual Scientific Meeting, October 2018; oral presentation, Case Report Category, Philippine General Hospital Department of Medicine Research Forum, November 2018; poster presentation, Asian Pacific Society of Cardiology Congress, Taipei, Taiwan, May 2018; and poster presentation, 20th Asia Pacific League of Associations for Rheumatology Congress, Kaohsiung, Taiwan, September 2018.

References

[1] L. O. C. Mocarzel, P. G. Lanzieri, R. A. Montes, R. A. O. C. Gismondi, and C. T. Mesquita, "Systemic lupus erythematosus: review of cardiovascular aspects," *Internacional Journal of Cardiovascular Sciences*, vol. 28, no. 3, pp. 251–261, 2015.

[2] A. Kurata, T. Kawakami, J. Sato, A. Sakamoto, T. Muramatsu, and K. Nakabayashi, "Aortic aneurysms in systemic lupus erythematosus: a meta-analysis of 35 cases in the literature and two different pathogeneses," *Cardiovascular Pathology*, vol. 20, no. 1, pp. e1–e7, 2011.

[3] B. H. Hahn, "Systemic lupus erythematosus," in *Harrison's Principles of Internal Medicine*, D. L. Longo, A. S. Fauci, D. L. Kasper, S. L. Hauser, J. L. Jameson, and J. Loscalzo, Eds., vol. 18e, p. 2124, McGraw-Hill, New York, NY, USA, 2012.

[4] E. Salido and H. Reyes, "Epidemiology of systemic lupus erythematosus in Asia," *Lupus*, vol. 19, no. 12, pp. 1365–1373, 2010.

[5] G. Slobodin, J. E. Naschitz, E. Zuckerman et al., "Aortic involvement in rheumatic diseases," *Clinical and Experimental Rheumatology*, vol. 24, no. 2, Supplement 41, pp. S41–S47, 2006.

[6] A. Guy, S. Tiosano, D. Comaneshter et al., "Aortic aneurysm association with SLE – a case–control study," *Lupus*, vol. 25, no. 9, pp. 959–963, 2016.

[7] C. S. Restrepo, D. Ocazionez, R. Suri, and D. Vargas, "Aortitis: imaging spectrum of the infectious and inflammatory conditions of the aorta," *RadioGraphics*, vol. 31, no. 2, pp. 435–451, 2011.

[8] H. Gornik and M. Creager, "Aortitis," *Circulation*, vol. 117, no. 23, pp. 3039–3051, 2008.

[9] V. Katabathina and C. Restrepo, "Infectious and noninfectious aortitis: cross-sectional imaging findings," *Seminars in Ultrasound, CT and MRI*, vol. 33, no. 3, pp. 207–221, 2012.

[10] R. B. Hsu and F. Y. Lin, "Risk factors for bacteraemia and endovascular infection due to non-typhoid *salmonella*: a reappraisal," *QJM: An International Journal of Medicine*, vol. 98, no. 11, pp. 821–827, 2005.

[11] Y. J. Chou, H.-W. Lin, C.-J. Yang et al., "Risk of recurrent non-typhoid *Salmonella* bacteremia in human immunodeficiency virus-infected patients with short-term secondary prophylaxis in the era of combination antiretroviral therapy," *Journal of Microbiology, Immunology and Infection*, vol. 49, no. 5, pp. 760–767, 2016.

[12] R. A. McPherson, M. R. Pincus, and J. B. Henry, *Henry's Clinical Diagnosis and Management by Laboratory Methods*, Saunders Elsevier, Philadelphia, PA, USA, 2007.

[13] C. F. Huang, P.-L. Chen, M.-F. Liu et al., "Nontyphoidal *Salmonella* bacteremia in patients with connective tissue diseases," *Journal of Microbiology, Immunology and Infection*, vol. 45, no. 5, pp. 350–355, 2012.

36

Patent Foramen Ovale Closure for Splenic Infarction: An Unusual Presentation and an Unusual Indication

Edgar Stroppa Lamas[1] **and Alan Vinicius Gamero Osti**[2]

[1]*Department of Interventional Cardiology, Intercor, Hospital 13 de Maio, Sorriso, Brazil*
[2]*Department of Interventional Cardiology, Intercor, Hospital Santo Antonio, Sinop, Brazil*

Correspondence should be addressed to Edgar Stroppa Lamas; edslamas@gmail.com

Academic Editor: Expedito E. Ribeiro

Background. Splenic infarction is a rare clinical condition. It is generally attributed to hematologic, vascular, cardioembolic, and infectious diseases or trauma. *Case Presentation.* We describe a rare case in an otherwise asymptomatic 41-year-old overweight woman with acute abdominal pain. Imaging work-up revealed splenic infarction. Common etiologies were excluded. A transesophageal echocardiography (TEE) revealed a patent foramen ovale (PFO). The patient was sent to closure with good outcome. *Conclusion.* Paradoxical embolism due to PFO can be a cause of splenic infarction, and its investigation and subsequent closure may be considered when there are no other causative disorders.

1. Introduction

Splenic infarction is a rare cause of acute abdominal pain which can mimic several other conditions. It is often the result of infiltrative hematologic disorders [1, 2]. Other conditions like hypercoagulable states, infective endocarditis, cardioembolic events, and more rarely, infectious mononucleosis may be associated [3].

Patent foramen ovale is encountered in about 25% of unselected patients [4]. Recent debates focus on its closure in cryptogenic stroke in young patients. Some reports describe other probably paradoxical cardioembolic events (renal, splenic) that may be benefited by patent foramen ovale closure [5, 6].

In this report, we present a rare cause of abdominal pain due to splenic infarction in which the etiology investigation points to paradoxical embolic infarction due to patent foramen ovale. Percutaneous closure was successfully done with good midterm outcome.

2. Case Presentation

A 41-year-old woman presented to the emergency department with acute epigastric pain radiating to the back associated with nausea. There was no history of diarrhea, fever, or trauma. There was no response to analgesics. Her medical history was unremarkable except class I obesity. On admission, the patient was apyrexial (36.7°C), eupneic at rest (respiratory rate of 14/min), and with a blood pressure of 130/80 mmHg and a pulse rate of 102 beats per minute. Cardiopulmonary examination was normal. There was localized left-sided and epigastric tenderness and no peritonism. Bowel sounds were normal.

An electrocardiogram (ECG) showed sinus tachycardia and no other abnormalities. Laboratory tests showed WCC $9.4 \times 109/L$, Hb 15 g/L, and CRP 24 mg/L. Serum levels of electrolytes, bilirubin, alkaline phosphatase, amilase, and creatinine were normal.

Abdominal ultrasound did not show any abnormalities. Abdominal magnetic resonance imaging (MRI) was performed and revealed a heterogeneous signal on a splenic topographic, low-intensity, and hypovascularized area with a cuneiform shape on its upper portion (Figure 1).

The patient was tested for the inherited thrombophilic factors including protein C, protein S, or antithrombin deficiency; hyperhomocysteinemia; lupus anticoagulant and anticardiolipin antibodies; activated protein C resistance;

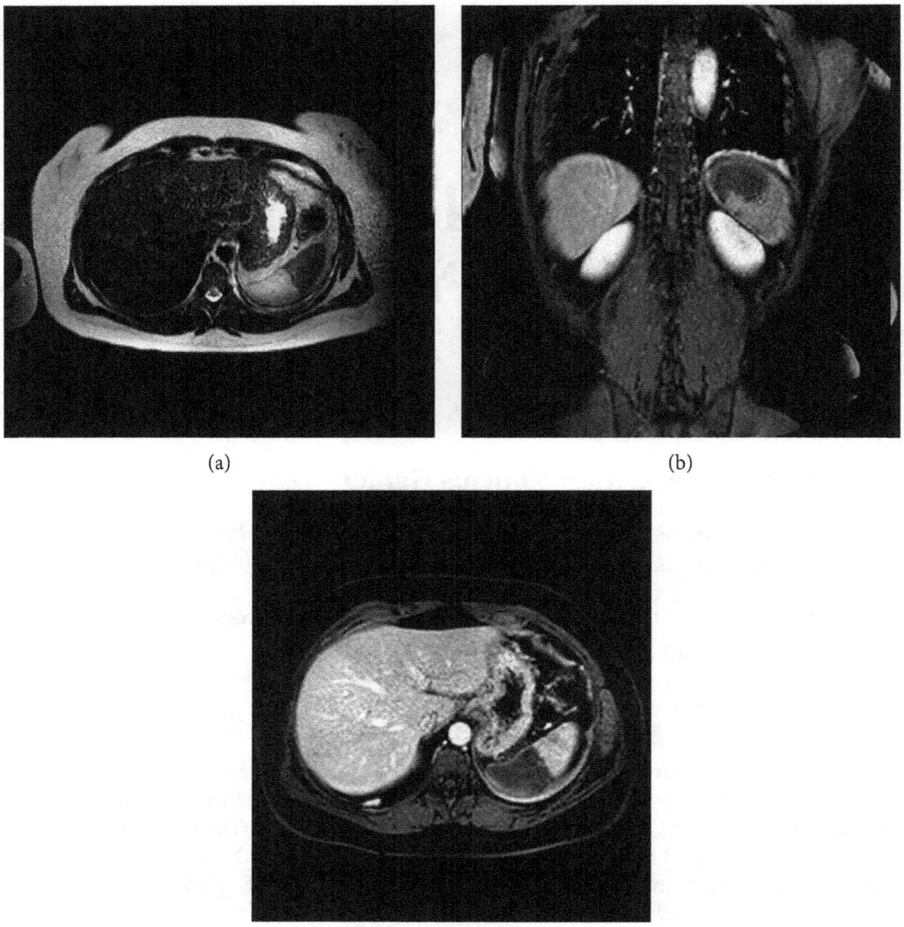

(a) (b)

(c)

Figure 1: Abdominal MRI. Axial T2-weighted image (a) showing a high-intensity signal in the upper splenic portion. Coronal (b) and axial (c) T1-weighted fat suppressed postcontrast image revealing a hypovascularized area in the corresponding area.

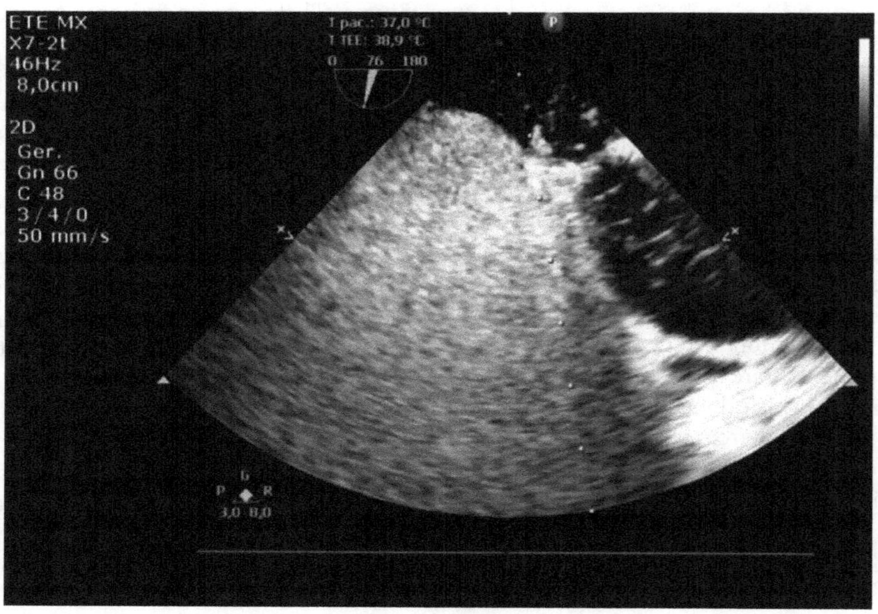

Figure 2: Transesophageal echocardiogram. Image revealing patent foramen ovale. After injection of agitated saline, a right-to-left shunt was observed.

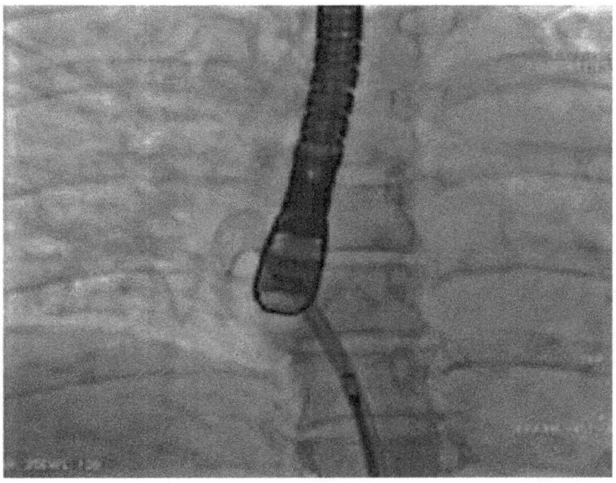

FIGURE 3: Percutaneous PFO closure with a Figulla Flex II PFO occluder. Right side portion of the device opened in the right atrium.

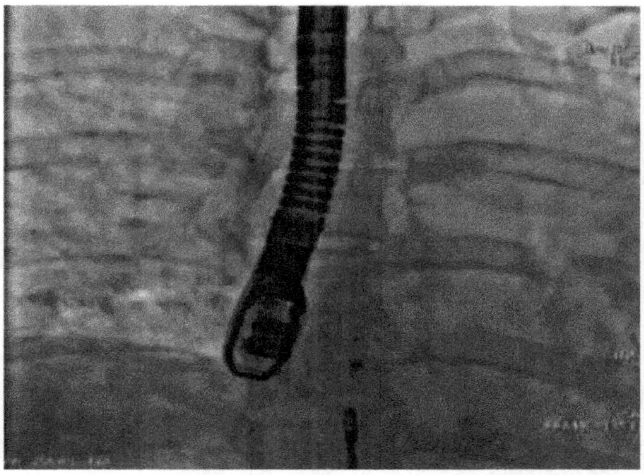

FIGURE 4: Percutaneous PFO closure with a Figulla Flex II PFO occluder. Left side portion of the device opened in the left right atrium.

and factor V Leiden mutation and prothrombin gene mutations. All tests were normal. A venous ultrasound of the lower limbs excluded deep venous thrombosis.

Therapeutic anticoagulation with enoxaparin (1 mg per kilogram subcutaneous) was started which provided a remarkable relief from the abdominal pain. Transthoracic echocardiogram was performed and revealed good biventricular function and no evidence of thrombus or valvular disease. The patient was then discharged asymptomatic with oral anticoagulation (rivaroxaban) prescribed.

On ambulatory follow-up one week later, the patient was on good evolution. Computed tomography angiography of the abdomen did not reveal any atherosclerotic patterns. Ambulatory monitoring with 24-hour Holter did not show paroxysmal atrial fibrillation or other significant supraventricular or ventricular arrhythmias.

A transesophageal echocardiogram (TEE) was done and revealed a patent foramen ovale with right-to-left shunt after agitated saline contrast injection during a Valsalva maneuver (Figure 2).

Based on these findings, the patient underwent percutaneous closure of the patent foramen ovale with insertion of a 23/25 mm self-expandable Figulla Flex II PFO occluder (Occlutech, Helsingborg, Sweden). The device was inserted using the right femoral approach. The procedure was done with TEE guiding. Immediate angiography and echocardiographic result was excellent (Figures 3 and 4).

Acetylsalicylic acid 100 mg/d and clopidogrel 75 mg/d were prescribed for three months, and thereafter, aspirin was continued alone following implantation. Rivaroxaban was suspended after the procedure.

Clinical and echocardiographic follow-ups were performed after one and six months and revealed good echocardiographic results and no clinical events or abnormalities.

3. Discussion

There is recent intense debate on the management of embolic cryptogenic stroke in the presence of patent foramen ovale. In specific subjects, patent foramen ovale closure may be considered over medical treatment [7]. Despite the low incidence, other potential sources of embolic damage should be remembered leading to the investigation of this etiology and consideration for patent foramen ovale closure.

Splenic infarction is a rare and difficult condition to recognize. Hematologic disorders especially Sickle cell disease and thrombophilic conditions are usually considered in this context. Like our case, after full investigation, particularly in a young patient, patent foramen ovale diagnostic workup and its respective closure may be considered.

Abbreviations

PFO: Patent foramen ovale
TEE: Transesophageal echocardiography
MRI: Magnetic resonance image.

Consent

Written informed consent was obtained from the patient for publication of this case report and any accompanying images.

References

[1] M. Nores, E. H. Phillips, L. Morgenstern, and J. R. Hiatt, "The clinical spectrum of splenic infarction," *The American surgeon*, vol. 64, p. 182, 1998.

[2] R. Parsons, G. Argoud, and D. L. Palmer, "Mixed bacterial infection of the pericardium," *Southern Medical Journal*, vol. 76, no. 8, pp. 1046–1048, 1983.

[3] M. Velez, V. Velez, and M. Auron, "A well-traveled clot: splenic infarct from a paradoxical embolism," *Journal of Hospital Medicine*, vol. 6, supplement 2, 2011.

[4] P. T. Hagen, D. G. Scholz, and W. D. Edwards, "Incidence and size of patent foramen ovale during the first 10 decades of life: an autopsy study of 965 normal hearts," *Mayo Clinic Proceedings*, vol. 59, no. 1, pp. 17–20, 1984.

[5] A. Dobrin, T. Thevenot, B. Alby, V. Di Martino, N. Sailley, and N. Meneveau, "A case of isolated splenic infarction associated with a foramen ovale and an interatrial septal aneurysm," *Gastroentérologie Clinique et Biologique*, vol. 32, no. 3, pp. 351–353, 2008.

[6] O. Khoma, A. Suppiah, and D. Martin, "Case report. Renal infarction by paradoxical embolism through the patent foramen ovale as an unusual cause of post-operative abdominal pain after sleeve gastrectomy," *International Journal of Surgery Case Reports*, vol. 26, pp. 47–49, 2016.

[7] H. Mir, R. A. C. Siemieniuk, L. C. Ge et al., "Patent foramen ovale closure, antiplatelet therapy or anticoagulation in patients with patent foramen ovale and cryptogenic stroke: a systematic review and network meta-analysis incorporating complementary external evidence," *BMJ Open*, vol. 8, no. 7, article e02376, 2018.

37

Antithrombotic Dilemmas after Left Atrial Appendage Occlusion Watchman Device Placement

Tania Ahuja,[1] **Scarlett Murphy,**[2] **and Daniel J. Sartori**[2]

[1]*New York University Langone Health, Department of Pharmacy, 550 First Avenue, New York, NY 10016, USA*
[2]*New York University Langone Health, Department of Medicine, 550 First Avenue, New York, NY 10016, USA*

Correspondence should be addressed to Tania Ahuja; tania.ahuja@nyumc.org

Academic Editor: Alfredo E. Rodriguez

Antithrombotic therapy for stroke prevention in patients with atrial fibrillation (AF) has dramatically shifted from warfarin, a vitamin K antagonist, to the direct oral anticoagulants (DOACs) such as dabigatran, apixaban, and rivaroxaban. In patients with contraindications to oral anticoagulation, left atrial appendage occlusion (LAAO) devices, such as the Watchman™ device, may be considered; however, temporary postimplantation antithrombotic therapy is still a recommended practice. We present a case of complex antithrombotic management, post LAAO device implantation, designed to avoid drug interactions with concomitant rifampin use and remained necessary secondary to subsequent device leak. This case highlights the challenges of antithrombotic therapy post LAAO device placement in a complex, but representative, patient.

1. Introduction

Antithrombotic therapy for stroke prevention in patients with atrial fibrillation (AF) has dramatically shifted from warfarin, a vitamin K antagonist, to the direct oral anticoagulants (DOACs) such as dabigatran, apixaban, and rivaroxaban [1–4]. In patients with contraindications to oral anticoagulation, left atrial appendage occlusion (LAAO) devices, such as the Watchman™ device (Boston Scientific Corporation; Natick, MA), may be considered [5, 6]. After device implantation, prevention of device-related thrombosis is essential during endothelialization. Prospective studies that investigated the Watchman™ device utilized antithrombotic strategies consisting of warfarin for 45 days post placement, followed by dual antiplatelet therapy (DAPT) for 6 months. However, DOACs, in conjunction with aspirin for 3 months, constitute an alternative regimen post device placement [7–10]. Indeed, real-life registry data reveal a spectrum of varied antithrombotic therapy currently in use, which is likely informed by a patient history of major bleeding or ineligibility for oral anticoagulation therapy [9]. The use of alternative anticoagulants, such as low-molecular-weight heparin (LMWH), post LAAO devices remains unknown. We present a case of complex antithrombotic management post Watchman™ device implantation designed to avoid drug interactions with concomitant rifampin use and subsequent device leak.

2. Case Report

The patient is a 70-year-old man, with a history of nonvalvular atrial fibrillation (NVAF) with prior stroke, chronic obstructive lung disease, hypertension, diabetes mellitus, chronic foot ulcers, and frequent falls, who initially presented with a fall 5 days after Watchman™ device placement. His history of NVAF was complicated by multiple episodes of syncope, despite various strategies including antiarrhythmic therapy. He was previously on dabigatran which resulted in severe bruising and rivaroxaban which was intolerable due to headaches. After discussion with his cardiologist, a Watchman™ device was placed given his high thrombotic risk and prior complications with oral antithrombotic therapy (CHADS2-VASC2 score of 6 and HAS-BLED score of 4) [11, 12]. After device placement, he was started on apixaban 5 mg twice daily plus aspirin 81 mg daily, with the plan for continuation for the following 45 days. However, 5 days after device placement, he presented to the emergency room after a fall, with lethargy, fever, and hypotension. He was found to be in septic shock from methicillin-resistant *staphylococcus aureus* (MRSA) bacteremia. His hemodynamics and mental status initially improved in the intensive care unit (ICU) on vasopressors, stress dose steroids, and broad-spectrum antibiotics, which were subsequently narrowed to intravenous vancomycin. In addition, his apixaban was transitioned to intravenous unfractionated heparin upon presentation to the ICU. In spite of hemodynamic improvement, his mental status worsened. Magnetic resonance imaging (MRI) of the brain revealed multiple acute small punctuate infarcts in the left corona radiata, right occipital cortex, and right frontal deep white matter. These multifocal strokes were thought to be cardioembolic, not septic in origin. Upon further questioning, the patient admitted to missing doses of apixaban post LAOO device placement. A transesophageal echocardiogram (TEE) was obtained; no thrombus in the left atrial appendage was noted, and there were no vegetations or patent foramen ovale. A well-positioned 27 mm Watchman™ device was visualized occluding the LAA orifice with a 1.3 mm paradevice leak, stable from prior. Given high concern for potential seeding of the newly implanted Watchman™ device, a six-week course of intravenous vancomycin plus oral rifampin was recommended by infectious disease consultants as a means of targeting MRSA and additionally preventing biofilm formation and device seeding. This was to be followed by a prolonged suppressive course of oral antibiotics.

The patient improved clinically with recovery of mental status and was deemed ready for transition from unfractionated heparin to an oral anticoagulant. Given the concerns about significant drug interactions with either warfarin or a DOAC with concomitant rifampin, a strong cytochrome (CYP) 3A4 inducer, strong permeability glycoprotein (Pgp) inducer, and moderate CYP2C9 inducer, a shared decision was reached to use weight-based LMWH with enoxaparin to complete the 45 days post Watchman™ device implantation.

The patient refused repeat TEE at 45 days, and anticoagulation therapy was continued with enoxaparin until the device could be evaluated. Two months after Watchman™ device placement, a repeat TEE was performed, revealing improvement in the paradevice leak from 1.3 mm to 1 mm, and the antithrombotic therapy was transitioned to DAPT with aspirin 81 mg daily and clopidogrel 75 mg daily. A repeat brain MRI obtained 4 months post LAOO device placement noted a right cerebellar chronic hemorrhage with numerous susceptibility foci distributed in the bilateral supratentorial and infratentorial compartment predominantly in the periphery of the brain parenchyma. Given the short interval since the prior MRI, the presence of these foci was concerning for microemboli of likely cardiac origin. A repeat TEE did not reveal a thrombogenic focus; however, there was persistence of paradevice leak at 1.3 mm. Anticoagulation therapy with apixaban was resumed, and DAPT was discontinued, due to the persistent device leak. The patient continues to struggle with worsening frequent falls; however, he remains functional at home with continued rehabilitation with physical therapy. He continues to take apixaban, living with the risks of associated bleeding that Watchman™ device placement was intended to reduce.

3. Discussion

The Watchman™ device, a LAAO device, has become an established alternative to oral anticoagulation in patients at risk for stroke with AF who have contraindications to anticoagulant therapy. Prevention of acute device-related thrombosis is critical following initial device placement, which paradoxically requires anticoagulant use. Although strategies vary, warfarin or a DOAC may be considered postimplant [7–9]. Low molecular weight heparins such as enoxaparin offer an attractive alternative to DOACs if oral anticoagulants are contraindicated. However, LMWHs have not been prospectively evaluated for the prevention of device related thrombosis. DAPT monotherapy constitutes a permissible alternative to oral anticoagulation, as real-world registry data reflects that patients with a history of major bleeding or other hard contraindications to anticoagulation therapy have received DAPT exclusively postimplant without an increase in device-related thrombosis [9].

In the case, rifampin was recommended as an adjunct to intravenous vancomycin in hopes of preventing biofilm formation of the Watchman™ device in the setting of known MRSA bacteremia, complicating anticoagulant selection. Due to the concerns of potential significant drug interaction between rifampin and the DOACs, these agents were initially deferred. Warfarin, a vitamin K antagonist, can be dose adjusted to overcome the induction from rifampin; however, there remains a risk of warfarin resistance, making this option challenging as well [13, 14]. This patient's course was further complicated by leakage into the left atrial appendage due to incomplete closure with the Watchman™. This complication has been noted in up to one-third of patients after placement [15]. Despite pervasive concerns about thrombosis, incomplete closure with the device may not lead to increase in thromboembolic events, according to a subanalysis of PROTECT AF [16]. However, given the gravity of possible stroke and systemic embolism with paradevice leaks, many clinicians prefer to continue anticoagulation therapy, as was seen in our case. Given the patient's high thrombotic risk ($CHADS_2$-$VASC_2$ of 6 and concomitant paradevice leak), a strategy of parenteral subcutaneous anticoagulation with enoxaparin was chosen for the postimplant period. He was later transitioned to DAPT, but as the leak reoccurred and the MRI revealed new foci, DAPT was replaced with a strategy of oral anticoagulation with apixaban selected as the patient was no longer receiving rifampin.

This case highlights the challenges with antithrombotic therapy post Watchman™ device placement, due to drug interactions and concern for stroke and systemic embolic due to device leak. A patient should carefully be selected for consideration for Watchman™ device placement, as anticoagulation therapy is often necessary at least temporarily after implantation and decision making regarding choice of anticoagulation may not always be able to be supported by the existing body of literature.

Consent

Informed consent was obtained prior to publication.

Authors' Contributions

T Ahuja, S Murphy, and DJ Sartori were all clinical providers for the patient and major contributors in writing the manuscript. All authors read and approved the final manuscript.

References

[1] S. J. Connolly, M. D. Ezekowitz, S. Yusuf et al., "Dabigatran versus warfarin in patients with atrial fibrillation," *The New England Journal of Medicine*, vol. 361, no. 12, pp. 1139–1151, 2009.

[2] W. I. Gonsalves, R. K. Pruthi, and M. M. Patnaik, "The new oral anticoagulants in clinical practice," *Mayo Clinic Proceedings*, vol. 88, no. 5, pp. 495–511, 2013.

[3] C. B. Granger, J. H. Alexander, J. McMurray et al., "Apixaban versus warfarin in patients with atrial fibrillation," *The New England Journal of Medicine*, vol. 365, no. 11, pp. 981–992, 2011.

[4] M. R. Patel, K. W. Mahaffey, J. Garg et al., "Rivaroxaban versus warfarin in nonvalvular atrial fibrillation," *The New England Journal of Medicine*, vol. 365, no. 10, pp. 883–891, 2011.

[5] B. Meier, Y. Blaauw, A. A. Khattab et al., "EHRA/EAPCI expert consensus statement on catheter-based left atrial appendage occlusion," *Europace*, vol. 16, no. 10, pp. 1397–1416, 2014.

[6] A. Tzikas, D. R. Holmes, S. Gafoor et al., "Percutaneous left atrial appendage occlusion: the Munich consensus document on definitions, endpoints and data collection requirements for clinical studies," *EuroIntervention*, vol. 12, no. 1, pp. 103–111, 2016.

[7] D. R. Holmes, V. Y. Reddy, Z. G. Turi et al., "Percutaneous closure of the left atrial appendage versus warfarin therapy for prevention of stroke in patients with atrial fibrillation: a randomised non-inferiority trial," *The Lancet*, vol. 374, no. 9689, pp. 534–542, 2009.

[8] D. R. Holmes Jr, S. Kar, M. J. Price et al., "Prospective randomized evaluation of the Watchman left atrial appendage closure device in patients with atrial fibrillation versus long-term warfarin therapy: the PREVAIL trial," *Journal of the American College of Cardiology*, vol. 64, no. 1, pp. 1–12, 2014.

[9] L. V. A. Boersma, B. Schmidt, T. R. Betts et al., "EWOLUTION: Design of a registry to evaluate real-world clinical outcomes in patients with AF and high stroke risk-treated with the WATCHMAN left atrial appendage closure technology,„ *Catheterization and Cardiovascular Interventions*, vol. 88, no. 3, pp. 460–465, 2016.

[10] Y. Enomoto, V. K. Gadiyaram, C. Gianni et al., "Use of non-warfarin oral anticoagulants instead of warfarin during left atrial appendage closure with the Watchman device," *Heart Rhythm*, vol. 14, no. 1, pp. 19–24, 2017.

[11] G. Y. H. Lip, R. Nieuwlaat, R. Pisters, D. A. Lane, and H. J. G. M. Crijns, "Refining clinical risk stratification for predicting stroke and thromboembolism in atrial fibrillation using a novel risk factor-based approach: the euro heart survey on atrial fibrillation," *Chest*, vol. 137, no. 2, pp. 263–272, 2010.

[12] G. Y. H. Lip, L. Frison, J. L. Halperin, and D. A. Lane, "Comparative validation of a novel risk score for predicting bleeding risk in anticoagulated patients with atrial fibrillation: the HAS-BLED (hypertension, abnormal renal/liver function, stroke, bleeding history or predisposition, labile INR, elderly, drugs/alcohol concomitantly) score," *Journal of the American College of Cardiology*, vol. 57, no. 2, pp. 173–180, 2011.

[13] J. A. Romankiewicz and M. Ehrman, "Rifampin and warfarin: a drug interaction," *Annals of Internal Medicine*, vol. 82, no. 2, pp. 224-225, 1975.

[14] L. D. Heimark, M. Gibaldi, W. F. Trager, R. A. O'Reilly, and D. A. Goulart, "The mechanism of the warfarin-rifampin drug interaction in humans," *Clinical Pharmacology and Therapeutics*, vol. 42, no. 4, pp. 388–394, 1987.

[15] V. Y. Reddy, H. Sievert, J. Halperin et al., "Percutaneous left atrial appendage closure vs warfarin for atrial fibrillation: a randomized clinical trial," *JAMA*, vol. 312, no. 19, pp. 1988–1998, 2014.

[16] J. F. Viles-Gonzalez, S. Kar, P. Douglas et al., "The clinical impact of incomplete left atrial appendage closure with the Watchman device in patients with atrial fibrillation: a PROTECT AF (percutaneous closure of the left atrial appendage versus Warfarin therapy for prevention of stroke in patients with atrial fibrillation) substudy," *Journal of the American College of Cardiology*, vol. 59, no. 10, pp. 923–929, 2012.

38

Left Atrial Ball-Shaped Thrombus with Concomitant Biatrial Appendage Thrombi in a Patient with Prior Mitral Valve Replacement

Kanako Akamatsu, Takahide Ito, Kazushi Sakane, Yumiko Kanzaki, Koichi Sohmiya, and Masaaki Hoshiga

Department of Cardiology, Osaka Medical College, Takatsuki, Osaka, Japan

Correspondence should be addressed to Takahide Ito; in3016@osaka-med.ac.jp

Academic Editor: Ertugrul Ercan

We reported a 67-year-old woman in whom large atrial thrombi were found by chance during discontinuation of therapeutic anticoagulation. The patient, with a history of mitral valve replacement surgery, had stopped anticoagulation for months because of intractable gastrointestinal bleeding, during which she was found to have 3 large thrombi in the atria on transesophageal echocardiography: left atrial free-floating ball-shaped thrombus, left atrial appendage thrombus, and right atrial appendage thrombus. One month following diagnosis, she still had the free-floating thrombus despite adequate anticoagulation. Free-floating ball-shaped thrombus is a rare finding observed on echocardiography in patients with mitral valve disease and an even rarer finding in case of appendage thrombi coexisting.

1. Introduction

Free-floating ball-shaped thrombus in the left atrium is a rare type of cardiac thrombus that may cause embolism, syncope, congestive heart failure, and sudden death [1–3]. It was first reported by Wood in 1814, who described an autopsy record in a 15-year-old girl with rheumatic mitral stenosis presenting recurrent syncope [3]. Since then, there have been a volume of reports on this entity particularly in the echocardiography era [4–11]. We herein reported a 67-year-old woman with prior mitral valve replacement surgery in whom multiple atrial thrombi, including a free-floating ball-shaped thrombus, were found on echocardiography.

2. Case Report

The woman was referred to the department of cardiology with consultation for left atrial masses detected by chance with follow-up echocardiography and computed tomography (Figure 1). Eight years ago, the patient had undergone mitral valve replacement surgery for rheumatic mitral stenosis. She had discontinued therapeutic anticoagulation for 4 months because she suffered from intractable gastrointestinal bleeding due to radiation therapy for peritoneal dissemination of uterine cancer. Her electrocardiogram showed atrial fibrillation with a heart rate of 84 bpm. Transthoracic echocardiography revealed a free-floating round-shaped mass in the left atrium that was not detected 5 months before. The left ventricular dimension (44 mm) and ejection fraction (62%) were normal, and the left atrial diameter was markedly increased (65 mm).

With the subsequent evaluation by transesophageal echocardiography, using an x8-2t transducer on an EPIQ 9 ultrasound machine (Philips Medical Systems, Andover, MA, USA), 2 atrial thrombi occupying the left and right atrial appendage cavities, respectively, in addition to the free-floating round-shaped mass were found (Figure 2). The left atrial appendage thrombus was fibrillated with cardiac beats while the right atrial appendage thrombus was immobile. There was a degree of spontaneous echo contrast

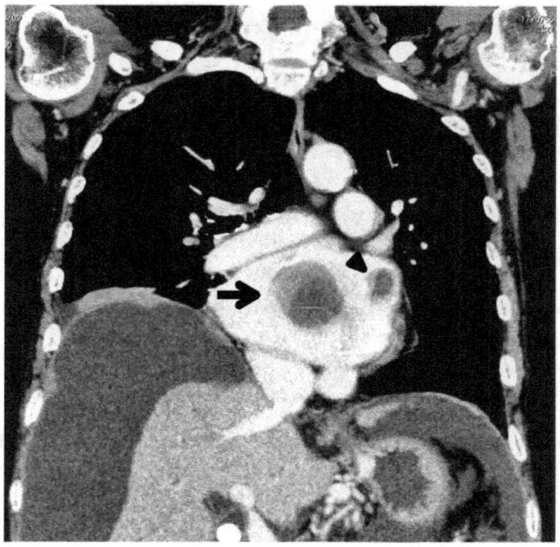

FIGURE 1: Computed tomography scan of the heart showing the free-floating ball-shaped thrombus (arrow) and appendage thrombus (arrow head). They look blurred due to movement within the left atrium.

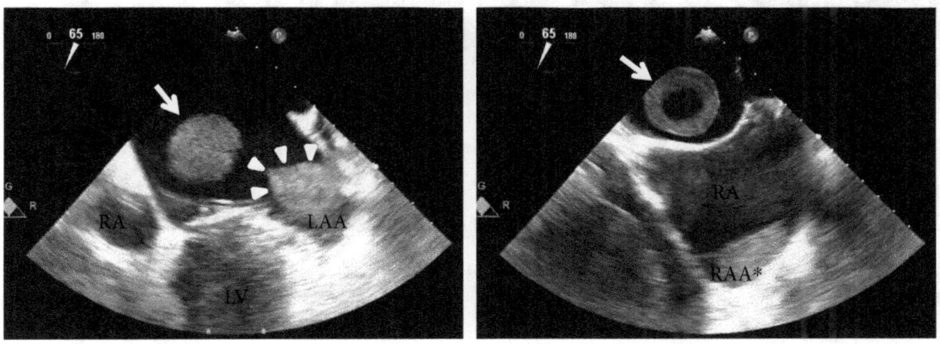

FIGURE 2: Two-dimensional transesophageal echocardiographic images of the free-floating ball-shaped mass (arrows), left (arrow heads), and right (*) atrial appendage thrombi. LA: left atrium; LAA: left atrial appendage; LV: left ventricle; RA: right atrium; RAA: right atrial appendage.

in both atria indicating a low-flow condition. A moderate degree of stenotic physiology was present across the mitral valve (9.0 mmHg of the mean pressure gradient). With the real-time 3-dimensional transesophageal echocardiographic imaging, the round-shaped mass was ascertained to be ball-shaped (Figure 3). The 3-dimensional images of both appendage thrombi are shown in Figure 4.

Based on her clinical history (long-standing atrial fibrillation and postprosthetic valve implantation), situations (discontinued anticoagulation and coexistence of appendage thrombi), and previous reports on similar cases [4–11], the ball-shaped free-floating mass was implied as a thrombus. Although a surgical procedure for the atrial thrombi was considered, the patient was determined to be managed conservatively with therapeutic anticoagulation, because she was diagnosed as having terminal cancer and thus in a malnourished condition. One month following anticoagulation, she still had the free-floating thrombus on transthoracic echocardiography. She died a few months after moving to another hospital for palliative care.

3. Discussion

Free-floating ball-shaped thrombus in the left atrium is a rare finding among patients with mitral valve disease with or without a history of valve replacement surgery [3–8]. This type of thrombus was reported to form in the absence of valve disease and also to recur despite adequate anticoagulation [10, 11]. The precise mechanism behind the occurrence of a free-floating ball-shaped thrombus remains uncertain. In the beginning, the thrombus is considered to be a small mural thrombus attached to the atrial wall [2]. The thrombus gradually grows and projects into the atrial cavity while connecting with the atrial wall via a thin stalk [9]. Then, as the thrombus becomes larger, the stalk becomes thinner and ultimately breaks off the atrial wall. The thrombus, becoming free, moves around in the atrial cavity, polishes itself by the circumjacent structures, and consequently, takes on a smooth, ball-shaped appearance.

Nevertheless, the mechanism for free-floating ball-shaped thrombus formation that we and others proposed

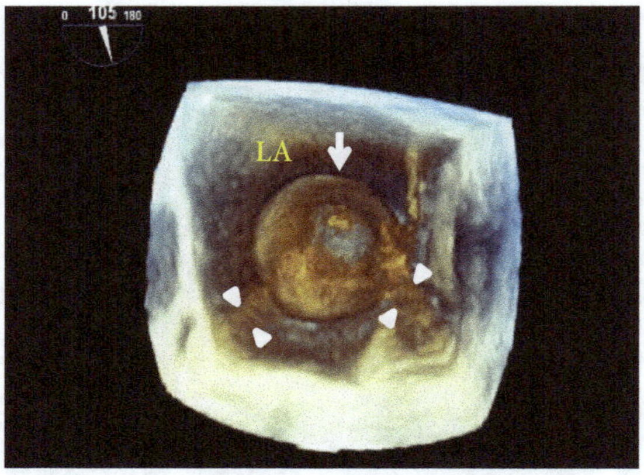

FIGURE 3: Three-dimensional transesophageal echocardiographic image of the free-floating ball-shaped mass (arrow) around which some sludge (arrow heads) is present suggesting a potential mechanism of its formation. Abbreviations are the same as in Figure 2.

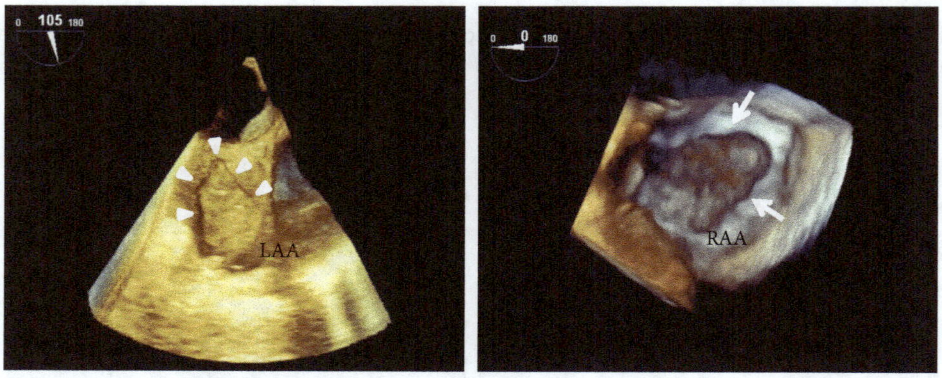

FIGURE 4: Three-dimensional transesophageal echocardiographic images of the left (arrow heads) and right (arrows) atrial appendage thrombi. Abbreviations are the same as in Figure 2.

above seems to differ from the observation by Wright-Smith et al., who demonstrated that the cut section of the ball-shaped thrombus resected from a patient with mitral stenosis represented a laminated and onionskin appearance with central cavitation [4]. Their findings of the thrombus were similar to ours in 2- and 3-dimensional echocardiographic findings with respect to its smooth surface and cavity forming [4], suggesting that such a thrombus grows to form ball-shaped, rather than attached to the atrial wall.

Because of the intricate clinical situation, the patient could not receive either surgery or thrombolytic therapy, although prompt surgical removal of the thrombus is generally preferred [2]. We restarted anticoagulation concerning about occurrence of complications such as systemic embolization and valve orifice obstruction. Consequently, no serious complications occurred on the patient until hospital discharge, but her clinical condition precluded histological presentation for the free-floating ball-shaped thrombus, which could have delineated an onionskin appearance as reported by Wright-Smith et al. [4].

Although similar cases were abundantly described [4–11], to the best of our knowledge, a free-floating ball-shaped thrombus with coexisting biatrial appendage thrombi imaged on echocardiography was the first reported case. In the only relevant report, Yoshioka et al. introduced a case of left atrial ball-shaped thrombus in conjunction with left atrial appendage thrombus [11]. For our case, in addition, other than anatomical and functional abnormalities of the left atrium, a low-output state associated with stenotic prosthetic valve might facilitate thrombosis in the appendages. Interestingly, compared to the left atrial appendage thrombus, the right appendage thrombus appeared to be organized to a more extent (Figure 4), presumably growing under a laminar blood flow condition specific to the right atrium.

4. Conclusion

This is the first report in which ball-shaped free-floating thrombus and biatrial appendage thrombi were coincidentally imaged on echocardiography. In this case, however, surgical removal of the thrombus was given up because of serious clinical conditions of the patient.

References

[1] D. Wrisley, A. Giambartolomei, I. Lee, and W. Brownlee, "Left atrial ball thrombus: review of clinical and echocardiographic manifestations with suggestions for management,"

American Heart Journal, vol. 121, no. 6, pp. 1784–1790, 1991.

[2] A. G. Fraser, G. D. Angelini, S. Ikram, and E. G. Butchart, "Left atrial ball thrombus: echocardiographic features and clinical implications," *European Heart Journal*, vol. 9, no. 6, pp. 672–677, 1988.

[3] J. T. Lie and M. L. Entman, ""Hole-in-one" sudden death: mitral stenosis and left atrial ball thrombus," *American Heart Journal*, vol. 91, no. 6, pp. 798–804, 1976.

[4] G. R. Wright-Smith, D. J. Burstow, R. Seymour, C. Smith, and M. F. O'Brien, "Mobile left atrial thrombus associated with mitral stenosis," *Circulation*, vol. 98, no. 9, pp. 931-932, 1998.

[5] T. Chen, T. H. LeJemtel, J. Garcia, G. M. Gordon, and D. M. Spevack, "Free-floating left atrial ball thrombus following mitral valve replacement," *Echocardiography*, vol. 22, no. 5, pp. 438–440, 2005.

[6] D. Osmonov, G. Durmuş, Y. Canga, and M. B. Karataş, "A huge ball-shaped pedunculated thrombus in the left atrium," *Türk Kardiyoloji Derneği Arşivi*, vol. 37, no. 7, p. 514, 2009.

[7] M. Ozkan, M. Ali Astarcioglu, A. Tuncer, and M. Yildiz, "Delineation of the free-floating left atrial ball mass with real time three-dimensional transesophageal echocardiography in a patient with mechanical mitral valve prosthesis," *Echocardiography*, vol. 29, no. 3, pp. E82–E84, 2012.

[8] T. P. Carrigan, S. Azam, C. Sullivan, and B. D. Hoit, "A billiard ball in the left atrium," *Echocardiography*, vol. 29, no. 7, pp. E153–E155, 2012.

[9] K. Demir, A. Avci, B. B. Altunkeser, and N. S. Ugras, "Is the thrombus truly free-floating? A case report," *Journal of Clinical Ultrasound*, vol. 42, no. 4, pp. 252–255, 2014.

[10] U. Gurcun, M. Boga, E. A. Ozkisacik, M. I. Badak, and B. Discigil, "Left atrial free-floating ball thrombus in a case of hyperthrophic cardiomyopathy," *Journal of Thrombosis and Thrombolysis*, vol. 20, no. 1, pp. 39–41, 2005.

[11] T. Yoshioka, T. Mori, Y. Taniguchi et al., "A case with recurrent free-floating ball thrombi in left atrium," *American Journal of Case Reports*, vol. 18, pp. 324–328, 2017.

Complete AV Block in Vaccinated COVID-19 Patient

Kevin Lee,[1] **Osman Rahimi**,[1] **Neelesh Gupta**,[2] **and Chowdhury Ahsan**[2]

[1]*Department of Internal Medicine, University of Nevada, Las Vegas, 1707 W Charleston Blvd, Suite 100, Las Vegas, NV 89102, USA*
[2]*Department of Cardiology, University of Nevada, Las Vegas, 1800 W Charleston Blvd, Las Vegas, NV 89102, USA*

Correspondence should be addressed to Kevin Lee; kevin.lee@unlv.edu

Academic Editor: Christopher S. Snyder

Background. Coronavirus 2019 (COVID-19) was initially identified approximately in December 2019 at Wuhan, China, as patients presented with vague prodromal and respiratory symptoms. With the developing investigation of its clinical manifestation, cardiac symptoms have been widely reported including acute coronary syndromes, myocarditis, arrhythmias, heart failure, and cardiac arrest. *Case Summary.* An 84 year-old male with history of coronary artery disease, hypertension, and hyperlipidemia presented to an outside urgent care with prodromal symptoms. The patient had received the second Pfizer vaccine three months prior. This presentation, he was found to be COVID-19 positive as well as bradycardic with a complete AV block. He was transferred to a tertiary center for further evaluation and management. However, after transfer, the patient refused further invasive cardiac interventions and after medical therapy was discharged home in complete AV block. *Discussion.* We report a novel case of a Pfizer-vaccinated patient whose initial presenting symptoms of COVID-19 included a complete AV block as well as the challenges and difficulties in approaching such patients. Although this patient's etiology of his complete AV block may result from multiple factors, given the acuity in setting of concurrent COVID-19 infections, top differentials include viral myocarditis, COVID-19-induced Takotsubo cardiomyopathy complicated by a complete AV-block, or a direct conduction pathway infection. Management of patients should focus on a multidisciplinary approach, and prevention is critical via vaccination.

1. Introduction

Severe acute respiratory syndrome coronavirus-2 (SARS-CoV-2) also known as coronavirus 2019 (COVID-19) was initially identified approximately in December 2019 at Wuhan, China, as patients presented with vague prodromal and respiratory symptoms. The virus rapidly progressed to a pandemic with surmountable casualties. With the developing investigation of its clinical manifestation, cardiac symptoms have been widely reported including acute coronary syndromes, myocarditis, arrhythmias, heart failure, and cardiac arrest [1].

We report a novel case of a Pfizer-vaccinated SARS-CoV-2 positive patient who presented with a complete AV block. Although previous high-degree AV blocks have been reported as a later complication of COVID-19 [2–4], this is the first documented case whose initial presenting symptom was a complete AV block in a vaccinated patient.

2. Case Presentation

An 84-year-old male with a history of coronary artery disease, hypertension, and hyperlipidemia presented to an urgent care in with body aches, malaise, fatigue, and dyspnea for three days. No other infectious symptoms were endorsed. At the outside facility, he was found to be bradycardic with a complete AV block. Total of atropine 1.0 mg was administered at that encounter. Afterwards, the patient went into a supraventricular tachycardia briefly with spontaneous return to a complete AV block. He was placed on transcutaneous pacing and transferred to our facility for further evaluation and management. Upon encounter, he denied any symptoms of lightheadedness, dizziness, palpitations, orthopnea, and chest pain. Patient also noted that he received both doses of the Pfizer vaccine at the beginning and end of April 2021, approximately six months prior to presentation. No booster doses were administered. Furthermore, he was recently seen by his cardiologist approximately a week prior with no abnormalities reported at the time. His previously known heart rate ranged between 77 and 99. Prior PR interval was 128. He had no history of tobacco, alcohol, or drug use. A possible culprit home medication was atenolol 50 mg daily which he reported taking as instructed. No other pertinent or new medications were noted in the patient's history.

On initial evaluation, he appeared comfortable and euvolemic. His blood pressure was 96/36 with an oxygen saturation of 82%. He was transcutaneously paced at a rate of 60 bpm at 70 mA. No audible bruits or murmurs were heard. The lungs were clear to auscultation. No peripheral edema was present. Underlying EKG without pacing showed an atrial rate of 128 bpm and a ventricular rate of 48 bpm (Figure 1). His previous EKG in May 2021 showed sinus rhythm with left bundle branch block and a prolonged QTc (Figure 2). Chest X-ray on admission showed pulmonary infiltrates without cardiomegaly (Figure 3). Initial troponin was 52 ng/L with a peak at 1699 ng/L six hours after. Pertinent labs were as follows: calcium 8.9 mg/dL, D-dimer 0.35 mg/L, ferritin 348.4 ng/L, LDH 263 U/L, and CRP 51.4 mg/L. Real-time RT-PCR COVID-19 test (DiaSorin Molecular) was positive. No significant electrolyte or other lab abnormalities were noted. Echocardiogram was performed and showed a new onset of reduced ejection fraction between 30 and 35%. He did not have a known history of reduced ejection fraction. His oxygen requirement was 2 L on nasal cannula saturating between 93 and 100%. He was moved to the CCU for further evaluation and management.

The patient was started on a low-dose dopamine infusion at 10 mcg/kg/min and dexamethasone 6 mg IV QD. Infectious disease team was consulted, and remdesivir was started based on a multidisciplinary team approach. Blood pressure remained between 140/76 and 162/62. The patient remained awake and comfortable. The patient was offered both cardiac catheterization and permanent pacemaker placement; however, after an extensive discussion with the patient and his son, the patient refused all invasive therapeutic intervention. The patient was discontinued off the dopamine infusion as well as transcutaneous pacing; however, he was continued on methylprednisolone and remdesivir. On posthospitalization day 6, his symptoms at onset had grossly improved, and given his aversion to testing, no follow-up imaging was conducted. He was discharged safely still in AV block with home oxygen.

3. Discussion

Complete AV block etiology is exhaustive including systemic diseases, ischemic heart disease, myocarditis, structural heart disease, and infectious disease. It has been reported in Takotsubo cardiomyopathy as well [5]. Arrhythmias and cardiovascular manifestation, including myocarditis and Takotsubo cardiomyopathy, has been seen in COVID-19 infections in approximately 17% hospitalized patients and 44% ICU patients. It may be attributed to multiple factors including hypoxia, electrolyte derangement, and cytokine surge [6].

Although this patient's etiology of his complete AV block may result from multiple factors, given the acuity in setting of concurrent COVID-19 infections, top differentials include viral myocarditis, COVID-19-induced Takotsubo cardiomyopathy complicated by a complete AV-block, or a direct conduction pathway infection. Ischemia cannot be completely ruled out as well. Due to his distant history, the patient did not know whether his right coronary artery was stented or diseased. No prior catheterization report was available as most recent catheterization was 16 years prior out-of-state. COVID-19 has been documented to infect cells via the angiotensin-converting enzyme-2 (ACE-2) receptor [7]. Therefore, a direct infection of the conduction pathway is plausible. Complete AV blocks are also clinical symptoms of myocarditis. Otherwise, vaccine-induced myocarditis complications should also be considered [8].

Management is complicated given the mortality rate of COVID-19. There has been a case report of transient high-grade AV blocks in COVID-19 infected patients [4]. Whether all patients with COVID-19 induced high-grade AV blocks require a pacemaker remains a question. Furthermore, in patients with increased probability of mortality, discussion should revolve around risks and benefits as well as quality of life even after a pacemaker placement. Palliative service consultation should also be considered. If the patient is stable with a seemingly irreversible complete AV block, a pacemaker should be recommended.

Throughout the pandemic, multiple medications have been investigated for treatment options. In particular, remdesivir has shown to decrease time to recovery in hospitalized patients as well as the rate of lower respiratory tract infection [9]. However, remdesivir has been associated with duration-dependent cardiac adverse effects due to mitochondrial toxicity and similarities of its active metabolite to adenosine triphosphate. These effects include SA node automaticity reduction, AV nodal abnormalities, QRS prolongation, and myocyte toxicity [10]. The discussion to administer remdesivir in COVID-19 patients with high-degree AV block should be approached in a multidisciplinary fashion.

With the rise of the new COVID-19 variants, vaccination and booster doses should be recommended for all patients without contraindication. It is possible that the virus may mutate to present with more cardiologic pathologies given the pathophysiology. Depending on the type of vaccine, individuals may benefit with protection from variants [11].

4. Conclusion

We present a case of a Pfizer-vaccinated COVID-19 infected individual whose initial presenting symptoms included a

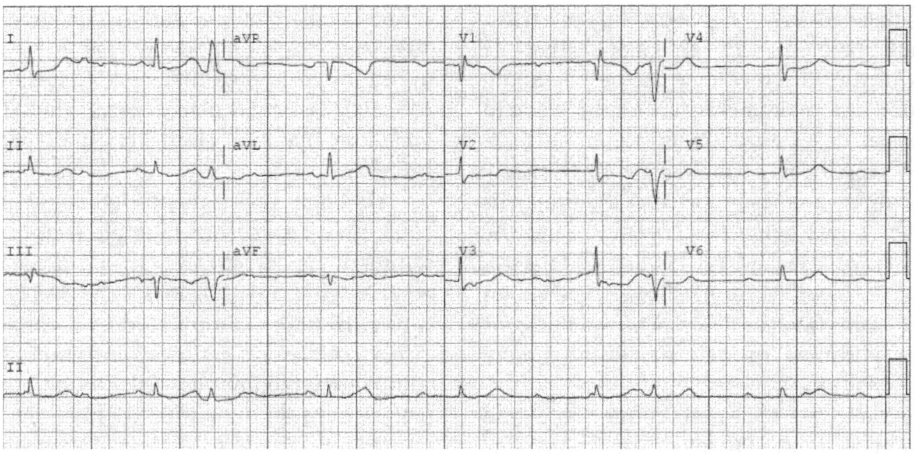

Figure 1: Initial presenting EKG.

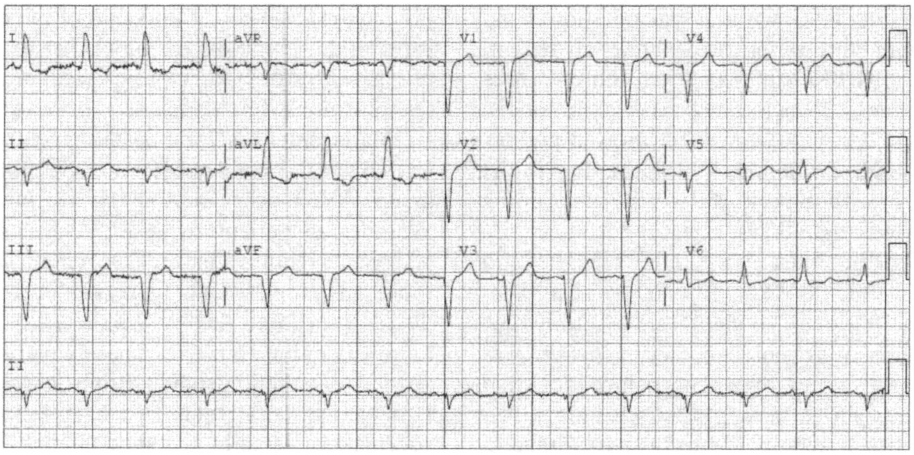

Figure 2: EKG 6 months prior to presentation.

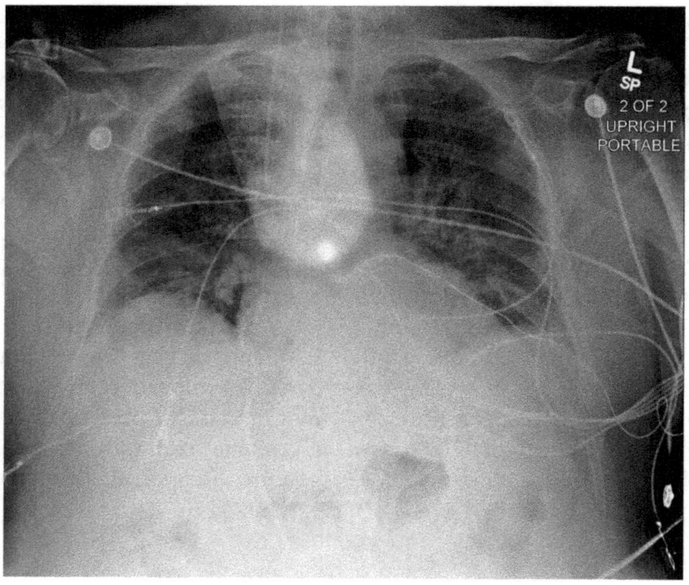

Figure 3: CXR on initial presentation.

complete AV block. To the author's knowledge, this is the first documentation of such case.

Consent

Consent has been obtained for report from patient.

References

[1] I. Basu-Ray, N. K. Almaddah, A. Adeboye, and M. P. Soos, "Cardiac manifestations of coronavirus (COVID-19)," *StatPearls*, 2021.

[2] F. I. Haddadin, T. E. Mahdawi, L. Hattar, H. Beydoun, F. Fram, and M. Homoud, "A case of complete heart block in a COVID-19 infected patient," *Journal of Cardiology Cases*, vol. 23, no. 1, pp. 27–30, 2021.

[3] T. Eneizat Mahdawi, H. Wang, F. I. Haddadin, D. Al-Qaysi, and J. V. Wylie, "Heart block in patients with coronavirus disease 2019: a case series of 3 patients infected with SARS-CoV-2," *Hear Case Reports*, vol. 6, no. 9, pp. 652–656, 2020.

[4] J. H. Chen, B. Robinson, P. Patel et al., "Transient complete heart block in a patient with COVID-19," *Cureus*, vol. 13, no. 6, 2021.

[5] N. F. N. Sakul, S. Shrestha, N. Balabbigari, and S. Talati, "Complete heart block: a rare complication of takotsubo syndrome," *Case Reports in Cardiology*, vol. 2019, 5 pages, 2019.

[6] B. Long, W. J. Brady, A. Koyfman, and M. Gottlieb, "Cardiovascular complications in COVID-19," *The American Journal of Emergency Medicine*, vol. 38, no. 7, pp. 1504–1507, 2020.

[7] B. Gyawali, B. Baral, S. Shah, S. Yadav, and C. M. Poudel, "A patient infected with SARS-CoV-2 presenting with complete heart block," *Case Reports in Cardiology*, vol. 2021, Article ID 5011294, 4 pages, 2021.

[8] N. Gautam, P. Saluja, M. Fudim, K. Jambhekar, T. Pandey, and S. Al'Aref, "A late presentation of COVID-19 vaccine-induced myocarditis," *Cureus*, vol. 13, no. 9, 2021.

[9] J. H. Beigel, K. M. Tomashek, L. E. Dodd et al., "Remdesivir for the treatment of COVID-19 — final report," *The New England Journal of Medicine*, vol. 383, no. 19, pp. 1813–1826, 2020.

[10] L. B. Day, H. Abdel-Qadir, and M. Fralick, "Bradycardia associated with remdesivir therapy for COVID-19 in a 59-year-old man," *Canadian Medical Association Journal*, vol. 193, no. 17, pp. E612–E615, 2021.

[11] C. J. Hemmer, M. Löbermann, and E. C. Reisinger, "COVID-19: epidemiology and mutations : an update," *Der Radiologe*, vol. 61, no. 10, pp. 880–887, 2021.

40

One 6-F Guiding Catheter and One Microcatheter to Accomplish a Retrograde Chronic Total Occlusion Approach: The "Reverse Tip-In" or "Introspect" Technique

Ata Firouzi, Zahra Hosseini, and Ehsan Khalilipur

Cardiovascular Intervention Research Center, Rajaie Cardiovascular Medical and Research Center, Iran University of Medical Sciences, Tehran, Iran

Correspondence should be addressed to Ehsan Khalilipur; ehsankhalilipur@gmail.com

Academic Editor: Mihaela Mocan

The retrograde approach has significantly increased the overall success rate of chronic total occlusion (CTO) percutaneous coronary intervention (PCI), up to 90% in the hands of experienced CTO operators. The "tip-in" technique involves inserting an antegrade microcatheter over the retrograde guidewire, allowing for antegrade intervention on the CTO segment. Through the presentation of the following case, we want to illustrate how to undertake a retrograde approach to bridge the occluded segment via the "reverse tip-in" or "introspect" technique, using a single guiding catheter with one microcatheter inside.

1. Introduction

The retrograde technique in chronic total occlusion (CTO) percutaneous coronary intervention (PCI) has considerably boosted the overall success rate, up to 90% in the hands of experienced CTO operators [1]. The "tip-in" technique, initially reported in 2015, was created to address some of the shortcomings of regularly used retrograde techniques in CTO PCI. The "tip-in" approach entails the insertion of an antegrade microcatheter over the retrograde guidewire, allowing for a subsequent antegrade intervention on the CTO segment. This technique enables the successful completion of a retrograde CTO treatment [2]. The wiring can be finished by inserting an antegrade wire through the retrograde microcatheter and crossing the CTO, a procedure referred to as "rendezvous."

Through the presentation of the following case, we seek to demonstrate how to perform a retrograde approach to cross the occlusion segment using a single guiding catheter with one microcatheter inside via the "reverse tip-in" or "introspect" technique.

2. Case Report

A 65-year-old man presented to a cardiology clinic with recent-onset typical exertional chest pain Canadian Cardiovascular Society (CCS) classes II-III. A gated exertional myocardial perfusion scan revealed moderate ischemia in the anterior territory. Despite optimized guideline-directed medical therapy, however, the patient had exertional chest pain (New York Heart Association functional classes II–III), as a result of which he underwent coronary angiography in another center. The procedure demonstrated total occlusion in the midpart of the left anterior descending artery (LAD) with retrograde and ipsilateral interventional collateral vessels (Rentrop grade III) (Figures 1(a) and 1(b)). Despite our explanation to the patient, he was not willing to proceed with coronary artery bypass graft (CABG) surgery, and he was, therefore, scheduled for PCI on LAD CTO in our center.

The first images proved the total occlusion in the LAD. The PCI procedure was started with a left extra-backup 6-F XB guide catheter and a Caravel 150 cm microcatheter (ASAHI Intecc Medical) through right common femoral

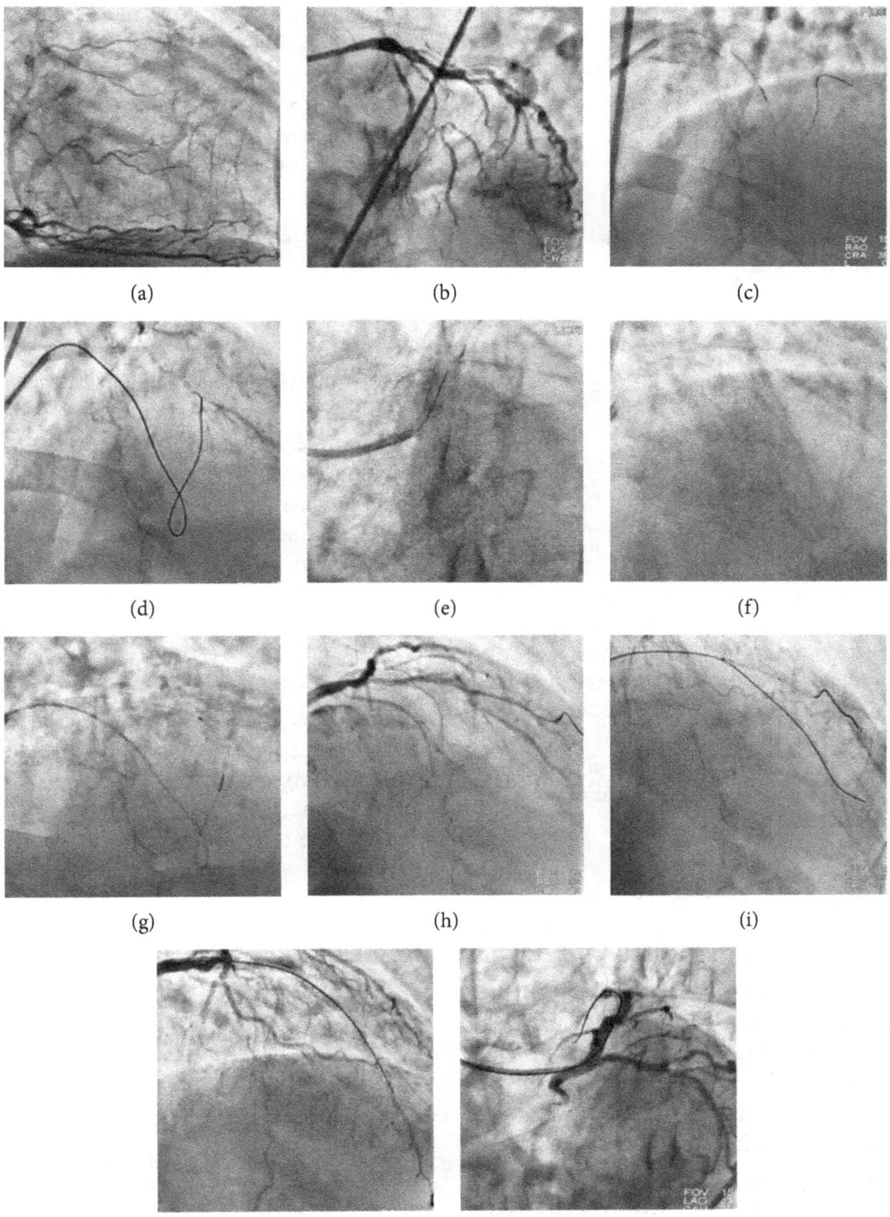

FIGURE 1: (a–k) Selective right coronary artery injection shows well-developed collateral vessels, which fill the left anterior descending artery (LAD) retrogradely (a). Selective left main injection shows a totally cut LAD at the midpart (at the trifurcation point) with an ambiguous cap and a lengthy occluded segment, with a good runoff (b). A large proximal septal branch fills the LAD antegradely. Hence, with the aid of a SUOH 03 wire (ASAHI Intecc Medical) and a Caravel 150 cm microcatheter (ASAHI Intecc Medical), septal surfing is performed (c). Once the wire reaches the distal cap, the microcatheter is advanced over it (d). Thereafter, with a Gaia second wire (ASAHI Intecc Medical), several attempts are made to puncture the distal cap but to no avail. Subsequently, with a Gladius wire (ASAHI Intecc Medical), the distal cap is crossed, the wire is tipped into the guide catheter, and the same microcatheter is passed over it (e). In this stage, a SION blue wire (ASAHI Intecc Medical) is advanced antegradely toward the retrograde microcatheter ("reverse tip-in"), creating a loop between the LAD and the septal branch (f). Afterward, the microcatheter is retracted, and predilation and LAD preparation are done antegradely (g). The wire is positioned antegrade to the diagonal branch at the site of the trifurcation (h). Under the guidance of a dual-lumen SASUKE microcatheter (ASAHI Intecc Medical) over the SION blue wire, the Gaia second wire is advanced toward the LAD (i). The LAD is then predilated, and stenting is performed, yielding good final results (j, k).

artery access. A Fielder XT-A wire (ASAHI Intecc Medical) was selected for the antegrade approach, but it failed to cross the CTO (trifurcated at the occluded segment with an ambiguous cap). As shown in Figure 1(b), there was one large septal branch at the proximal segment of the LAD with one good collateral vessel to the midportion of the LAD. Accordingly, a decision was made to cross the CTO via a retrograde septal-to-LAD approach using the same microcatheter and a SUOH 03 wire (ASAHI Intecc Medical) with a view to surfing this septal segment to the midportion of

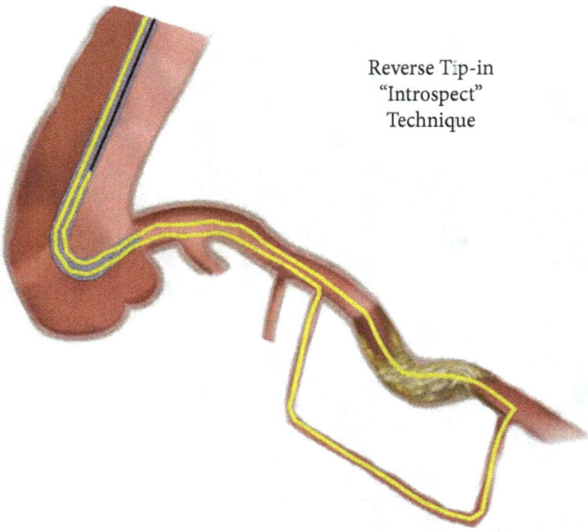

FIGURE 2: The image depicts the "reverse tip-in" technique. Primarily, the first retrograde wire crosses the lesion and with "introspect technique" the position of the microcatheter inside the guiding catheter as depicted in this figure; the antegrade wire from guiding catheter is tipped into the microcatheter and then with simultaneous pulling backward the microcatheter and retrograde wire and withdrawing the antegrade wire forward; the lesion could be passed via antegrade wire, and with final position of the antegrade wire distal to the lesion, predilation of CTO segment could be performed.

the LAD. Once the distal cap was accessed (Figure 1(d)), the wire was substituted with a Gaia second wire (ASAHI Intecc Medical) to puncture the distal cap but to no avail. Subsequently, with a Gladius wire (ASAHI Intecc Medical), the occluded segment was crossed, and the microcatheter was passed to the proximal part of the LAD over the Gladius wire and then into the same guiding catheter. In this step, with a workhorse SION blue wire (ASAHI Intecc Medical) from the guiding catheter, the wire was inserted into the tip of the microcatheter (the "reverse tip-in" technique) before it was passed distal to the occluded segment (Figures 1(e) and 1(f)). Afterward, the microcatheter was pulled back, and the wire was positioned antegrade to the diagonal branch at the site of the trifurcation (Figure 1(g)). Next, under the guidance of a dual-lumen SASUKE microcatheter (ASAHI Intecc Medical) over the SION blue wire, the Gaia second wire was advanced toward the LAD (Figure 1(i)). Through the gradual escalation of the balloon size (i.e., from a 1.5 balloon to a 2.5 semicompliant balloon), the CTO segment was successfully predilated. Thereafter, a 3×38 drug-eluting stent was implanted, and it was postdilated with a 3.5 noncompliant balloon, conferring good final results (Figures 1(j) and 1(k)).

The patient was transferred to a cardiac care unit and was discharged the following day.

3. Discussion

Kahn and Hartzler conducted the first retrograde CTO PCI in 1990, since which time other retrograde techniques have been added to the armamentarium [3]. The technology has advanced swiftly, resulting in a higher rate of initial success, a shorter duration of the procedure, and less radiation exposure [4, 5]. Because of the difficulty and risk associated with the retrograde approach, however, it is often drawn upon when antegrade crossing attempts fail or increase anticipated risks. Numerous operators advise that an antegrade crossing be attempted first as antegrade preparation is inevitably required to complete a retrograde crossing [6]. Externalization of wires is the step most frequently taken following a retrograde wire crossing since it enables subsequent equipment deliveries.

In this case, we employed a 6-F guide catheter and a single Caravel 150 cm microcatheter to perform the antegrade and retrograde approaches. When the antegrade route failed, we utilized the retrograde septal-to-septal pathway to bypass the CTO segment. Via the retrograde wire escalation technique, we succeeded in passing the occluded segment, inserting the tip of the microcatheter into the same guide, and creating a loop of microcatheter inside the guide. To our knowledge, we are the first to report the use of this "reverse tip-in" or "introspect" technique (Figure 2) in this stage with the intention to insert a workhorse wire into the loop of the microcatheter. We, thereafter, pulled back the retrograde wire and placed the antegrade workhorse wire distal to the CTO segment (Figure 1(e)). We also managed to overcome the obstacle of trifurcation at the distal cap using a double-lumen microcatheter. Notably, in many cases, finding a distal septal branch could obviate this step. We think that this strategy could reduce the need for dual access and the use of two microcatheters and two sets of wires and devices, as well as the risk of complications.

References

[1] M. N. Vo, A. Ravandi, and E. S. Brilakis, ""Tip-in" technique for retrograde chronic total occlusion revascularization," *The Journal of Invasive Cardiology*, vol. 27, no. 5, pp. E62–E64, 2015.

[2] M. Megaly, A. Ali, M. Saad et al., "Outcomes with retrograde versus antegrade chronic total occlusion revascularization," *Catheterization and Cardiovascular Interventions*, vol. 96, no. 5, pp. 1037–1043, 2020.

[3] J. K. Kahn and G. O. Hartzler, "Retrograde coronary angioplasty of isolated arterial segments through saphenous vein bypass grafts," *Catheterization and Cardiovascular Diagnosis*, vol. 20, no. 2, pp. 88–93, 1990.

[4] S. Rathore, O. Katoh, H. Matsuo et al., "Retrograde percutaneous recanalization of chronic total occlusion of the coronary arteries," *Circulation. Cardiovascular Interventions*, vol. 2, no. 2, pp. 124–132, 2009.

[5] M. Kimura, O. Katoh, E. Tsuchikane et al., "The efficacy of a bilateral approach for treating lesions with chronic total occlusions: the CART (controlled antegrade and retrograde subintimal tracking) registry," *JACC. Cardiovascular Interventions*, vol. 2, no. 11, pp. 1135–1141, 2009.

[6] M. Megaly, I. Xenogiannis, N. Abi Rafeh et al., "Retrograde approach to chronic total occlusion percutaneous coronary intervention," *Circulation. Cardiovascular Interventions*, vol. 13, no. 5, article e008900, 2020.

41

Zero-Contrast Left Main Bifurcation PCI in an Elderly Patient with Chronic Kidney Disease

Prathap Kumar, Stalin Roy, Blessvin Jino, Manu Rajendran, and Sandheep G. Villoth

Meditrina Hospital, Kollam, Kerala, India

Correspondence should be addressed to Prathap Kumar; prathapndr@gmail.com

Academic Editor: Yigit Canga

Patients with chronic kidney disease develop acute kidney injury (AKI) following percutaneous coronary intervention (PCI). We report a case highlighting the benefits of zero-contrast left main bifurcation PCI in an 82-year-old male with non-ST elevation myocardial infarction and contrast-induced AKI following coronary angiography. The patient was on routine follow-up, and he was stable and asymptomatic at nine months follow-up.

1. Introduction

Percutaneous coronary intervention (PCI) in patients with significant renal dysfunction poses multiple challenges. The advent of image-guided zero or ultralow contrast angioplasty is beneficial for patients who were previously considered ineligible or at "high risk" for routine coronary angioplasty [1]. Although zero-contrast PCI is a new emerging method in the field of coronary interventions, complex interventions such as PCI for left main coronary artery, difficult chronic total occlusions (CTO), [2], and severely calcified lesion subtypes [3] pose significant challenges when performed without using contrast media/agents. On the other hand, contrast-induced nephropathy (CIN) significantly impacts the long-term prognosis of patients undergoing PCI, and it is independently associated with higher mortality in patients with diabetes [4].

In general, contrast volume should be restricted to twice or thrice the estimated glomerular filtration rate (eGFR). The maximum acceptable contrast dose (MACD) is calculated as 5 ml × body weight (kg)/baseline serum creatinine (mg/dl) [5]. The MACD is validated, and contrast use within the cut-off value reduces the incidence of CIN [6]. Recently, a stringent cut-off MACD value of 3.7 x eGFR has been proposed and endorsed by the Society for Cardiovascular Angiography and Interventions consensus statement [7, 8]. Intravascular ultrasound- (IVUS-) guided PCI significantly reduces the contrast volume compared to the conventional PCI ("Angiography only" approach). Herein, we present a case of zero-contrast left main bifurcation PCI in a patient with non-ST elevation acute coronary syndrome (NSTE ACS) and contrast-induced acute kidney injury (CI-AKI) following coronary angiography (CAG). To the best of our knowledge, this is the first case report of zero-contrast left main bifurcation PCI.

2. Case Report

An 82-year-old male patient with diabetes, hypertension, and chronic kidney disease (CKD) stage III-b (eGFR: 39 ml/min/1.73 m^2) presented to a primary hospital with NSTE ACS. Coronary angiography revealed critical three-vessel disease involving the ostium of the left anterior descending (LAD), left circumflex (LCX) arteries (medina 0,1,1), and proximal right coronary artery (RCA; Figure 1). However, 48 hours after CAG, serum creatinine levels increased from 178 μmol/l to 290 μmol/l (eGFR, 19 ml/min/1.73 m^2), indicating CI-AKI. The patient was given the option of coronary artery bypass grafting (CABG)/left main bifurcation PCI and referred to our centre for further management.

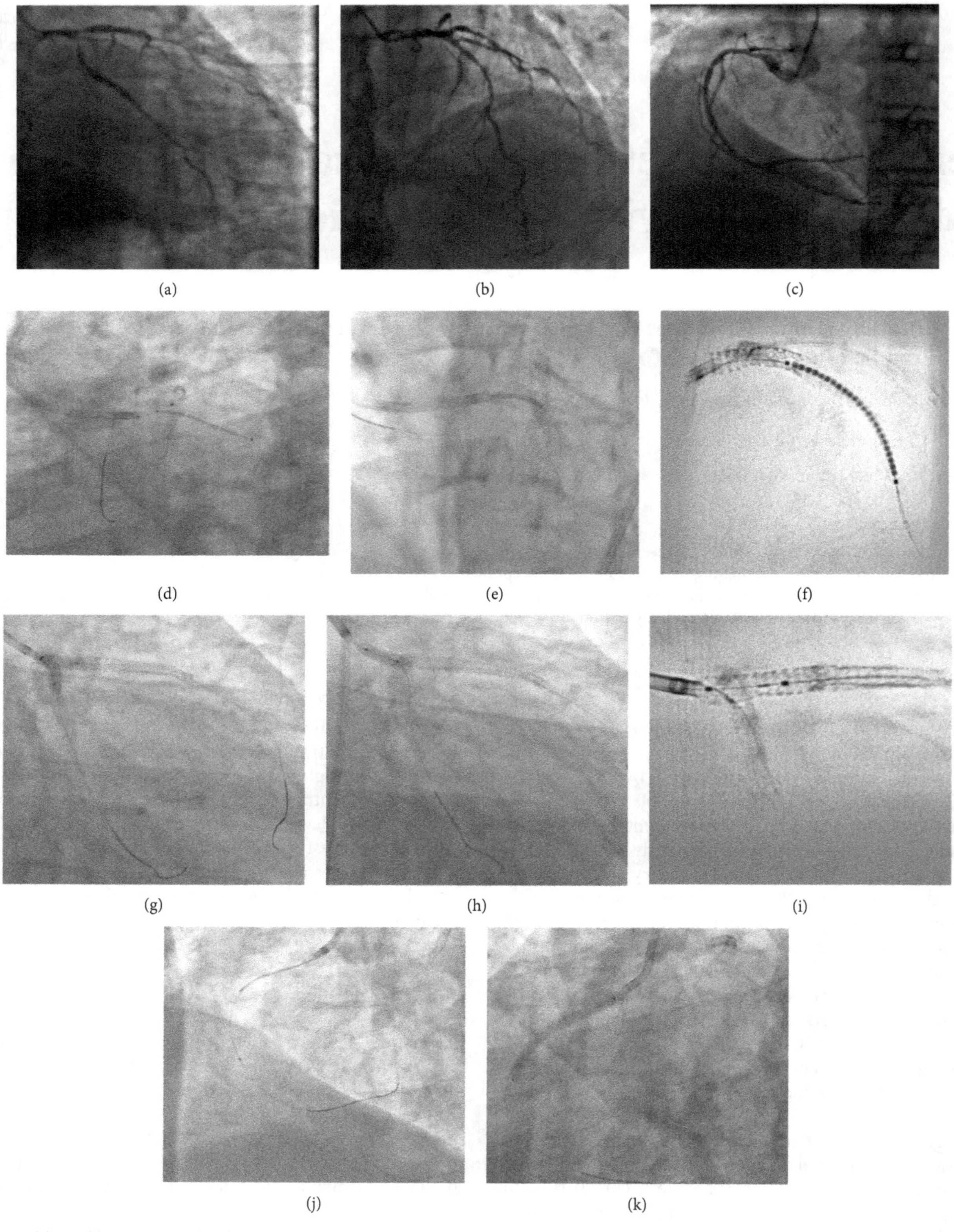

FIGURE 1: (a) Medina 0,1,1 disease. (b) Significant disease in proximal-mid LAD. (c) RCA proximal-mid disease. (d) Ostial LCX stent. (e) Sepal wire technique for ostial LMCA stent. (f) CLEARstent image of LAD stent. (g) FKBI (h) POT. (i) CLEARstent of bifurcation. (j) IVUS evaluation of RCA disease. (k) Ostial RCA stent.

Diagnostic CAG films available from primary centre were reviewed. The patient presented with a SYNTAX score of 25 and a high STS II score (25% morbidity/mortality) and hence was advised to undergo zero-contrast left main bifurcation PCI. The other main factor for choosing PCI over CABG is due to significant past experience in performing ultralow and zero-contrast PCI at our centre. Post consent, the procedure was performed via the femoral approach using

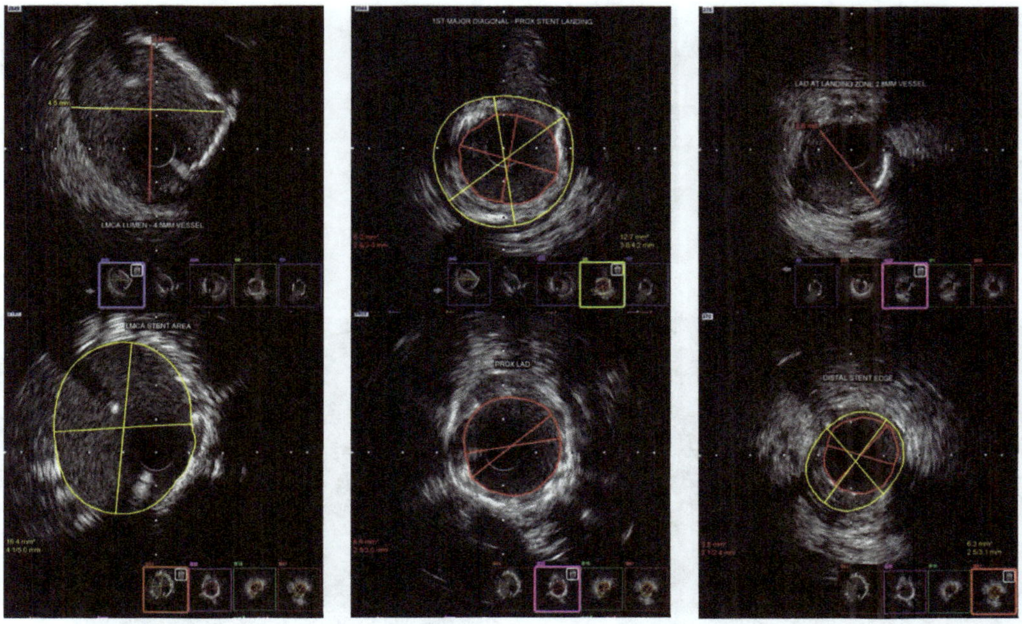

(a) (b) (c)

Figure 2: (a) Pre-poststenting images of LMCA. (b) Proximal LAD pre-poststenting. (c) Distal landing zone and stent edge.

a 7Fr 3.5 EBU guide catheter, three days after CAG. Distal landing zones and measurements were obtained from the IVUS runs from LCX and LAD to LMCA (Figures 2 and 3(a)–3(c)). Although LMCA disease was not observed, ostial disease of both LAD and LCX was noted. The LCX and LAD lesions were subsequently predilated with multiple noncompliant (NC) balloons.

Minicrush technique was proposed for the LMCA bifurcation as described in the European Bifurcation Club consensus document [9]. The lesion length in the LCX-OM segment was 21 mm, and the reference luminal diameter at the distal landing zone was 2.9 mm. Hence, a 3 × 24 mm drug-eluting stent (DES) was used for LCX. The stent was placed in the LCX ostium using a balloon in the LMCA-LAD as a marker. The balloon placed in the main vessel (LMCA-LAD) helps us identify the ostium of the side branch (LCX) precisely, so that the LCX stent was deployed at the ostium with minimal protrusion into the LMCA (proximal stent edge positioned just touching the balloon in the LMCA). Then the LCX guidewire was removed. The stent was then crushed using the balloon in the LMCA-LAD. The LMCA-LAD stent chosen was a 4 × 16 mm DES, as the LAD vessel diameter was 4 mm up to the first diagonal branch, and the length from the LMCA ostium to the diagonal was 14.5 mm (Figures 3(d) and 3(e)).

Aorto-ostial stenting is a difficult procedure especially when performed without using contrast media/agents to check the exact stent position while deploying. We used marker wire technique (sepal technique) for optimal positioning of the stent in ostial LMCA and RCA [10]. In this technique of ostial stenting, a second guide wire was placed in the aortic root to mark the ostium of the coronary vessel (LMCA). When the guide catheter is maximally advanced with the secondary guidewire in the aorta, it stops exactly at the ostium of the coronary artery (as further advancement is prevented by the guidewire which is floating in the aorta) (Figure 1(e)). Hence, the tip of the guide catheter serves as the marker for the coronary ostium, from which point the LMCA-LAD stent was deployed; the middistal LAD lesion was reassessed using IVUS for deciding the second stent in LAD. The distal reference diameter was 2.75 mm, and the myocardial bridge was observed distal to the lesion. The length of the lesion from the stent edge was 31 mm. Hence, a 2.75 × 32 mm DES was selected to avoid landing in the myocardial bridge segment, and a precise, minimal overlap was done to ensure entire lesion coverage using the "CLEARstent" technology from Siemens.

The minicrush procedure was completed with proximal optimization technique (POT) followed by recross into the LCX. Subsequently, final kissing balloon inflation (FKBI) was carried out. Final POT was performed using a 4.5 × 8 mm NC balloon followed by IVUS runs of the LAD and LCX arteries. The LMCA ostium was well covered, and there was no malapposition or edge dissection. A few areas of underexpansion were noted in the LAD stent, and the ostial area of LCX was only 4.72 mm^2. Therefore, postdilatation of these regions was performed again using high-pressure NC balloons. Bifurcation PCI was completed by redoing FKBI, followed by a POT (Figure 1).

Right coronary intervention was subsequently performed; after engaging the RCA, IVUS was done, which showed significant disease starting from the ostioproximal to mid-RCA with a lesion length of 31.5 mm. A 3.5 × 37 mm DES was used. Using the sepal wire technique, the stent was positioned in the RCA ostium and deployed. Postdilatation was performed, and final IVUS showed a well-expanded stent with no edge dissection or malapposition, covering the RCA ostium.

It is difficult to identify the exact stent position and perform aorto-ostial stenting without contrast media. We used the marker wire technique for precise positioning of the

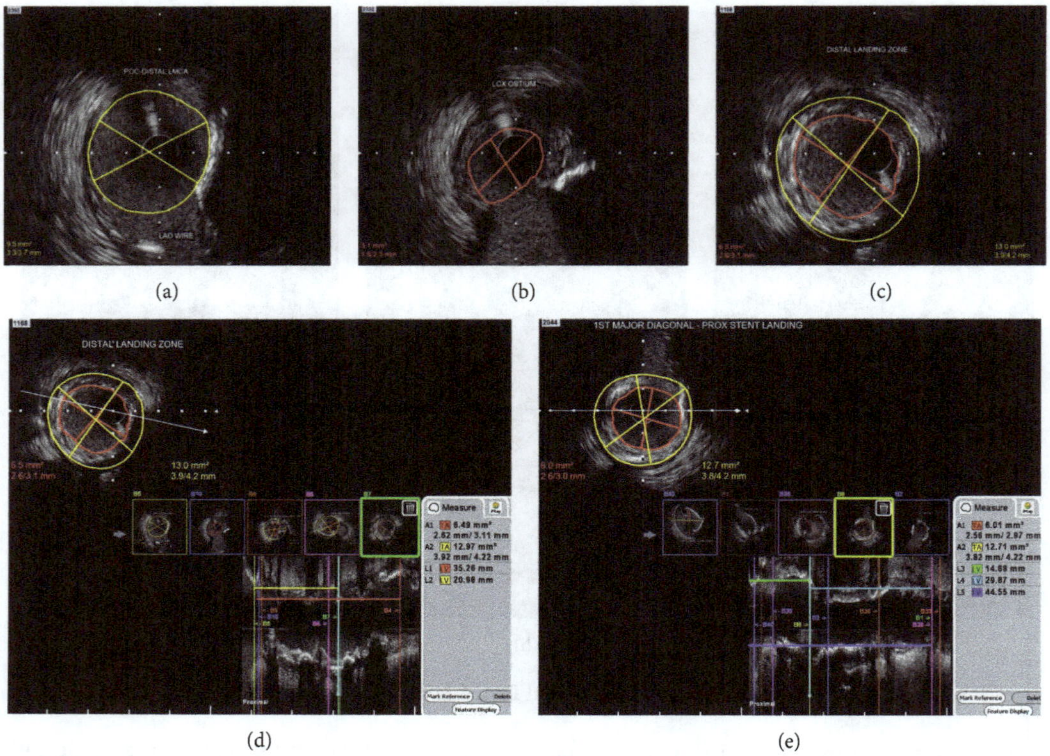

Figure 3: (a) Distal LMCA IVUS. (b) Significant disease at LCX ostium. (c) Distal landing zone in major OM. (d) IVUS image in LCX for assessing stent length. (e) IVUS in LM-LAD to decide proximal and distal stent lengths.

LMCA and RCA ostial stents. The procedure was completed at a total fluoroscopy time of 36.9 minutes and a radiation dosage of 4434 milligray (mGy) with 0 ml of contrast medium/agents. The patient was discharged 72 hours later, after creatinine levels reduced from 290 μmol/l to 253 μmol/l. The post-PCI eGFR was 23 m/min/1.73 m^2. No renal replacement therapy was required before or during the hospital stay. The patient visited the hospital periodically for routine evaluation, and after three months, he was totally asymptomatic. His serum creatinine levels stabilized at around 177 μmol/l without the need for hospitalization or renal replacement therapy.

3. Discussion

To the best of our knowledge, this is the first case report describing zero-contrast IVUS-guided left main bifurcation PCI. This case substantiates the role of image and physiology-guided zero-contrast PCI in managing highly complex interventions for critical conditions such as left main bifurcation disease. Experts in this area can help in alleviating angina associated with coronary artery disease in patients having significant renal impairment and are ineligible for undergoing PCI for fear of worsening renal function.

Larger catheters are preferred for zero-contrast PCI, as simultaneous use of multiple guidewires and imaging is required. Catheter engagement was confirmed by passing the guidewire using previous roadmaps and comparing the course of the wire in the coronary vessel. Other techniques for confirming guide catheter engagement are injection of cold saline (10–20 ml) and identification of electrocardiogram changes. The saline injection induces T-wave inversion or increases its amplitude along with ST-segment depression or elevation if catheter is properly inserted [3]. During wiring of coronary vessels, the same projections taken in the diagnostic study are used, and reference images are always kept side by side. This step may be challenging when the diagnostic study is performed at a different centre and images cannot be displayed while performing the procedure. This limitation is overcome using additional monitor screens in the Cath Lab.

Intravascular imaging is an important component of zero-contrast PCI. Expertise in IVUS image interpretation, as well as strict vigilance in anticipating, identifying, and successfully managing complications, is of paramount importance. It is recommended that only highly trained IVUS interpreters attempt such complex procedures [2]. The IVUS catheter can be manually positioned at the proximal and distal reference segments, with dry cine taken and used as landmarks for stent deployment. Other techniques for identifying the stent position are using marker wires in major branches and measuring the lengths of such branching points from the stent-landing zone using "marker wire" or "metallic silhouette" technique [11].

The threshold for using contrast in the event of a suspected complication should be extremely low. For clinical signs such as chest pain, ECG changes, or hypotension, a low-contrast check angiogram should be performed immediately, considering the safety of the patient. Poststenting IVUS should be done and reviewed meticulously to check for complications. It is mandatory to use transthoracic echocardiogram immediately postprocedure to evaluate for the presence of pericardial effusion. Finally, fractional flow reserve (FFR) is a highly beneficial tool for confirming the accuracy of PCI.

4. Conclusion

Imaging-guided left main bifurcation PCI without the use of contrast was feasible and safe in a patient presenting with multivessel coronary artery disease and CI-AKI. This technique can be used safely in patients who are at high risk for CI-AKI in centres with expertise in complex PCI with intravascular imaging guidance.

Additional Points

Learning Objectives. Intravascular ultrasound-guided zero-contrast PCI is very difficult to accomplish, especially when the left main coronary artery bifurcation is involved. However, steps such as identification of the exact vessel dimensions, lesion length, and planning stent deployment by marking the landing zone using dry cine angiograms while keeping the IVUS catheter, when done by those with significant expertise in IVUS-guided left main interventions, can immensely benefit CKD patients with significant angina.

Acknowledgments

We thank BioQuest Solutions Pvt Ltd for providing editorial support for the manuscript.

References

[1] Z. A. Ali, K. Karimi Galougahi, T. Nazif et al., "Imaging- and physiology-guided percutaneous coronary intervention without contrast administration in advanced renal failure: a feasibility, safety, and outcome study," *European Heart Journal*, vol. 37, no. 40, pp. 3090–3095, 2016.

[2] R. Hatem, M. T. Finn, R. F. Riley et al., "Zero contrast retrograde chronic total occlusions percutaneous coronary intervention: a case series," *European Heart Journal - Case Reports*, vol. 2, no. 2, pp. 1–5, 2018.

[3] J. Sacha, M. Gierlotka, P. Feusette, and D. Dudek, "Ultra-low contrast coronary angiography and zero-contrast percutaneous coronary intervention for prevention of contrast-induced nephropathy: step-by-step approach and review," *Postepy Kardiol Interwencyjnej*, vol. 15, no. 2, pp. 127–136, 2019.

[4] E. Nikolsky, R. Mehran, D. Turcot et al., "Impact of chronic kidney disease on prognosis of patients with diabetes mellitus treated with percutaneous coronary intervention," *The American Journal of Cardiology*, vol. 94, no. 3, pp. 300–305, 2004.

[5] R. G. Cigarroa, R. A. Lange, R. H. Williams, and L. D. Hillis, "Dosing of contrast material to prevent contrast nephropathy in patients with renal disease," *The American Journal of Medicine*, vol. 86, no. 6, pp. 649–652, 1989.

[6] J. R. Brown, J. F. Robb, C. A. Block et al., "Does safe dosing of iodinated contrast prevent contrast-induced acute kidney injury?," *Circulation. Cardiovascular Interventions*, vol. 3, no. 4, pp. 346–350, 2010.

[7] W. K. Laskey, C. Jenkins, F. Selzer et al., "Volume-to-creatinine clearance ratio: a pharmacokinetically based risk factor for prediction of early creatinine increase after percutaneous coronary intervention," *Journal of the American College of Cardiology*, vol. 50, no. 7, pp. 584–590, 2007.

[8] S. S. Naidu, H. D. Aronow, L. C. Box et al., "SCAI expert consensus statement: 2016 best practices in the cardiac catheterization laboratory: (Endorsed by the cardiological society of india, and sociedad Latino Americana de Cardiologia intervencionista; Affirmation of value by the Canadian Association of interventional cardiology–Association canadienne de cardiologie d'intervention)," *Catheterization and Cardiovascular Interventions*, vol. 88, no. 3, pp. 407–423, 2016.

[9] F. Burzotta, J. F. Lassen, T. Lefèvre et al., "Percutaneous coronary intervention for bifurcation coronary lesions. The 15th Consensus Document from the European Bifurcation Club," *EuroIntervention*, 2020.

[10] C. K. Chan and R. C. Fung, ""Sepal wire technique"–a novel technique for aorto-ostial left main stenting," *The Journal of Invasive Cardiology*, vol. 23, no. 5, pp. 211-212, 2011.

[11] J. Sacha, "Marking wire technique for zero-contrast percutaneous coronary interventions," *Advances in Interventional Cardiology*, vol. 14, no. 2, pp. 204-205, 2018.

42

Ticagrelor-Induced Prolongation of the QTc Interval

Avik Ray,[1] **Ahmad Najmi**,[1] **Gaurav Khandelwal**,[2] **and Balakrishnan Sadasivam**[1]

[1]*Department of Pharmacology, All India Institute of Medical Sciences Bhopal, Saket Nagar, Bhopal 462020, Madhya Pradesh, India*
[2]*Department of Cardiology, All India Institute of Medical Sciences Bhopal, Saket Nagar, Bhopal 462020, Madhya Pradesh, India*

Correspondence should be addressed to Avik Ray; avik.jrpharma18@aiimsbhopal.edu.in

Academic Editor: Man-Hong Jim

Background. Ticagrelor has been accepted as a class I antiplatelet agent in patients undergoing percutaneous coronary angioplasty (PTCA). There have been cases reported on ticagrelor being associated with various cardiac conduction defects. But there is no evidence of QTc prolongation associated with the drug as of yet. *Case Presentation.* A 64-year-old male who underwent PTCA was given ticagrelor. A baseline electrocardiogram (ECG) showed a QTc of 402 ms. He returned after 1.5 months with complaints of shortness of breath. An ECG revealed a prolonged QTc of 468 ms. Ticagrelor was discontinued in view of ticagrelor-induced dyspnea and the patient was started on clopidogrel. The other medications were kept unchanged. The patient returned after a month without any complaints. A follow-up ECG showed a reduced QTc of 425 ms. *Conclusion.* We present a case of ticagrelor-induced QTc prolongation. To our knowledge, this is the first case to be reported on the same. The Naranjo algorithm for causality assessment gave a total score of 6 indicating that the adverse drug reaction falls under the *probable* category.

1. Introduction

QTc prolongation is defined as the QTc (QT interval corrected by the RR interval) ≥ 460 ms in men and ≥ 480 ms in women [1], although this definition varies depending on the source. It can lead to the development of torsades de pointes (TdP) which might be associated with episodes of ventricular fibrillation, cardiac arrest and sudden death. The risk of developing TdP increases with QTc intervals being more than 500 ms. Various risk factors for QTc prolongation include bradycardia, structural cardiac defects, females, old age (≥ 65 years), metabolic abnormalities, traumatic brain injury (TBI) and the presence of any QTc prolonging agent [1].

Drug-induced QTc prolongation is the most common reason for the condition [2]. Medicines that increase the interval are proposed to do so by interfering or inhibiting the action of delayed rectifier potassium channels [3]. Several antiarrhythmics, antihistamines, antimicrobials, antidepressants and prokinetic agents are known to cause QTc prolongation [3].

Since the approval of Ticagrelor as an antiplatelet agent by the US Food and Drug Administration (USFDA) on July 20, 2011, there has not been a single recorded case report or evidence of it being associated with QTc prolongation. We hereby report a case of probable ticagrelor-induced QTc prolongation.

2. Case Report

A 64-year-old male with a medical history of hypertension, diabetes mellitus and hyperlipidemia and a chronic smoker presented with complaints of chest pain which was sharp, continuous in nature and was aggravated by slight walking or lifting of heavy loads. The patient also had complaints of shortness of breath of Grade 4 according to the Medical Research Council (MRC) Dyspnoea Scale [4]. He had a body mass index (BMI) of 25.8 Kg/m^2. The baseline HbA1c% value was 10.8 gm%. He underwent coronary angiography at the discretion of the concerned cardiologist. A diagnosis of Acute Coronary Syndrome (ACS) with Non-ST elevation Myocardial Infarction (NSTEMI) with an occlusion of 99%

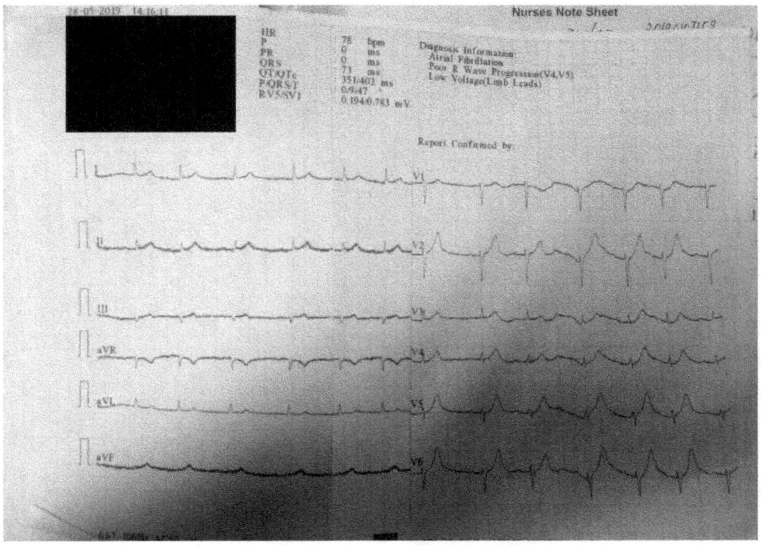

FIGURE 1: Electrocardiogram showed atrial fibrillation with poor progression of the R wave in leads V4 and V5 along with a QTc of 402 ms.

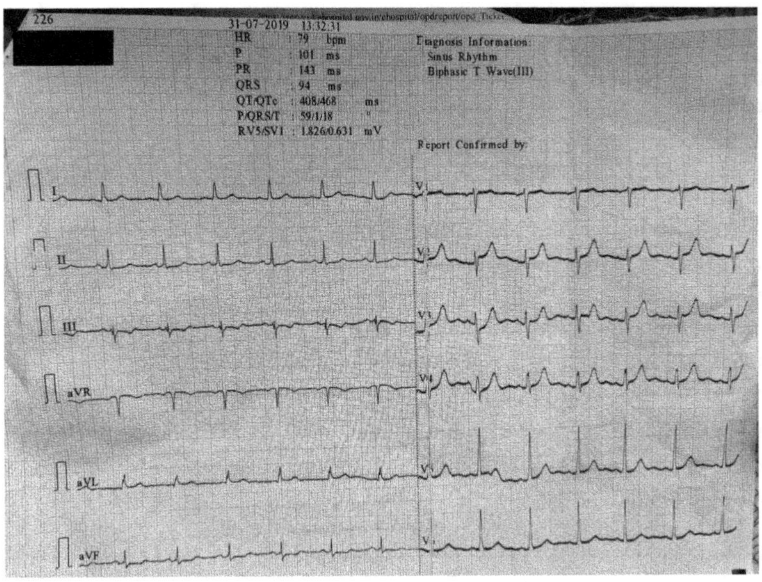

FIGURE 2: Electrocardiogram revealed a sinus rhythm with biphasic T wave in lead III and a QTc of 468 ms.

in the left circumflex artery (LCX) was made. Percutaneous Coronary Angioplasty (PTCA) was performed on the same day with the placement of one everolimus eluting coronary stent in the LCX.

A loading dose of 180 mg of ticagrelor was given to the patient just before the PTCA was performed. A thrombolysis in myocardial infarction (TIMI) 3 flow was achieved post the procedure. Blood flow distal to the stent was achieved and the procedure was concluded successfully. The post procedural ejection fraction (EF) was 45%. Post procedural electrocardiogram (ECG) was also performed and it showed a QTc of 402 ms with atrial fibrillation and poor progression of the R wave in leads V4 and V5 (Figure 1). He got discharged after 2 days with an advice of 180 mg ticagrelor, 75 mg aspirin, 20 mg atorvastatin, 25 mg metoprolol, 25 mg spironolactone, 10 mg furosemide and 1000 mg of metformin daily. He was advised to visit the out-patient department (OPD) of Cardiology after 2 months or the ED in case of any emergency.

The patient came to the OPD after 1.5 months with complaints of severe shortness of breath (MRC Dyspnoea Scale Grade 5) along with infrequent bouts of coughs. Vitals were measured and the blood pressure was 104/60 mm Hg, with the pulse being 68/min. On auscultation, no bronchopulmonary abnormality could be inferred. Bilateral clear breath sounds were obtained. A BMI of 24.6 Kg/m^2 was recorded. In view of ticagrelor induced dyspnea, ticagrelor was discontinued and 75 mg clopidogrel once daily was started while rest of the medications were kept unchanged. An ECG was obtained and it showed a QTc of 468 ms (16.4% increase) with biphasic T wave in Lead III (Figure 2). He was advised to visit the Cardiology OPD after 1 month or the ED in case of any emergency.

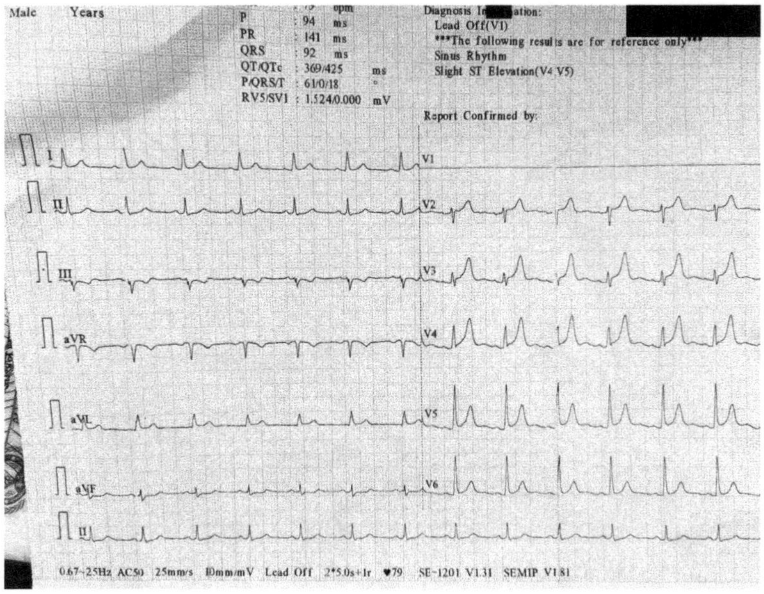

Figure 3: Electrocardiogram revealed a sinus rhythm with slight ST elevation in leads V4 and V5. The QTc was 425 ms, a reduction of 9.2% as compared to the previous reading.

Table 1: The Naranjo algorithm to assess the causality. Total score categories are defined as follows: Adverse Drug Reaction (ADR) is: certain >9; probable 5-8; possible 1-4; unlikely 0.

Question	Yes	No	Do not know	Score
Are there previous conclusive reports on this reaction?	+1	0	0	0
Did the adverse event appear after the suspected drug was administered?	+2	-1	0	+2
Did the adverse reaction improve when the drug was discontinued or a specific antagonist was administered?	+1	0	0	+1
Did the adverse reaction reappear when the drug was re-administered?	+2	-1	0	0
Are there alternative causes (other than the drug) that could solely have caused the reaction?	-1	+2	0	+2
Was the drug detected in the blood (or other fluids) in a concentration known to be toxic?	-1	+1	0	0
Was the reaction more severe when the dose was increased, or less severe when the dose was decreased?	+1	0	0	0
Did the patient have a similar reaction to the same or similar drugs in any previous exposure?	+1	0	0	0
Was the adverse event confirmed by objective evidence?	+1	0	0	+1
Total score				**6**

The patient came back after one month for follow-up. He had no complaints of shortness of breath or cough this time. Vitals were measured and blood pressure was 114/78 mm Hg with a pulse rate of 66/min. HbA1c% came out to be 9.6 gm%. An ECG was done and it showed a drastic reduction of the QTc to 425 ms (9.2% reduction) (Figure 3) with slight ST elevation in leads V4 and V5. An echocardiography was also performed and the EF came out to be 50%.

3. Discussion

A literature search was conducted to find out any report or evidence of QTc prolongation associated with ticagrelor use. A PubMED search was done using the keywords *ticagrelor, QTc prolongation, cardiac, conduction defects, torsades de pointes* and *arrhythmia*.

A single study concluding that a single oral dose of ticagrelor does not prolong the QT interval in health subjects could be found [5]. The association of ticagrelor use with other conduction defects such as atrioventricular block [6, 7] is well known. During a phase IIb dose-ranging safety trial, an unexpected high number of incidences of ventricular pauses was seen in patients receiving ticagrelor [8]. The pivotal trial PLATO monitored for such conduction related adverse events via continuous ECG monitoring on over 3000 patients in the form of a sub-study. Ticagrelor was associated with an increased rate of ventricular pauses ≥3 seconds (5.8% vs. 3.6%, RR: 1.61; 95% CI, 1.14–2.26) [9].

Latest studies have discovered that ticagrelor prevents the uptake of adenosine by the red blood cells in patients of ACS, leading to an increased adenosine plasma concentration (APC), similar to the observation obtained for dipyridamole [10]. Adenosine exerts cardiological effects by acting on the A1 receptors. It has got negative chronotropic effects by suppressing the automaticity of the pacemaker cells and a negative dromotropic effect by inhibiting the atrioventricular bundle [11]. The effect of ticagrelor on the adenosine concentration conveys unique properties to this drug as compared to other P2Y12 antagonists namely clopidogrel, cangrelor and prasugrel.

On performing causality assessment using the Naranjo algorithm [12], a total score of 6 was obtained indicating that the adverse drug reaction falls under the *probable* category (Table 1). The case was reported on the national pharmacovigilance portal.

Other non-pharmacological causes of QTc prolongation such as hypothyroidism [13] and hypocalcemia [14] were ruled out in this patient. As mentioned earlier, the patient was a known case of type 2 diabetes mellitus which has been found to be associated with prolongation of the QTc interval [15]. Since the initial QTc interval was normal and it came back to the normal range after discontinuation of ticagrelor, we can rule out this factor as well. Everolimus has been associated with QTc prolongation in renal transplant patients where it has been used as an immunosuppressant [16]. The drug is usually undetectable in blood 30 days after the implantation of the everolimus-eluting stent. It has been seen that only when a patient has the maximum number of four stents, it is possible to achieve a plasma drug concentration similar to that with oral treatment [17]. This helps us to rule out any possible causality between everolimus and the observed QTc prolongation in this case.

We were hence able to identify a temporal and causal relationship between the initiation and discontinuation of ticagrelor and the development of QTc prolongation. To our knowledge, this is the first case to be reported on the same. The mechanism by which it causes QTc prolongation and whether it differs from the usual mechanism of interference with the action of the delayed rectifier potassium channels and thus extending the duration of phase 3 of myocardial repolarization needs to be investigated [3]. Clinicians should be made aware about this so that cardiac monitoring in the form of an ECG can be considered at the baseline and at the subsequent follow-up visits, especially in patients with multiple risk factors for QTc prolongation.

References

[1] B. J. Drew, M. J. Ackerman, M. Funk et al., "Prevention of torsade de pointes in hospital settings: a scientific statement from the American Heart Association and the American College of Cardiology Foundation," *Circulation*, vol. 121, no. 8, pp. 1047–1060, 2010.

[2] D. Pickham, E. Helfenbein, J. A. Shinn et al., "High prevalence of corrected QT interval prolongation in acutely ill patients is associated with mortality: results of the QT in Practice (QTIP) Study," *Critical Care Medicine*, vol. 40, no. 2, pp. 394–399, 2012.

[3] Y. G. Yap and A. J. Camm, "Drug induced QT prolongation and torsades de pointes," *Heart*, vol. 89, no. 11, pp. 1363–1372, 2003.

[4] J. C. Bestall, E. A. Paul, R. Garrod, R. Garnham, P. W. Jones, and J. A. Wedzicha, "Usefulness of the Medical Research Council (MRC) dyspnoea scale as a measure of disability in patients with chronic obstructive pulmonary disease," *Thorax*, vol. 54, no. 7, pp. 581–586, 1999.

[5] K. Butler, C. Wei, and R. Teng, "Single-dose ticagrelor does not prolong the QT interval in healthy subjects," *International Journal of Clinical Pharmacology and Therapeutics*, vol. 48, no. 10, pp. 643–651, 2010.

[6] M. Ünlü, S. Demirkol, A. O. Yildirim, Ş. Balta, C. Öztürk, and A. Iyisoy, "Atrioventricular block associated with ticagrelor therapy may require permanent pacemaker," *International Journal of Cardiology*, vol. 202, pp. 946-947, 2016.

[7] M. Sharma and D. A. N. Mascarenhas, "Ticagrelor Associated Heart Block: The Need for Close and Continued Monitoring," *Case Reports in Cardiology*, vol. 2017, Article ID 5074891, 4 pages, 2017.

[8] C. P. Cannon, S. Husted, R. A. Harrington et al., "Safety, tolerability, and initial efficacy of AZD6140, the first reversible oral adenosine diphosphate receptor antagonist, compared with clopidogrel, in patients with non–ST-segment elevation acute coronary syndrome: primary results of the DISPERSE-2 trial," *Journal of American College of Cardiology*, vol. 50, pp. 1844–1851, 2007.

[9] B. M. Scirica, C. P. Cannon, H. Emanuelsson et al., "The incidence of bradyarrhythmias and clinical bradyarrhythmic events in patients with acute coronary syndromes treated with ticagrelor or clopidogrel in the PLATO (platelet inhibition and patient outcomes) trial: results of the continuous electrocardiographic assessment substudy," *Journal of American College of Cardiology*, vol. 57, pp. 1908–1916, 2011.

[10] M. Cattaneo, R. Schulz, and S. Nylander, "Adenosine-mediated effects of ticagrelor: evidence and potential clinical relevance," *Journal of the American College of Cardiology*, vol. 63, no. 23, pp. 2503–2509, 2014.

[11] L. Bonello, M. Laine, N. Kipson et al., "Ticagrelor increases adenosine plasma concentration in patients with an acute coronary syndrome," *Journal of the American College of Cardiology*, vol. 63, no. 9, pp. 872–877, 2014.

[12] S. A. Zaki, "Adverse drug reaction and causality assessment scales," *Lung India*, vol. 28, no. 2, pp. 152-153, 2011.

[13] K. H. Kweon, B. H. Park, and C. G. Cho, "The effects of L-thyroxine treatment on QT dispersion in primary hypothyroidism," *Journal of Korean Medical Science*, vol. 22, no. 1, pp. 114–116, 2007.

[14] S. Nijjer, A. K. Ghosh, and S. W. Dubrey, "Hypocalcaemia, long QT interval and atrial arrhythmias," *Case Reports*, vol. 2010, article bcr0820092216, 2010.

[15] S. Giunti, G. Gruden, P. Fornengo et al., "Increased QT interval dispersion predicts 15-year cardiovascular mortality in type 2 diabetic subjects: the population-based Casale Monferrato study," *Diabetes Care*, vol. 35, no. 3, pp. 581–583, 2012.

[16] B. Ikitimur, K. Cosansu, B. Karadag et al., "Long-Term Impact of Different Immunosuppressive Drugs on QT and PR Intervals in Renal Transplant Patients," *Annals of Noninvasive Electrocardiology*, vol. 20, no. 5, pp. 426–432, 2015.

[17] A. Saez and R. Moreno, "Everolimus-eluting coronary stents," *Medical Devices: Evidence and Research*, vol. 3, pp. 51–56, 2010.

Transcatheter Tricuspid Valve-in-Valve Replacement using a J-Valve System for a Failed Tricuspid Bioprosthesis

Mingkui Zhang, Hui Xue, Lifu Miao, Xiujie Tang, and Yanbin Shao

Heart Center, First Hospital of Tsinghua University, No. 6 1st Street, Jiuxianqiao, Chaoyang District, Beijing 100016, China

Correspondence should be addressed to Mingkui Zhang; mingkuizhang@163.com

Academic Editor: Yuli Huang

Background. Redo operation for failed tricuspid bioprosthetic valves is associated with high morbidity and mortality. Transcatheter tricuspid valve-in-valve implantation has become an acceptable option for high-risk patients with a failed tricuspid bioprosthesis. We present a case of successful tricuspid valve-in-valve implantation using a J-valve in a failed tricuspid bioprosthesis position. *Case Summary.* A 48-year-old male, who had a failed tricuspid bioprosthesis, presented with right-side heart failure, right-to-left shunting at the atrial level, severe dyspnea, cyanosis, peripheral edema, hepatauxe, and ascites. After the interdisciplinary assessment, we successfully performed transcatheter tricuspid valve-in-valve implantation with the J-valve system. At 34-month postoperative follow-up, the patient had no symptoms of heart failure and the echocardiogram showed good valve position and well hemodynamic status. *Conclusions.* This case demonstrated that the J-valve system may be a new option for high-risk patients with a failed tricuspid bioprosthetic valve.

1. Introduction

The bioprosthetic valve has become the main choice for tricuspid valve replacement because of its advantages such as low incidence of thrombosis and avoidance of complications associated with anticoagulation [1, 2]. However, bioprosthetic valve failure is inevitable in the long term due to degeneration and calcification [3]. Reoperation is the standard treatment for failed bioprosthetic valves, but it may carry significant risks of adverse perioperative events [4]. The first-in-man tricuspid valve-in-valve (VIV) was reported in 2011 using the off-label Edwards SAPIEN valve (Edwards Lifesciences). Since then, transcatheter tricuspid VIV implantation has become an acceptable alternative for high-risk patients with a failed tricuspid bioprosthesis [5–8]. The J-valve system (Jiecheng Medical Technology Co., Ltd., Suzhou China) is a new second generation of transcatheter heart valves and has been an adequate option for the treatment of high-risk patients with aortic valve stenosis and regurgitation [9]. We describe a man with severe bioprosthetic tricuspid valve (TV) stenosis who underwent transcatheter tricuspid valve-in-valve with the use of a J-valve system.

2. Case Presentation

In August 2019, a 48-year-old male presented at our hospital due to severe dyspnea (NYHA III), cyanosis, dizziness, peripheral edema, hepatauxe, and massive ascites. He had a history of the congenital ventricular septal defect, infective endocarditis, heart valve infective vegetation, and severe tricuspid valve regurgitation and undergone ventricular septal defect repair, aortic valve repair, pulmonary valve repair, and the tricuspid valve replacement with a 29 mm bioprosthesis (Edwards Lifesciences, LLC; Irvine, California) in another hospital in 2005. Severe postoperative pulmonary infection complications occurred and required tracheotomy and ventilator-assisted therapy for more than seven days. From the beginning of 2017, he gradually started to present heart failure symptoms and underwent multiple hospital admissions for severe dyspnea, peripheral edema, and recurrent ascites. The current physical examination revealed lethargy, cyanotic lips, jugular vein distension, a grade of 2/6

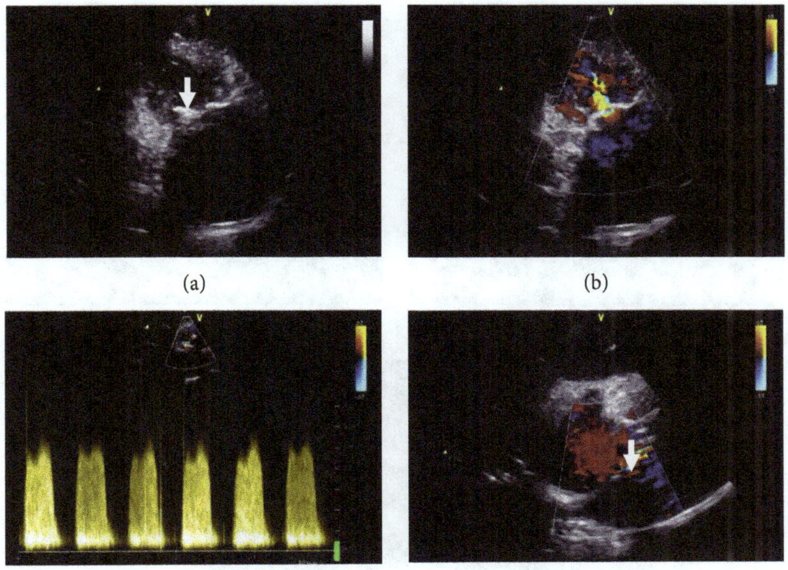

(a) (b) (c) (d)

FIGURE 1: Transthoracic echocardiography (TTE) and Doppler before the operation: bioprosthetic tricuspid valve calcification (white arrow) and stenosis (a, b). Bioprosthetic maximal velocity 2.7 m/s (c). The foramen ovale opening (white arrow) (d).

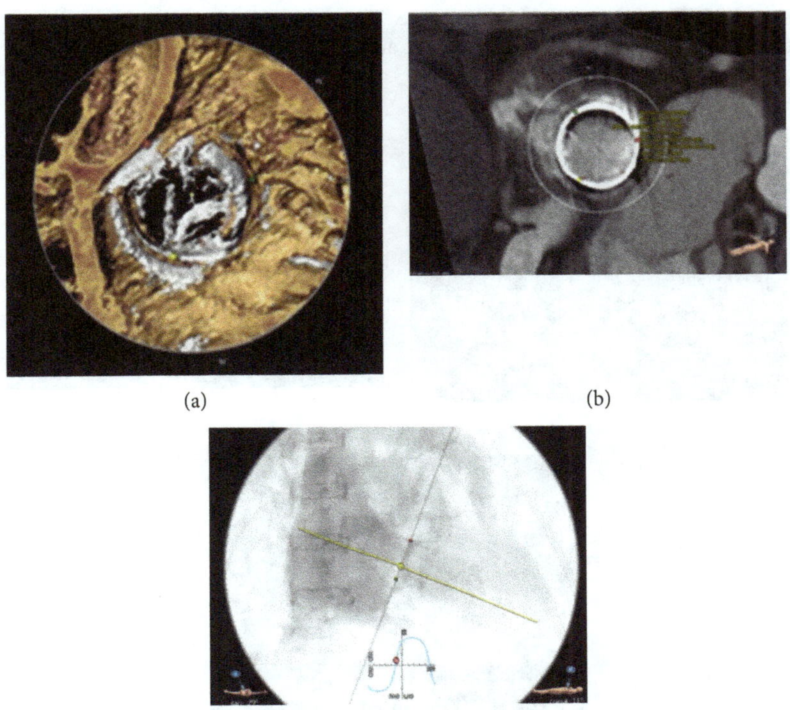

(a) (b) (c)

FIGURE 2: Cardiac computed tomography images: distribution of severe bioprosthetic leaflet calcification (a). Inner diameter of the bioprosthetic valve (26.3 mm) (b). The best projection angles (c).

diastolic murmur at the left lower sternal border, hepatauxe, and massive ascites. Blood gas analysis shows that oxygen pressure is 56.8 mmHg, oxygen saturation is 88.2%, carbon dioxide is 27.6 mmHg, and hemoglobin is 231 g/L.

Transthoracic echocardiography revealed bioprosthetic TV stenosis (Figure 1). The mean transvalvular gradient pressure and peak transvalvular gradient pressure were 21 mmHg and 33 mmHg, respectively. The aortic valve had mild regurgitation, foramen ovale opening (6 mm), and right-to-left shunting. The right atrial and ventricular volumes were enlarged. The tricuspid annular plane systolic excursion was 8 mm, and the fractional area change (FAC) was 40%. The distribution of severe calcification in the bioprosthetic valve and the bioprosthesis annulus's diameter

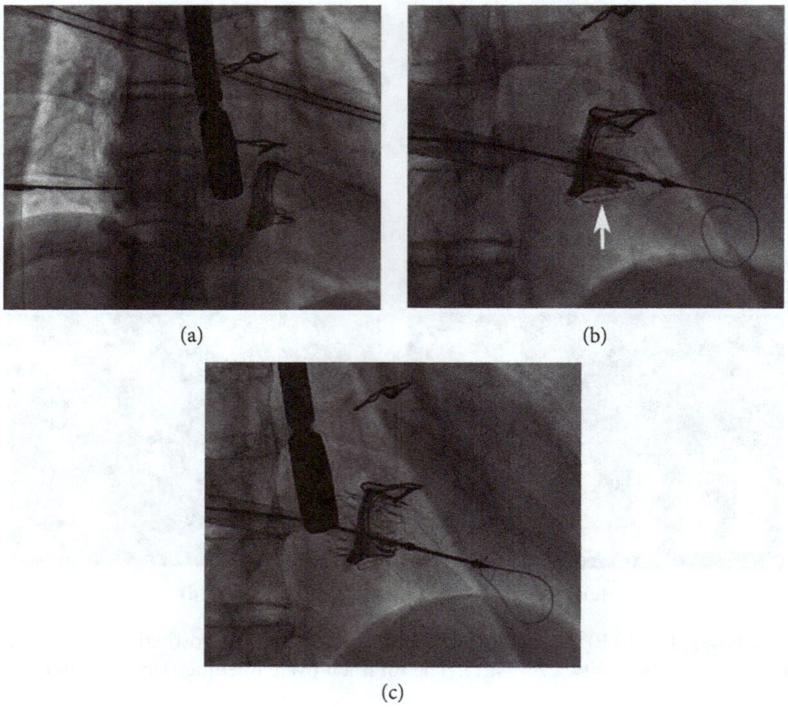

Figure 3: Step-by-step transatrial TVIV implantation of the J-valve. The right atrium puncture according to the coaxial position of the tricuspid annulus (a). The three "U-shape graspers" were released and embraced the prior bioprosthetic struts (white arrow) (b). Full deployment of the J-valve (c).

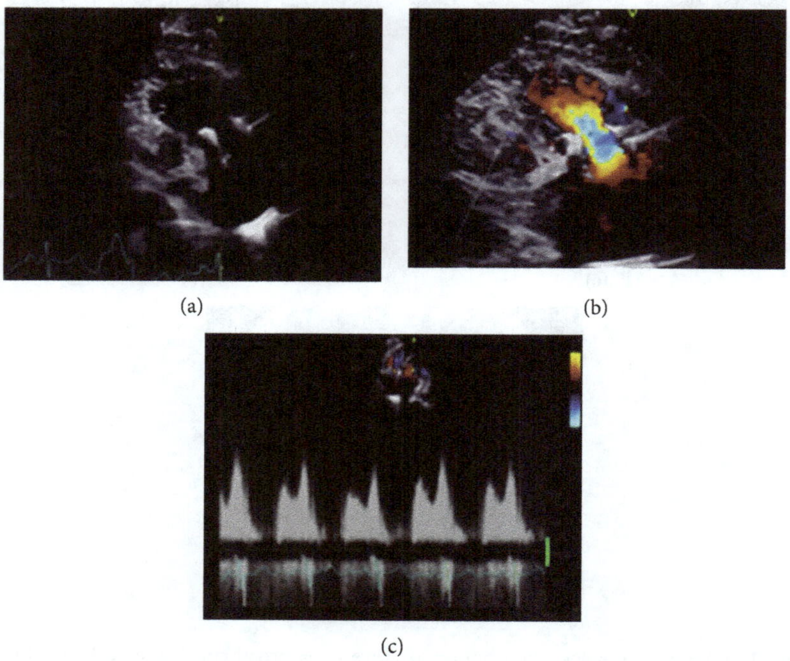

Figure 4: The transthoracic echocardiogram images during the 34-month follow-up period: TTE showed optimal valve position and well hemodynamic status (a, b). TTE with color flow showed a maximal velocity of 1.6 m/s (c).

were determined by multidetector computed tomography (MDCT) (Figure 2). Diagnostic cardiac catheterization examination showed that the superior vena cava pressure, the inferior vena cava pressure, and the right atrial pressure were 29/12/19 mmHg, 28/20/23 mmHg, and 29/16/21 mmHg, respectively. These findings were consistent with a severe stenosis of the bioprosthesis in the tricuspid position.

After the interdisciplinary assessment, the heart team decided to perform transcatheter tricuspid VIV implantation using the J-valve system because of a significantly increased surgical risk for conventional redo surgery: the estimated surgical risks (EuroSCORE II) were 12.4%. Based on MDCT measurements, the 27 mm J-valve was suitable for valve-in-valve replacement in the tricuspid position.

After confirmed consent and Hospital Ethics Committee approval (no. 20190009) were obtained, the procedure was performed in a hybrid operating room under general anesthesia with a double-lumen endotracheal tube. Transesophageal echocardiogram (TEE) was used for the evaluation of the valve pathology and operation result. Both the right femoral artery and vein were exposed for emergency cardiopulmonary bypass. The left radial artery and right internal jugular vein puncture catheterization was performed for measurement of blood pressure and central venous pressure. A right minithoracotomy in the fourth intercostal space and the right atrial double purse-string sutures were performed according to the coaxial position of the tricuspid annulus. Heparin was administered to keep the activated clotting time at more than 300 seconds. After the right atrium puncture, a soft guide wire and then a superstiff guide wire were used to cross the bioprosthetic valve and into the right ventricle. The valvuloplasty (balloon inflated to 22 mm, Percutaneous Transluminal Valvuloplasty Catheter Z-MED II™, NuMED, CAN) was performed without rapid ventricular pacing. The J-valve was reversely loaded on the conveyor system and successfully implanted into the degenerated bioprosthesis. The three "U-shape graspers" were released and embraced the prior bioprosthetic struts (Figure 3). Intraoperative transesophageal echocardiograms confirmed the correct position, no periprosthetic leakage, right-to-left intracardiac shunt vanishment at the atrial level, and excellent function of the tricuspid bioprosthetic valve, with maximal pressure gradient 12 mmHg. Artery oxygen saturation and hemodynamic status were improved shortly.

Postoperatively, oral warfarin anticoagulation was used to maintain an internationalization ratio of 2.0-2.5 for three months. Transthoracic echocardiography and electrocardiogram were performed regularly for postoperative evaluation. Thirty-four months after surgery, the patient was free of heart failure symptoms and the echocardiogram suggested excellent hemodynamics of the bioprosthetic valve (Figure 4).

3. Discussion

Transcatheter VIV implantation has become an attractive option for failed aortic and mitral bioprostheses. The American Food and Drug Administration approved the mitral VIV procedure with the Edwards SAPIEN system in 2017 [10]. Recent publications reported good results following implanted stent valves in the aortic or mitral position [11, 12]. Since the first case of tricuspid valve-in-valve using an off-label Edwards SAPIEN valve (Edwards Lifesciences Corporation, Irvine, CA, USA) was reported, the literature on VIV implantation in failed tricuspid bioprostheses is reported in small case series and case reports [5, 13, 14]. Recently, registry data was reported by McElhinney, demonstrating that transcatheter tricuspid VIV implantation was hemodynamically and clinically beneficial in patients of various ages and underlying disease states. The adverse TVIV-related outcomes (TV dysfunction, endocarditis, and leaflet thrombosis) were relatively uncommon in 306 patients, and valve function remained excellent in the majority of patients in three-year follow-up results [15].

The J-valve is a new generation self-expendable valve and has previously been shown to be effective for the treatment of both serve aortic valve stenosis and aortic regurgitation. A J-valve multicenter study, which enrolled 107 high-risk patients with aortic valve stenosis, aortic valve regurgitation, or bicuspid aortic valve (BAV), demonstrated a lower rate of complications and mortality at 1-year follow-up [16]. The J-valve has several advantages: firstly, it is a short stent-valve frame that avoids the right ventricular outflow tract obstruction. Secondly, the unique 3 U-shaped graspers facilitate anchoring and avoid displacement after deployment. Thirdly, the shortest distance through the right atrium access facilitates the coaxiality of the implanted valve and is easy to manipulate. For this patient, the off-label procedure was the last resort to improve his quality of life, and the decision was made after a full discussion between the patient and the heart team. At the 34-month postoperative follow-up, the patient had no symptoms of heart failure and the echocardiogram showed good valve hemodynamics.

4. Conclusion

Transcatheter tricuspid VIV implantation has become an acceptable alternative to conventional open surgery for patients with a failed tricuspid bioprosthesis. This case demonstrated that transcatheter VIV replacement using a J-valve system may be a new option for the failed tricuspid bioprosthesis patients.

References

[1] P. Liu, W. H. Qiao, F. Q. Sun et al., "Should a mechanical or biological prosthesis be used for a tricuspid valve replacement? A meta-analysis," *Journal of Cardiac Surgery*, vol. 31, no. 5, pp. 294–302, 2016.

[2] A. Anselmi, V. G. Ruggieri, M. Harmouche et al., "Appraisal of long-term outcomes of tricuspid valve replacement in the current perspective," *The Annals of Thoracic Surgery*, vol. 101, no. 3, pp. 863–871, 2016.

[3] N. Côté, P. Pibarot, and M. A. Clavel, "Incidence, risk factors, clinical impact, and management of bioprosthesis structural valve degeneration," *Current Opinion in Cardiology*, vol. 32, no. 2, pp. 123–129, 2017.

[4] C. Chen, M. Ge, J. Ye et al., "The risk and outcomes of reoperative tricuspid valve replacement surgery," *The Heart Surgery Forum*, vol. 23, no. 5, pp. E658–E664, 2020.

[5] L. A. Van Garsse, R. M. Ter Bekke, and V. G. van Ommen, "Percutaneous transcatheter valve-in-valve implantation in stenosed tricuspid valve bioprosthesis," *Circulation*, vol. 123, no. 5, pp. e219–e221, 2011.

[6] D. B. McElinney, A. K. Cabalka, J. A. Aboulhosn et al., "Transcatheter tricuspid valve-in-valve implantation for the treatment of dysfunctional surgical bioprosthetic valves," *Circulation*, vol. 133, no. 16, pp. 1582–1593, 2016.

[7] F. Praz, I. George, S. Kodali et al., "Transcatheter tricuspid valve-in-valve intervention for degenerative bioprosthetic tricuspid valve disease," *Journal of the American Society of Echocardiography*, vol. 31, no. 4, pp. 491–504, 2018.

[8] M. Chandavimol, T. Ngernsritrakul, K. Meemook et al., "Transcatheter tricuspid valve-in-valve implantation for degenerative surgical bio-prosthesis using SAPIEN 3: a case series," *Clinical Case Reports*, vol. 9, no. 11, article e05029, 2021.

[9] X. Luo, X. Wang, X. Li et al., "Transapical transcatheter aortic valve implantation using the J-Valve system: a 1-year follow-up study," *The Journal of Thoracic and Cardiovascular Surgery*, vol. 154, no. 1, pp. 46–55, 2017.

[10] A. Shivaraju, J. Michel, A. H. Frangieh et al., "Transcatheter aortic and mitral valve-in-valve implantation using the Edwards Sapien 3 heart valve," *Journal of the American Heart Association*, vol. 7, no. 14, article e007767, 2018.

[11] M. Gallo, D. Dvir, S. Demertzis, G. Pedrazzini, D. Berdajs, and E. Ferrari, "Transcatheter valve-in-valve implantation for degenerated bioprosthetic aortic and mitral valves," *Expert Review of Medical Devices*, vol. 13, no. 8, pp. 749–758, 2016.

[12] M. Ghosh-Dastidar, A. Narayana, R. Boix, and V. Bapat, "Mitral valve-in-valve and valve-in-ring for failing surgical bioprosthetic valves and rings," *The Journal of Cardiovascular Surgery*, vol. 57, no. 3, pp. 372–380, 2016.

[13] D. M. Filsoof, D. F. Snipelisky, and B. P. Shapiro, "Use of a melody pulmonary valve in transcatheter valve-in-valve replacement for tricuspid valve bioprosthesis degeneration," *Texas Heart Institute Journal*, vol. 41, no. 5, pp. 511–513, 2014.

[14] C. Rogkakou, P. Braun, M. Kullmer, and W. Schöls, "Transfemoral implantation of Edwards SAPIEN-XT® transcatheter heart valve in a degenerated tricuspid bioprosthesis," *Journal of Cardiology Cases*, vol. 16, no. 4, pp. 131–133, 2017.

[15] D. B. McElhinney, J. A. Aboulhosn, D. Dvir et al., "Mid-term valve-related outcomes after transcatheter tricuspid valve-in-valve or valve-in-ring replacement," *Journal of the American College of Cardiology*, vol. 73, no. 2, pp. 148–157, 2019.

[16] M. Tung, X. Wang, F. Li et al., "A versatile transapical device for aortic valvular disease: one-year outcomes of a multicenter study on the J-Valve system," *Journal of Cardiology*, vol. 72, no. 5, pp. 377–384, 2018.

Percutaneous Aspiration of a Mobile Infected Thrombus from the Right Ventricular Outflow Tract using the AngioVac System

Justin Ugwu,[1] Umbreen Hussein,[2] Sampson Alliu,[3] and Ravi Gurujal[4]

[1]*Department of Hospital Medicine, Miami Valley Hospital, Dayton, Ohio, USA*
[2]*Cardiovascular Disease Fellowship, Wright State University, Dayton, Ohio, USA*
[3]*Department of Cardiovascular Medicine, Maimonides Medical Center, Brooklyn, New York, USA*
[4]*Department of Cardiology, Miami Valley Hospital, Dayton, Ohio, USA*

Correspondence should be addressed to Justin Ugwu; ugwujustin@yahoo.com

Academic Editor: Man-Hong Jim

The AngioVac system was invented in 2012 and was originally designed for the removal of thrombi from the venous system. It has been successfully used in the management of iliocaval and right endocardial thrombi but is reportedly less effective in the management of pulmonary emboli (PE). Since its advent, there has been interest in its application towards other medical situations. One of the most revolutionary uses thus far has been for percutaneous debridement of valvular and cardiac electronic device-associated vegetations. In most instances, the AngioVac device has been used to obviate the need for surgery in high-risk patients. Here, we describe a novel use of this device in the successful retrieval of a large, mobile, infected thrombus from the right ventricular outflow tract in a high surgical-risk patient.

1. Introduction

An isolated right ventricular (RV) outflow mass is a rare finding in clinical practice. The differential diagnosis of a mass appearing six days after a negative transesophageal echocardiogram (TEE) in this location includes thrombus, embolus, tumor embolus, and endocardial vegetation. Frequently, initial management options are conservative, including anticoagulation for thrombus/embolus and antibiotics for vegetations. When surgical intervention is indicated, thrombectomy, embolectomy, or vegetectomy is usually invasive and associated with increased morbidity and mortality. As described in several case reports, the AngioVac catheter has proven to be a suitable alternative to surgery in these scenarios [1–3].

2. Case Description

Our patient is a 64-year-old African American male with a past medical history significant for coronary artery disease status post percutaneous coronary intervention in the setting of a non-ST elevation myocardial infarction, hypertension, hyperlipidemia, diabetes mellitus type 2, chronic kidney disease stage III, and prior bariatric surgery. He presented to the emergency department with complaints of fatigue and progressive drainage from a left foot wound with associated pain. The patient was hypotensive (blood pressure 89/53 mmHg) and bradycardic (43 beats/minute) with complete heart block noted on telemetry monitoring and confirmed on 12-lead electrocardiogram. Initial laboratory tests were significant for leukocytosis (white blood cell count 32.1 K/mm^3), anemia (hemoglobin 9.5 g/dl), and elevated BUN (51 mg/dl) and creatinine (3.6 mg/dl) from baseline. A temporary transvenous pacemaker was placed emergently in the cardiac catheterization laboratory. The patient was subsequently hospitalized for the management of septic shock, wet gangrene of the left second toe, and complete heart block. Empiric antibiotic therapy was initiated with vancomycin and piperacillin/tazobactam, and he underwent urgent toe amputation followed by left ankle disarticulation. Postoperatively, the patient developed respiratory failure requiring intubation. Initial blood cultures grew MRSA. Given persistent hemodynamic instability despite presumed infectious source control, echocardiography was performed to rule out infective endocarditis. Transthoracic echocardiogram (TTE) on hospital day 1 and TEE on day 3 were, however, noncontributory (Figure 1). Bacteremia was persistent through the second week of hospitalization on multiple sets of blood cultures, and antibiotic regimen was changed to ceftaroline. Due to the persistent bacteremia, a whole-body 18-florodeoxyglucose positron emission tomography/computed tomography (18F-FDGPET/CT) scan was then obtained on hospital day 8 which revealed multiple PET-avid lung nodules and cavitary lesions concerning for septic pulmonary emboli (SPE). TEE was then repeated on hospital day 9 revealing a highly mobile echodensity in the right ventricular outflow tract (RVOT) measuring 3.4 cm by 1.6 cm (Figure 2) without valve leaflet or chordae involvement. The patient was evaluated for surgical vegetectomy; however, his surgical risk was deemed prohibitive in the acute setting, and thus conservative management was pursued with antibiotic therapy alone. Infection control was not successfully achieved. From a Heart Team approach, the decision was made to attempt an AngioVac evacuation of the RV mass on hospital day 12.

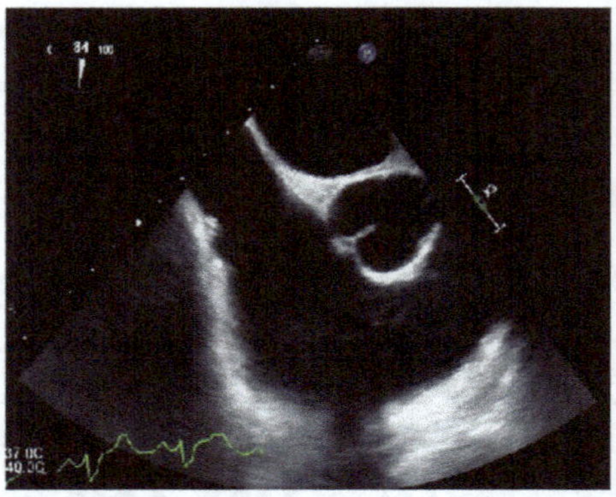

Figure 1: Midesophageal short axis view obtained on transesophageal echocardiogram performed on hospital day 3 with a focus on the right atrium, tricuspid valve, and RVOT. There was no clear, identifiable source of infection on this initial evaluation.

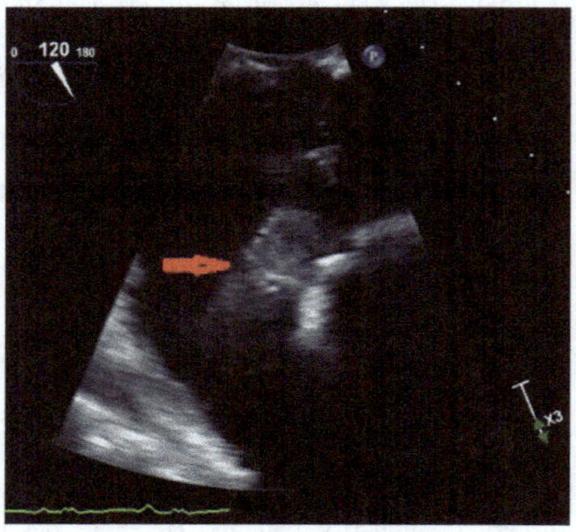

Figure 2: Focused midesophageal view of the RVOT on repeat TEE performed on hospital day 9. Note the large echodense structure measuring 3.4 cm × 1.6 cm that is independent of the tricuspid valve apparatus and is highly mobile with a narrow peduncle. The temporary pacemaker lead is also independent of this structure.

Venous access was obtained at both femoral venous sites with 6-French sheaths, and a right internal jugular access was obtained for the replacement of a temporary pacemaker. The left 6-French sheath was changed out with a 17-French cannula after serial dilatation while the right sheath was replaced with a number 26 DrySeal Sheath. Using a Swan-Ganz catheter, a Swan wire was positioned into the right pulmonary artery (PA). Using an MPA catheter, a Lunderquist wire was positioned in the right PA. The AngioVac return cannula was then attached with a wet-to-wet seal to the perfusion pump. The return cannula was loaded over the Lunderquist wire after removing air from the cannula. Under TEE guidance, the return cannula was advanced into the right atrium. When the return cannula could not be advanced further into the RV outflow tract, it was pulled back and the Lunderquist wire was repositioned into the left PA using the MPA catheter. It was then possible to advance the aspiration catheter back and forth, and this resulted in the return of a large amount of material visually consistent with clots. Activated clotting time was maintained above 300 seconds throughout the procedure with heparin. Postprocedure TEE showed up to 90% resolution of the mass (Figure 3). Aspirated blood sampled from the PA was positive for MRSA. Antibiotic therapy was continued, and subsequent blood cultures were sterile. Resolution of complete heart block was verified on continued telemetry monitoring, and the temporary pacemaker was removed. The patient was eventually discharged in stable condition on hospital day 27.

3. Discussion

In the case presented here, persistent MRSA bacteremia and SPE on 18F-FDG PET/CT heightened the suspicion for endocardial infection. The RV outflow mass seen on repeat TEE appeared within 6 days of initial negative TEE and was suspected to be an infected thrombus or vegetation. The recommended initial management of right endocardial infection is antibiotics [4]. Surgical intervention is considered in specific situations. In our patient, persistent bacteremia for more than 7 days despite adequate antibiotic therapy was an indication for surgery. As is often the case in endocardial infections, our patient was too unstable clinically to undergo surgery. Recent reports have suggested that AngioVac aspiration could be a minimally invasive alternative to surgery and the decision was made to pursue this option.

The AngioVac venous drainage system, invented in 2012, was developed for the removal of fresh, soft thrombi or emboli from the vascular system. It was intended to be used as an alternative to anticoagulation, catheter-directed thrombolysis, mechanical thrombectomy, pharmacomechanical thrombectomy, or open surgical embolectomy [5, 6]. In a single-center analysis of 16 procedures, AngioVac aspiration achieved the removal of more than 70% of thrombi/masses

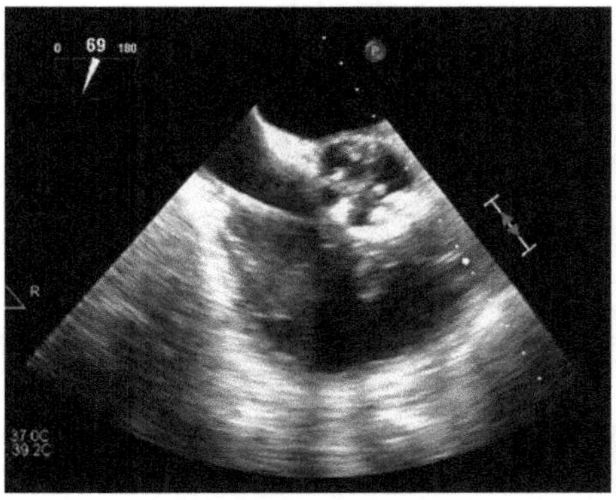

FIGURE 3: Midesophageal RVOT-focused view on intraoperative TEE immediately postaspiration using the AngioVac system (catheter can be visualized in this image.) Although residual vegetation is visible, there is approximately 90% resolution postaspiration.

with 67% and 100% success rate for the right atrial and iliocaval sites, respectively [7]. Similarly, Worku et al. analyzed case reports involving 56 procedures which showed the removal of 100% of material in 87% and 82% of iliocaval and intracardiac thrombus, respectively. On the other hand, the success rate for the removal of PE was remarkably low at 12.5% [8]. Pasha et al. had alternatively reported successful management of an acute massive PE in a hemodynamically unstable patient using the AngioVac system [9]. Other novel applications of the AngioVac catheter have been explored. Abubakar et al. published a detailed compilation of case reports including 65 procedures, noting an increasing popularity of AngioVac aspiration for vegetation debulking from right endocardial locations including the right atrium, tricuspid valve, pulmonic valve, and intracardiac device leads. In nearly all cases, successful vegetectomy led to infection control and clinical improvement [10]. In some cases, the AngioVac device has been used as a bridge to surgery [11, 12]. The most serious reported complication associated with the device is access site hematoma [8, 13].

With the finding of a large RV outflow mass initially suspected to be an infected thrombus or vegetation, we concluded that this was the source of persistent bacteremia and SPE. We decided that urgent thrombectomy or vegetectomy was the most viable option for infection control and for preventing further potentially catastrophic embolization into the pulmonary vasculature. Since our patient was at prohibitive perioperative risk, we elected to attempt retrieval by AngioVac aspiration. Following successful extraction of 90% of material visibly consistent with thrombus, we were able to achieve rapid control of the infection. To the best of our knowledge, this is the first report detailing successful AngioVac aspiration of a large infected thrombus from the RV outflow tract without serious complications.

4. Conclusion

When a right endocardial mass of any etiology is encountered in clinical practice, consideration should be given to the use of the AngioVac device if evacuation is desired. Use of this new device may be a safer alternative to surgical vegetectomy, particularly when the perioperative risk is prohibitive.

References

[1] N. Patel, T. Azemi, F. Zaeem et al., "Vacuum assisted vegetation extraction for the management of large lead vegetations," *Journal of Cardiac Surgery*, vol. 28, no. 3, pp. 321–324, 2013.

[2] A. K. Thiagaraj, M. Malviya, W. W. Htun et al., "A novel approach in the management of right-sided endocarditis: percutaneous vegectomy using the AngioVac cannula," *Future Cardiology*, vol. 13, no. 3, pp. 211–217, 2017.

[3] B. Nickel, T. McClure, and J. Moriarty, "A novel technique for endovascular removal of large volume right atrial tumor thrombus," *CardioVascular and Interventional Radiology*, vol. 38, no. 4, pp. 1021–1024, 2015.

[4] G. Habib, P. Lancellotti, M. J. Antunes et al., "2015 ESC guidelines for the management of infective endocarditis: The Task Force for the Management of Infective Endocarditis of the European Society of Cardiology (ESC). Endorsed by: European Association for Cardio-Thoracic Surgery (EACTS), the European Association of Nuclear Medicine (EANM)," *European Heart Journal*, vol. 36, no. 44, pp. 3075–3128, 2015.

[5] Angiodynamics, "AngioVac Cannula and Circuit," http://www.angiovac.com/wp-content/uploads/2017/10/AngioVac-Product-Brochure-ANGB-257-US-Rev-02.pdf.

[6] G. Behrens and H. Bjarnason, "Venous thromboembolic disease: the use of the aspiration thrombectomy device AngioVac," *Seminars in Interventional Radiology*, vol. 32, no. 4, pp. 374–378, 2015.

[7] J. M. Moriarty, R. al-Hakim, A. Bansal, and J. K. Park, "Removal of caval and right atrial thrombi and masses using the AngioVac device: initial operative experience," *Journal of Vascular and Interventional Radiology*, vol. 27, no. 10, pp. 1584–1591, 2016.

[8] B. Worku, A. Salemi, M. D. D'Ayala, R. F. Tranbaugh, L. N. Girardi, and I. M. Gulkarov, "The AngioVac device: understanding the failures on the road to success," *Innovations: Technology and Techniques in Cardiothoracic and Vascular Surgery*, vol. 11, no. 6, pp. 430–433, 2016.

[9] A. K. Pasha, M. D. Elder, D. Khurram, B. A. Snyder, and M. R. Movahed, "Successful management of acute massive pulmonary embolism using Angiovac suction catheter technique in a hemodynamically unstable patient," *Cardiovascular Revascularization Medicine*, vol. 15, no. 4, pp. 240–243, 2014.

[10] H. Abubakar, A. Rashed, A. Subahi, A. S. Yassin, M. Shokr, and M. Elder, "AngioVac system used for vegetation debulking in a patient with tricuspid valve endocarditis: a case report and review of the literature," *Case Reports in Cardiology*, vol. 2017, Article ID 1923505, 7 pages, 2017.

[11] A. A. Divekar, T. Scholz, and J. D. Fernandez, "Novel percutaneous transcatheter intervention for refractory active endocarditis as a bridge to surgery-angiovac aspiration system," *Catheterization and Cardiovascular Interventions*, vol. 81, no. 6, pp. 1008–1012, 2013.

[12] G. Makdisi, T. Casciani, T. C. Wozniak, D. W. Roe, and Z. A. Hashmi, "A successful percutaneous mechanical vegetation debulking used as a bridge to surgery in acute tricuspid valve endocarditis," *Journal of Thoracic Disease*, vol. 8, no. 1, pp. E137–E139, 2016.

[13] J. Salsamendi, M. Doshi, S. Bhatia et al., "Single center experience with the AngioVac aspiration system," *Cardio-Vascular and Interventional Radiology*, vol. 38, no. 4, pp. 998–1004, 2015.

45

Parallel Mapping and Catheter Ablation of Polymorphic Premature Ventricular Contractions: A New Feature for Activation Mapping

Moritz Nies[1,2] **Ruben Schleberger**[1] **Leon Dinshaw**[1] **Andreas Rillig**[1] **Andreas Metzner**[1] **and Christian Meyer**[1,2,3,4]

[1]*Department of Cardiology, University Heart and Vascular Center, University Medical Center Hamburg-Eppendorf, Martinistraße 52, 20246 Hamburg, Germany*
[2]*DZHK (German Center for Cardiovascular Research), Partner Site Hamburg/Lübeck/Kiel, Berlin, Germany*
[3]*Division of Cardiology, EVK Düsseldorf, cNEP, Cardiac Neuro- and Electrophysiology Research Consortium, Kirchfeldstraße 40, 40217 Düsseldorf, Germany*
[4]*cNEP, Cardiac Neuro- and Electrophysiology Research Consortium, Institute for Neural and Sensory Physiology, Heinrich Heine University Düsseldorf, Medical Faculty, Düsseldorf, Germany*

Correspondence should be addressed to Moritz Nies; m.nies@uke.de and Christian Meyer; christian.meyer@evk-duesseldorf.de

Academic Editor: Celestino Sardu

We report the case of an 80-year-old female presenting with polymorphic premature ventricular contractions, nonischemic cardiomyopathy, and severe, secondary mitral regurgitation. Despite a low intraprocedural PVC burden, activation mapping and successful ablation of different morphologies were achieved using a novel mapping tool, which facilitates simultaneous mapping of different PVC morphologies.

1. Introduction

For symptomatic patients with a high burden of polymorphic premature ventricular contractions, catheter ablation is a viable treatment option (1). So far, during activation mapping with a three-dimensional electroanatomical mapping system, only PVCs matching the pattern of the currently active map are registered. Other morphologies have to be addressed sequentially in separate mapping approaches, challenging the effective treatment of polymorphic PVCs with low intraprocedural prevalence. A novel algorithm (CARTO III Software Version 7, Carto Prime, Biosense Webster, Diamond Bar, CA, USA) facilitates simultaneous mapping of different morphologies and offers enhanced mapping opportunities in cases with rare, polymorphic PVCs.

2. Case Presentation

2.1. History of Presentation. We report the case of an 80-year-old female who presented to our outpatient clinic with recurrence of polymorphic PVCs, resulting in palpitations and dyspnea. Preexisting medical conditions included dilated, nonischemic cardiomyopathy with a reduced left ventricular ejection fraction of 40%. Furthermore, a severe, secondary mitral regurgitation was observed in transthoracic echocardiography. Apart from arterial hypertension and grade I obesity (BMI 31), no cardiovascular risk factors were identified (2).

After unsuccessful treatment with beta-blockers (bisoprolol, nebivolol), two ablation procedures of PVCs had been performed before: ablation in the right ventricular outflow tract and right coronary cusp (2018, initial reduction of PVC-

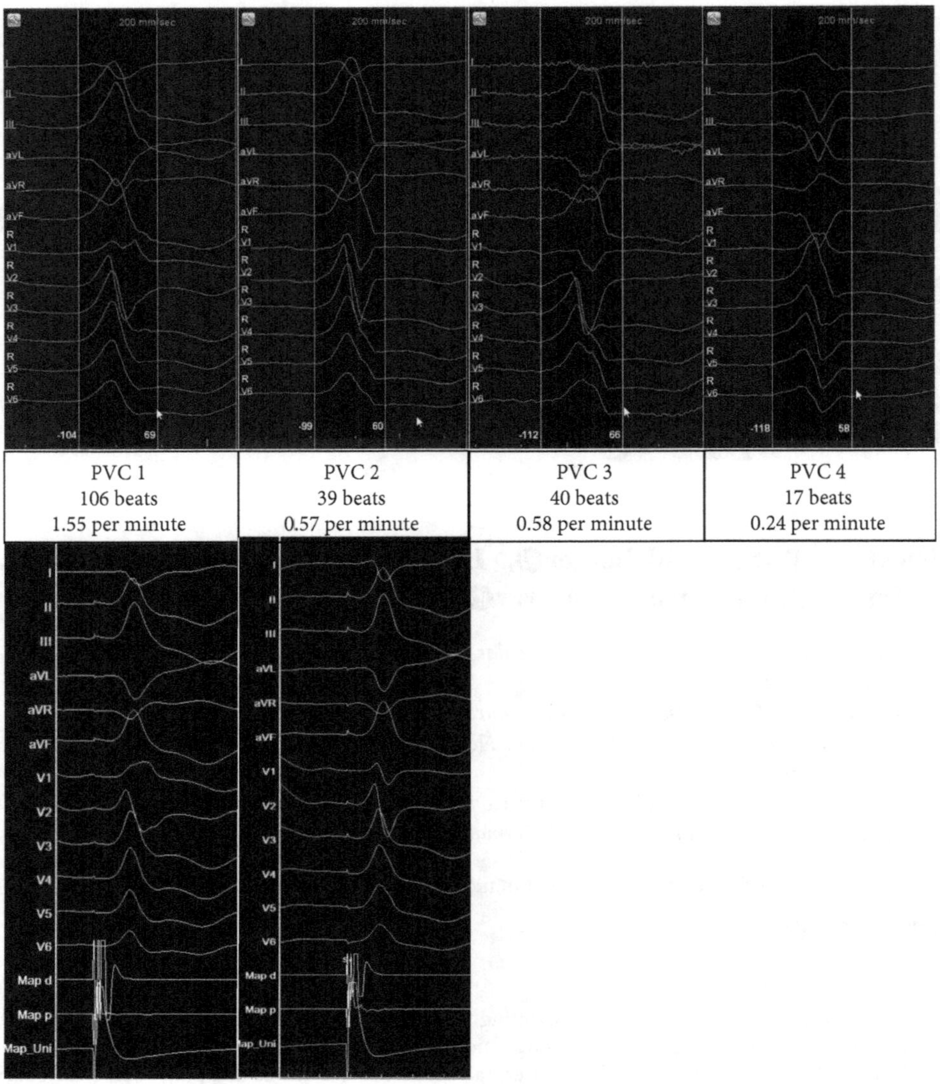

FIGURE 1: Mapped morphologies. Templates of mapped morphologies of premature ventricular contractions (upper panels), intraprocedural burden, and corresponding pacemaps (lower panels), 200 mm/sec.

burden from 32% to <1%) and ablation from the left coronary cusp and distal great cardiac vein (2019) had led to suppression of initially predominant morphologies. However, previous low-frequency PVCs with different morphologies had gained in burden. On presentation to our outpatient clinic, Holter-ECG documented a high burden of polymorphic PVCs (52%).

2.2. Differential Diagnosis. Aside from idiopathic dilated cardiomyopathy, two reasons were identified as potential causes for the aforementioned left ventricular dilation: first, PVCs in a clinically significant number may cause an arrhythmia-induced cardiomyopathy, mimicking dilated cardiomyopathy (3). Second, severe mitral regurgitation might lead to volume overload and thus to heart failure and dyspnea (4).

2.3. Ablation Procedure. Conscious sedation with fentanyl and propofol led to an immediate decrease in the prevalence of PVCs, refractory to provocation with orciprenaline, and after cessation of sedative agents.

With most PVCs showing a morphology indicating a left ventricular origin (Figure 1), a retrograde left ventricular access via the right femoral artery was established. This access proved sufficient for mapping and ablation in this case.

Clinical PVCs remained scarce during the procedure, which is evident in the low number of PVCs ($n = 202$) registered during a total mapping time of 68 : 23 minutes (2.9 PVCs per minute).

Parallel activation mapping of different morphologies was performed using a novel mapping software (CARTO 3, Software Version 7, Biosense Webster, Diamond Bar, CA, USA). Considering their low intraprocedural burden, the different morphologies were mapped simultaneously to record a higher number of PVCs for each respective map.

Four different morphologies were mapped, three of which were deemed clinically significant. Even though morphologies 2 and 3 (Figure 1) had a very low burden of 0.57 and 0.58 PVCs per minute, the three-dimensional map was sufficient for correct identification of the PVC origin. For PVCs 1-3, the earliest activation was recorded at different

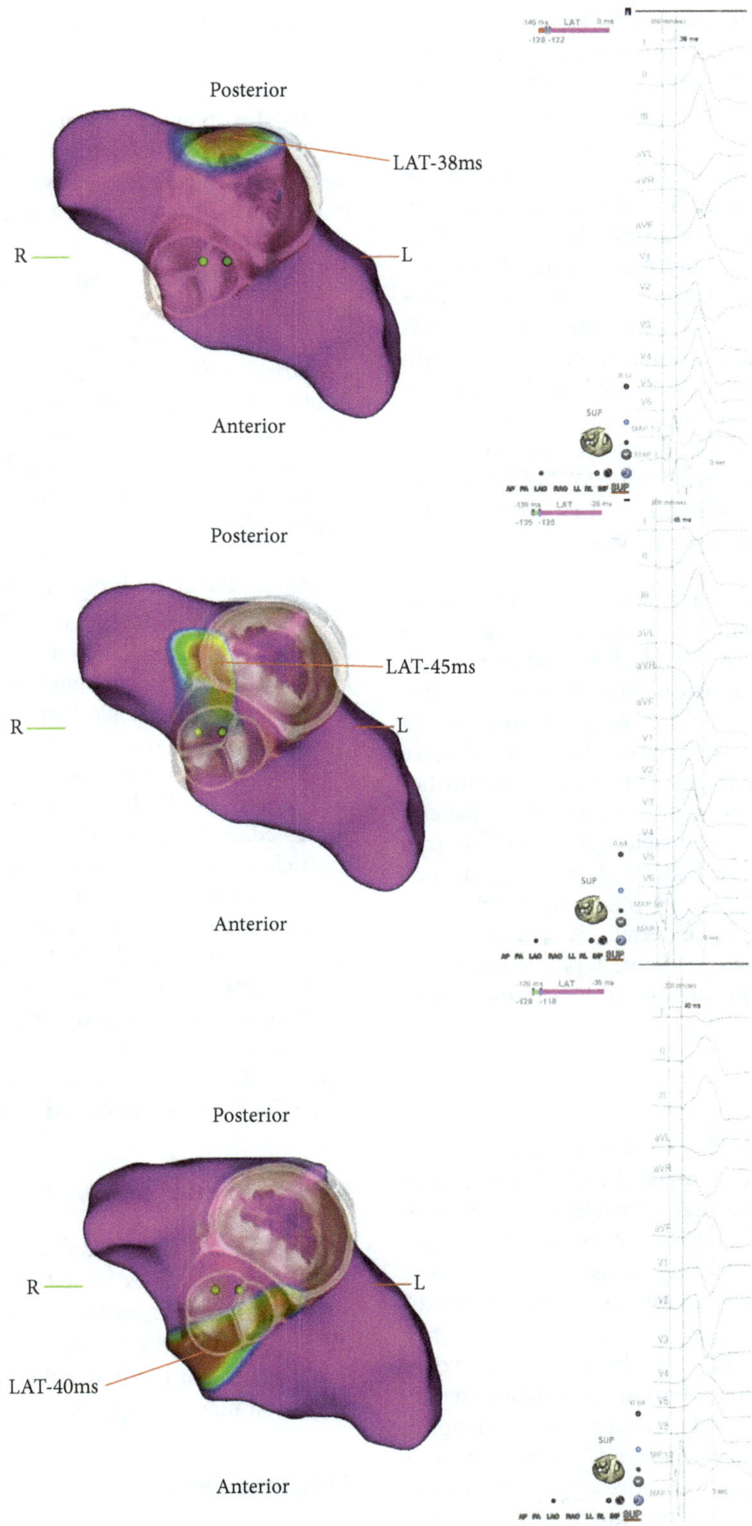

Figure 2: Activation maps. Simultaneously recorded activation maps of polymorphic premature ventricular contractions with corresponding surface ECG and intracardial signals. Partial maps of the left ventricle showing the aortomitral continuity/basal left ventricle, superior view. Color-coded visualization of local activation time (LAT) with the red area indicating the earliest activation. The overlay shows the approximate location of mitral and aortic valve.

locations in close proximity to the aortomitral continuity (AMC, Figure 2). For morphologies 1 and 2, pacemapping was performed and showed a match of 96% (in 12/12 ECG-leads) for both morphologies in their respective area of earliest activation. Regarding morphology 3, several spontaneous PVCs occurred in a short time with an early local activation time prior to ablation. Therefore, the ablation target was viewed as sufficiently localized, and pacemapping was not deemed necessary to confirm its localization while pacemapping can result in slight movements of the catheter itself. Also, to use the PVC disappearance as a success indicator/"procedural" endpoint, any delay to ablation was to be avoided, and no pacemapping was performed.

Consecutive RFC-ablation at the corresponding site of the earliest activation led to acute suppression of all targeted morphologies. To consolidate the ablation lesion for PVC 1, complimentary ablation via the distal great cardiac vein was performed. For mapping and ablation, a 3.5 mm tip catheter was used (Navistar D-Curve, 7 F, Biosense Webster, Diamond Bar, CA, USA). In total, 20 pulses were applied with a cumulative ablation time of 1375 seconds and titration to a maximum energy of 35 Watts for ablation in the left ventricle and 20 Watts for ablation in the distal great cardiac vein. Considering its very low burden (0.24 PVCs per minute) and remote location of origin, PVC was not addressed with catheter ablation in this intervention.

2.4. Follow-Up. In a follow-up visit three months after ablation, the patient reported a significant improvement of dyspnea and palpitations. A 24-hour Holter-ECG documented a reduction of the PVC-burden to <1%. The occasional episodes of peripheral edema and intermittent dyspnea were still observed. In light of these residual symptoms, transcatheter mitral valve implantation was performed later on, leading to further improvement of the clinical functional status of the patient. Conventional surgery was not a viable option for this frail patient, and valve calcification had ruled out percutaneous mitral valve repair. During a 9-month follow-up, no clinically significant burden of PVCs was detected. Echocardiography showed a good result after mitral valve replacement and a stable left ventricular ejection fraction of 40% despite treatment of mitral regurgitation.

3. Discussion

In patients with polymorphic PVCs and low intraprocedural burden, successful treatment is especially challenging since both of these features are associated with a lower success rate (5, 6). A lack of clinical PVCs during ablation procedure is a well-described phenomenon and can be caused by different factors, such as circadian fluctuations or administration of sedative agents (7, 8).

If activation mapping is impeded by a low intraprocedural burden of PVCs, pacemapping can be a viable alternative, as studies have shown satisfactory results for mapping and ablation relying solely on pacemaps (7). However, activation mapping has a superior spatial resolution compared to pacemapping (9) and is therefore widely accepted as the preferred strategy whenever possible.

With sequential activation mapping, PVCs not matching the singular active pattern are often ignored and lost to mapping, which may further impede the construction of a satisfactory map. In contrast, parallel mapping continuously includes all preregistered PVCs into a corresponding map and thereby simplifies the activation mapping of PVCs with low intraprocedural burden. Furthermore, consecutive activation mapping and ablation of different morphologies can be time-consuming. Parallel mapping might reduce the total procedure and fluoroscopy time as well as the dosage of sedative agents, limiting the risk for associated complications (10).

The feasibility of this approach is supported by the here presented case. However, no final conclusions regarding the usefulness of parallel activation mapping of polymorphic PVCs can be drawn from a single case and further studies are warranted.

The interplay between polymorphic premature ventricular contractions, nonischemic cardiomyopathy, and severe, secondary mitral regurgitation can challenge clinical decision making (11): while polymorphic PVCs are a common finding in patients with congestive heart failure (12) and the burden may increase as a result of a progressing cardiomyopathy (11), they can also be the cause for significant deterioration or development of heart failure (11). This renders the decision difficult which pathology should be treated primarily. Several considerations let to the decision to address the arrhythmia primarily in this case:

Given the high burden of PVC in this case, it was reasonable to suspect that PVCs also affected the evaluation of the functional mitral valve regurgitation, making it appear more severe in this pathologic hemodynamic state. Secondly, the patient's clinical status correlated well with PVC-burden, making this treatment most likely to improve her symptoms. Still, it seemed likely that both pathologies needed to be addressed. For catheter ablation, a transseptal access to the left ventricle might be necessary. Even though small studies have shown the feasibility of this approach after valve intervention (13), this is challenging after mitral valve replacement or percutaneous valve repair. Finally, catheter ablation of PVCs is the less invasive procedure and facilitated more effective cardiac recovery in this case, thereby lowering the risk of the more invasive mitral valve intervention. Considering both options, repeat catheter ablation seemed to be the more reasonable choice for the primary intervention in this case.

4. Conclusion

Our case report illustrates that parallel mapping of polymorphic PVCs facilitates simultaneous activation mapping of different morphologies for patients with low intraprocedural PVC-burden, in which the construction of conclusive activation maps might be challenging and time consuming with a sequential mapping approach.

Abbreviations

PVC: Premature ventricular contraction
ECG: Electrocardiogram
RFC: Radiofrequency current.

Additional Points

Teaching Points. In conventional, sequential activation mapping of polymorphic PVCs, the construction of the map is limited to one PVC morphology at a time. Other occurring morphologies are lost to the activated map, hampering the localization of ablation targets and prolonging the procedure time. Using a novel mapping software, simultaneous registration of different PVC morphologies is feasible and allows the parallel creation of activation maps of different PVC morphologies. Parallel activation mapping offers the opportunity to successfully localize and ablate the origins of rare polymorphic PVCs for which a sequential mapping approach might not offer sufficient information.

Disclosure

This research did not receive any specific grants from funding agencies in the public, commercial, or not-for-profit sectors.

References

[1] E. M. Cronin, F. M. Bogun, P. Maury et al., "2019 HRS/EHRA/APHRS/LAHRS expert consensus statement on catheter ablation of ventricular arrhythmias," *J Arrhythm.*, vol. 35, no. 3, pp. 323–484, 2019.

[2] C. Sardu, G. Carreras, S. Katsanos et al., "Metabolic syndrome is associated with a poor outcome in patients affected by outflow tract premature ventricular contractions treated by catheter ablation," *BMC Cardiovascular Disorders*, vol. 14, no. 1, p. 176, 2014.

[3] R. Gopinathannair, S. P. Etheridge, F. E. Marchlinski, F. G. Spinale, D. Lakkireddy, and B. Olshansky, "Arrhythmia-induced cardiomyopathies: mechanisms, recognition, and management," *Journal of the American College of Cardiology*, vol. 66, no. 15, pp. 1714–1728, 2015.

[4] R. A. Nishimura, A. Vahanian, M. F. Eleid, and M. J. Mack, "Mitral valve disease–current management and future challenges," *Lancet*, vol. 387, no. 10025, pp. 1324–1334, 2016.

[5] K. Baser, H. D. Bas, M. Yokokawa, R. Latchamsetty, F. Morady, and F. Bogun, "Infrequent intraprocedural premature ventricular complexes: implications for ablation outcome," *Journal of Cardiovascular Electrophysiology*, vol. 25, no. 10, pp. 1088–1092, 2014.

[6] S. H. Sheldon, R. Latchamsetty, F. Morady, and F. Bogun, "Catheter ablation in patients with pleomorphic, idiopathic, premature ventricular complexes," *Heart Rhythm*, vol. 14, no. 11, pp. 1623–1628, 2017.

[7] Y. Shirai, J. J. Liang, P. Santangeli et al., "Catheter ablation of premature ventricular complexes with low intraprocedural burden guided exclusively by pace-mapping," *Journal of Cardiovascular Electrophysiology*, vol. 30, no. 11, pp. 2326–2333, 2019.

[8] A. H. Mullis, K. Ayoub, J. Shah et al., "Fluctuations in premature ventricular contraction burden can affect medical assessment and management," *Heart Rhythm*, vol. 16, no. 10, pp. 1570–1574, 2019.

[9] F. Bogun, M. Taj, M. Ting et al., "Spatial resolution of pace mapping of idiopathic ventricular tachycardia/ectopy originating in the right ventricular outflow tract," *Heart Rhythm*, vol. 5, no. 3, pp. 339–344, 2008.

[10] N. S. Gerstein, A. Young, P. M. Schulman, E. C. Stecker, and P. M. Jessel, "Sedation in the Electrophysiology Laboratory: a multidisciplinary review, *Journal of the American Heart Association*, vol. 5, no. 6, 2016.

[11] L. Laplante and B. S. Benzaquen, "A review of the potential pathogenicity and management of frequent premature ventricular contractions," *Pacing and Clinical Electrophysiology*, vol. 39, no. 7, pp. 723–730, 2016.

[12] P. J. Podrid, R. I. Fogel, and T. T. Fuchs, "Ventricular arrhythmia in congestive heart failure," *The American Journal of Cardiology*, vol. 69, no. 18, pp. 82G–95G, 1992, discussion G-6G.

[13] K. Hayashi, C. H. Heeger, S. Mathew et al., "Antegrade-transseptal approach for left ventricular tachyarrhythmia in patients with previous Mitraclip implantation," *Europace*, vol. 20, no. 9, pp. 1527–1534, 2018.

Preoperative Noninvasive Mapping Allowed Targeted Concomitant Surgical Ablation and Revealed COVID-19 Infection

Constantin Mork,[1] Luca Koechlin,[1] Matthias Streif,[2] Alexa Hollinger,[3,4] Martin Siegemund,[3,4] Friedrich Eckstein,[1] and David Santer[1]

[1] *Department of Cardiac Surgery, University Hospital Basel, Basel, Switzerland*
[2] *Department of Radiology, University Hospital Basel, Basel, Switzerland*
[3] *Intensive Care Unit, University Hospital Basel, Basel, Switzerland*
[4] *Department of Clinical Research, University of Basel, Basel, Switzerland*

Correspondence should be addressed to David Santer; david.santer@usb.ch

Academic Editor: Christopher S. Snyder

In March 2020, a 64-year-old female with mitral valve insufficiency and persistent atrial fibrillation underwent preoperative noninvasive mapping for developing an ablation strategy. In the computed tomography (CT) scan, typical signs of COVID-19 were described. Since the consecutive polymerase chain reaction (PCR) test was negative, the severely symptomatic patient was planned for urgent surgery. Noninvasive mapping showed that atrial fibrillation was maintained by left atrial structures and pulmonary veins only. On admission day, the preoperative routine COVID-19 PCR test was positive, and after recovery, uneventful mitral valve repair with cryoablation of the left atrium and pulmonary veins was performed. Our case describes the potential benefit of preoperative noninvasive mapping for the development of a surgical ablation strategy, as well as the challenges in managing urgent surgical patients during the COVID-19 pandemic and the corresponding diagnostic relevance of CT.

1. Introduction

For concomitant surgical ablation, full Cox-Maze IV is the gold-standard set; however, most cardiac surgeons still prefer isolated pulmonary vein and left atrial ablation to reduce time of surgery [1]. Preoperative noninvasive mapping is a new low-risk option to plan targeted surgical ablation, which might limit surgical ablation to the maintaining sources of atrial fibrillation as well as improve efficiency and outcome of the procedure.

2. Case Presentation

We report the case of a 64-year-old woman who had been suffering from dyspnoea, dry cough, and New York Heart Association III for one and a half years and presented to the emergency department in January 2020 with dysphasia and sensory disturbances in the right hand and a left side facial paresis. A computed tomography (CT) scan revealed an acute ischaemic media infarct, wherefore lysis was administered immediately. Anticoagulation was continued with apixaban (Eliquis®, 2×5 mg/d, Bristol-Myers Sqibb SA, Steinhausen, Switzerland). In the electrocardiogram (ECG), a de novo persisting tachycardiac atrial fibrillation (AF; Figure 1(a)) was detected. Transoesophageal echocardiography (TTE) showed a left ventricular ejection fraction of 60% with flail leaflet of the posterior mitral valve with tendon rupture, resulting in a severe mitral valve insufficiency with an extrinsic jet and backflow into the pulmonary veins (peak gradient: 8 mmHg; mean gradient: 3 mmHg). The coronary

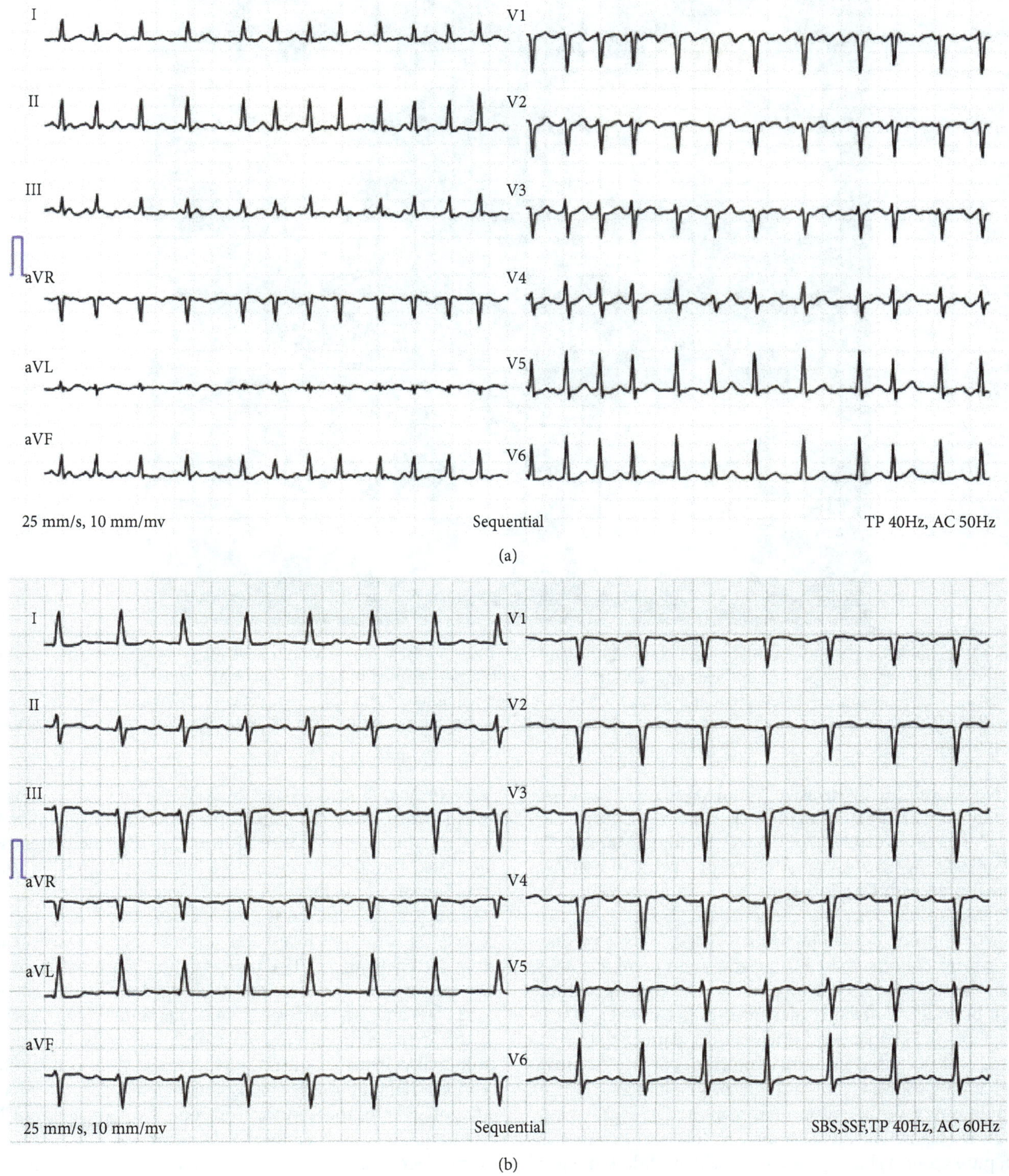

FIGURE 1: (a) The first detection (January 2020) of fibrillation with tachycardia at 142 bpm, a small QRS complex, and normal QT interval. (b) At discharge, the patient showed a sinus rhythm with an AV block I° (PQ = 264 ms), 88 bpm, small QRS complex, and normal QT interval.

arteries were free from any relevant stenoses. The Heart Team recommended minimally invasive surgical mitral valve repair via right anterolateral thoracotomy, concomitant surgical ablation, and closure of the left atrial appendage after completion of neurologic rehabilitation. In February 2020, the patient was transferred to the emergency department because of a new onset sensory disturbance in the right hand. Magnetic resonance imaging (MRI) disclosed a small new infarct in the medial thalamus. After neurological evaluation, the secondary prophylaxis was continued with apixaban. After discharge from neurological rehabilitation, the patient denied any neurological symptoms and was therefore

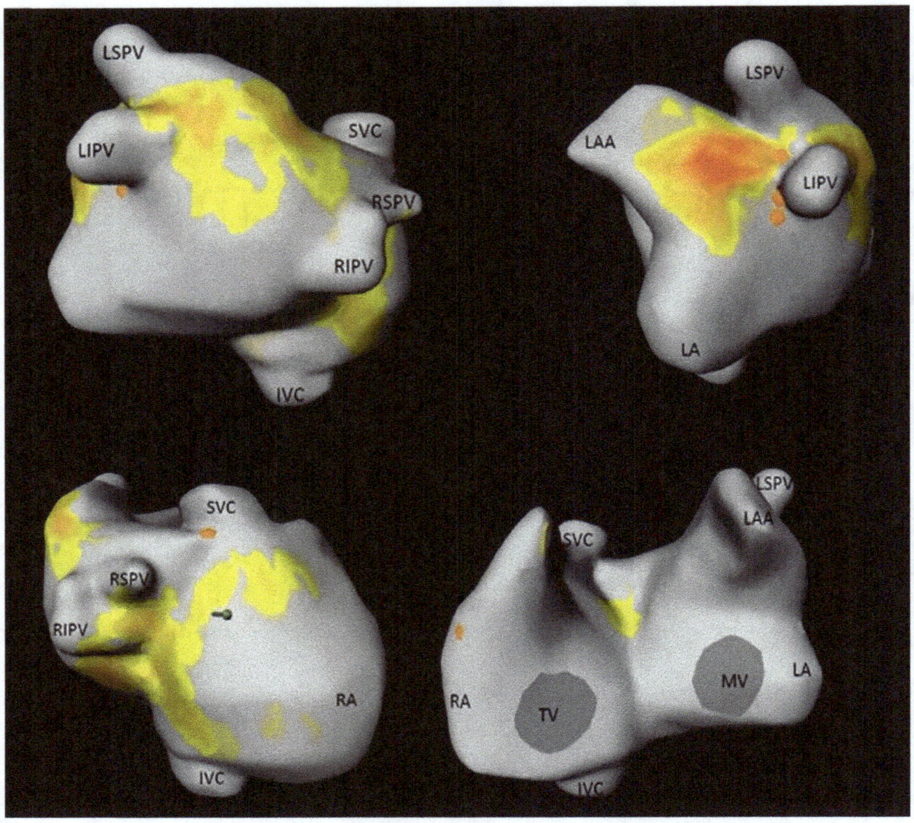

FIGURE 2: Preoperative noninvasive mapping with CardioInsight™-3D Mapping technology. Noninvasive mapping showed rotors and foci originating mainly from the pulmonary veins and left atrium; the right atrium seemed to be free from major sources of AF. IVC: inferior vena cava; LA: left atrium; LAA: left atrial appendix; LIPV: left inferior pulmonary vein; LSPV: left superior pulmonary vein; MV: mitral valve; RA: right atrium; RIPV: right inferior pulmonary vein; RSPV: right superior pulmonary vein; SVC: superior vena cava; TV: tricuspid valve.

referred for minimally invasive mitral valve repair and concomitant surgical ablation to the Department of Cardiac Surgery, University Hospital Basel, Switzerland, in March 2020.

For defining an ablation strategy, preoperative noninvasive mapping with CardioInsight™-3D Mapping technology (CIT, Medtronic SA, Münchenbuchsee, Switzerland) was performed in our outpatient clinic. This noninvasive mapping system collects chest ECG signals and combines these signals with CT scan data to produce and display simultaneous, biatrial and biventricular three-dimensional (3D) cardiac maps. A 3D epicardial image of the patient's atria was created with localization of foci and rotors of AF. Noninvasive mapping showed rotors and foci originating mainly from the pulmonary veins and the left atrium. The right atrium was clear (Figure 2). Furthermore, in this preoperative CT scan, pure ground glass opacities with a consolidation typical for COVID-19 were observed in the left lung (Figure 3(a) and (b)) [2]. The patient reported persisting dry cough, dyspnoea, and intermittent elevated temperature over the past few weeks. However, these were the same symptoms she had been experiencing for the past months and therefore could be explained by symptomatic mitral valve insufficiency. Nevertheless, the patient was requested to undergo immediate polymerase chain reaction (PCR) test (SARS-CoV-2 Reverse Transcription Quantitative Nucleic Acid Testing (RT-QNAT) targeting specific viral sequences of the spike-glycoprotein S-gene (Basel SCo V2-S-111 bp)) [3], which was performed by the general practitioner the day after the CT scan. Since the PCR result was negative, the patient was admitted for surgery seven days later. On March 26, 2020, the day of admission, the patient was normothermic, and the oxygen saturation was 96%. However, routine preoperative SARS-CoV2 PCR test was positive, and the patient was transferred to the COVID-19 isolation ward. Because she was asymptomatic, she was discharged from the hospital one day after to undergo home quarantine. On April 8, 2020, after two negative SARS-CoV2 test results, uneventful minimally invasive mitral valve repair with concomitant endocardial pulmonary vein isolation, left atrial cryoablation (CryoICE cryoprobe, Atricure Europe B.V., Amsterdam, The Netherlands), and endocardial suture of the left atrial appendage was performed via right anterolateral minithoracotomy. After surgery, the patient was transferred to the intensive care unit and underwent continuous atrial pacing for 24 hours. She was extubated on the day of the operation, transferred to the cardiac surgical ward on the second postoperative day, and discharged into rehabilitation on postoperative day 7. At discharge, the TTE showed a normal ejection fraction (60%), with a minimal residual mitral valve insufficiency. The patient was in sinus rhythm with first degree AV block (Figure 1(b)). After three months (July 2020), TTE showed a normotrophic left ventricle with an

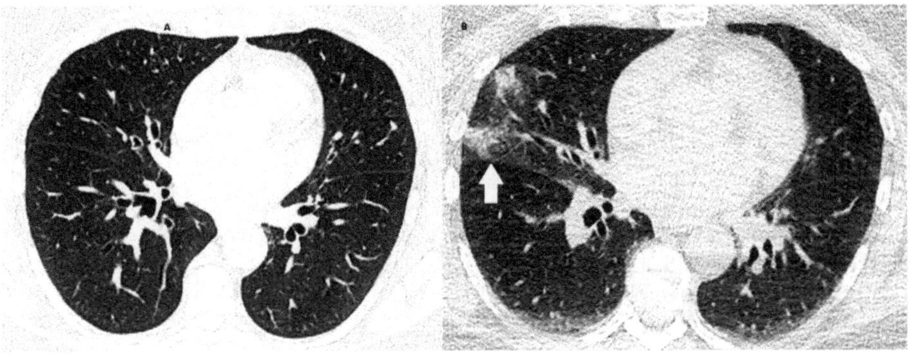

(a) (b)

Figure 3: (a) CT thorax scan (December 2019) showed inconspicuous lung emphysema in comparison with the preoperative (b) CT scan (March 2020) with typical ground glass opacities (arrow) in the medial lobe.

ejection fraction of 60% and mild mitral valve regurgitation. Holter ECG-detected sinus rhythm with a heart rate of 81 beats per minute was observed, with a small QRS complex and no detection of atrial fibrillation. The patient denied dyspnoea and palpitations, and the persisting dry cough had also stopped. In the lung function test, pulmonary static and dynamic volumes and capacities were normal. The residual restricted haemoglobin-corrected diffusion capacity was interpreted in the context of a postviral condition. In comparison to January 2020, there had been an improvement of the forced expiratory volume (+680 ml), the total lung capacity (+470 ml), and the diffusion capacity (+12%) in July 2020. The X-ray also showed a regression of the ventilation disorder. Neurologically, the patient had recovered very well with slightly discrete pyramidal stroke residuals in the right arm. She denied cognitive impairment and problems with alertness or language deficits.

3. Discussion

This case describes the option of targeted surgical ablation by preoperative noninvasive mapping, as well as the complexity in managing a patient with symptomatic mitral valve regurgitation and signs of a COVID-19 infection in a preoperative CT scan with a false-negative COVID-19 test. We want to underline four main messages from this case: (1) The decision of when to operate on urgent cardiac surgical patients with a recent or active COVID-19 infection is difficult to reach during an evolving pandemic. Recommendations for cardiac surgery during COVID-19 have been published suggesting not deferring surgery in case of severe mitral valve regurgitation [4]. Yet, since the patient was stable, we decided to defer the operation for another two weeks after the positive COVID-19 test result so that she could recover from her infection. However, the operation could have certainly not been postponed. If the patient would have been unstable, the surgery would have been performed as recommended [4]. (2) The Basel SCoV2- S-111 bp test with an analytical sensitivity and specificity of 99.68% (95% CI, 95%–100%) and 98.99% (95% CI, 91%–100%), respectively, was performed [3]. However, the CT scan offered a more reliable result than the standard PCR test [5]. Since the patient has been suffering from dry cough for over 18 months due to her mitral valve insufficiency, and since the primary PCR test was false-negative for unknown reasons, the COVID-19 infection was perfectly masked. (3) Although the full Cox-Maze IV is the gold-standard set for surgical ablation, most surgeons prefer isolated pulmonary vein and left atrial ablation to reduce complexity and cardiopulmonary bypass time [1]. Therefore, in our specific case, preoperative noninvasive mapping offered efficient preoperative guidance, which allowed performing targeted ablation on existing rotors and foci. According to our noninvasive mapping results, a full Cox-Maze IV with right atrial ablation retrospectively could be considered overtreatment. After three months, the patient is still in sinus rhythm with complete cardiopulmonary and neurological recovery. (4) Finally, in our case, the preoperative CT revealed unexpected but essential data and probably reduced the risk for postoperative complications. This shows again that preoperative routine CT scan should be discussed prior cardiac surgery [6]. Before the patient underwent a CT scan, the reasonable explanation for her symptoms was the progressive course of the mitral valve insufficiency. Therefore, the patient was prioritized for surgery in the first place despite the COVID-19 pandemic. Retrospectively, it can be seen that the COVID-19 infection might have been responsible for the accentuation of the symptoms and was masked by the symptomatic mitral valve disease.

In winter 2020, the uncontrolled COVID-19 pandemic is still ongoing, and common viral infections are upcoming during the winter months. Therefore, although testing tools have tremendously improved within the last few months, the challenge to rule out concomitant COVID-19 infection in periods of seasonal concomitant viral infections such as the flu and in the context of comorbidities with similar symptoms remains high. In conclusion, the current pandemic demands an increased awareness for cardiac symptoms which might be either masked or exacerbated by COVID-19 and vice versa.

Consent

We obtained written consent of our patient to report his case.

Authors' Contributions

CM, AH, MSt, MS, FE, and DS managed the patient. CM and DS prepared the original draft. AH, LK, MS, and FS reviewed and edited the manuscript. All authors have read and agreed to the published manuscript.

Acknowledgments

We thank Selina Ackermann, PhD, for kind proofreading of our manuscript.

References

[1] C. Ruaengsri, M. R. Schill, A. J. Khiabani, R. B. Schuessler, S. J. Melby, and R. J. Damiano, "The Cox-Maze IV procedure in its second decade: still the gold standard?," *European Journal of Cardio-Thoracic Surgery*, vol. 53, supplement_1, pp. i19–i25, 2018.

[2] J. Wu, J. Pan, D. Teng, X. Xu, J. Feng, and Y. C. Chen, "Interpretation of CT signs of 2019 novel coronavirus (COVID-19) pneumonia," *European Radiology*, vol. 30, no. 10, pp. 5455–5462, 2020.

[3] K. Leuzinger, T. Roloff, R. Gosert et al., "Epidemiology of severe acute respiratory syndrome coronavirus 2 emergence amidst community-acquired respiratory viruses," *The Journal of Infectious Diseases*, vol. 222, no. 8, pp. 1270–1279, 2020.

[4] V. Patel, E. Jimenez, L. Cornwell et al., "Cardiac surgery during the coronavirus disease 2019 pandemic: perioperative considerations and triage recommendations," *Journal of the American Heart Association*, vol. 9, no. 13, p. e017042, 2020.

[5] Y. Fang, H. Zhang, J. Xie et al., "Sensitivity of chest CT for COVID-19: comparison to RT-PCR," *Radiology*, vol. 296, no. 2, pp. E115–E117, 2020.

[6] A. Merlo, K. Chen, S. Deo, and A. Markowitz, "Does routine preoperative computed tomography imaging provide clinical utility in patients undergoing primary cardiac surgery?," *Interactive Cardiovascular and Thoracic Surgery*, vol. 25, no. 4, pp. 659–662, 2017.

Shock in the Setting of Diamond-Blackfan Anemia Relapse

Metri Haddaden,[1] Samir Husami,[2] Modar Alom,[3] Yifan Pang,[4] Zaid Imam,[5] and Daniel Keena[6]

[1]*MedStar Health, Department of Internal Medicine, Baltimore, Maryland, USA*
[2]*Department of Medicine, Division of Nephrology, Washington University School of Medicine, St. Louis, Missouri, USA*
[3]*National Cancer Institute, National Institutes of Health, Bethesda, Maryland, USA*
[4]*Department of Medicine, University of Toledo-College of Medicine and life Sciences Toledo, OH, USA*
[5]*William Beaumont Hospital, Department of Internal Medicine, Royal Oak, Michigan, USA*
[6]*William Beaumont Hospital, Division of Pulmonary and Critical Care, Department of Internal Medicine, Royal Oak, Michigan, USA*

Correspondence should be addressed to Zaid Imam; zaid.imam@beaumont.org

Academic Editor: Ertugrul Ercan

Adult intensivists have increasing exposure to individuals with congenital diseases surviving into adulthood. Solid knowledge bases and early recognition of the possible sequelae of congenital disorders are crucial in caring for these patients. We present a challenging case of shock and relapse of Diamond-Blackfan anemia in a 42-year-old man lost to follow-up for 18 years and highlighted the importance of healthcare transitions into adulthood and the challenges faced by health care systems to develop new strategies successfully transitioning complex pediatric patients to adult care.

1. Introduction

Diamond-Blackfan anemia (DBA) is a rare hereditary disorder secondary to a ribosomal protein gene mutation resulting in erythropoiesis failure, cancer predisposition, and associated congenital anomalies [1]. The incidence rate is 7 in 1,000,000 and is inherited mostly in an autosomal dominant fashion [1]. DBA presents within the first year of life with moderate to severe macrocytic anemia associated with mental retardation, hypertelorism, flat nasal bridge, high arched or cleft palate, triphalangeal thumb, and cardiac abnormalities [1–3].

The improvement in treatment modalities and diagnostics has improved the survival of patients with rare congenital diseases into adulthood by threefold between 2006 and 2016 [4–6]. Increased healthcare complexity highlighted the importance of transitions of care in decreasing hospital readmissions, system-wide financial burdens, and improving patients' outcomes [4]. In patients with rare diseases, these transitions of care are even more important as these patients' transition into adulthood [7].

Hereby, we report a case of high output cardiac failure and subsequent shock secondary to a relapse of DBA in a patient with a history of a repaired Tetralogy of Fallot lost to follow-up for 18 years highlighting the importance of close follow-up and transitions between pediatric and adult providers.

2. Case Presentation

A 42-year-old Caucasian male presented with worsening fatigue and dyspnea for 2 weeks. His medical history included a diagnosis of childhood Diamond-Blackfan anemia (DBA), for which he received corticosteroids until the age of 24 when he was lost to follow-up, and a Tetralogy of Fallot (TOF) with pulmonary atresia repaired at the age of 3 years with a right ventricle-pulmonary artery conduit. He denied any bleeding, and a complete review of systems was

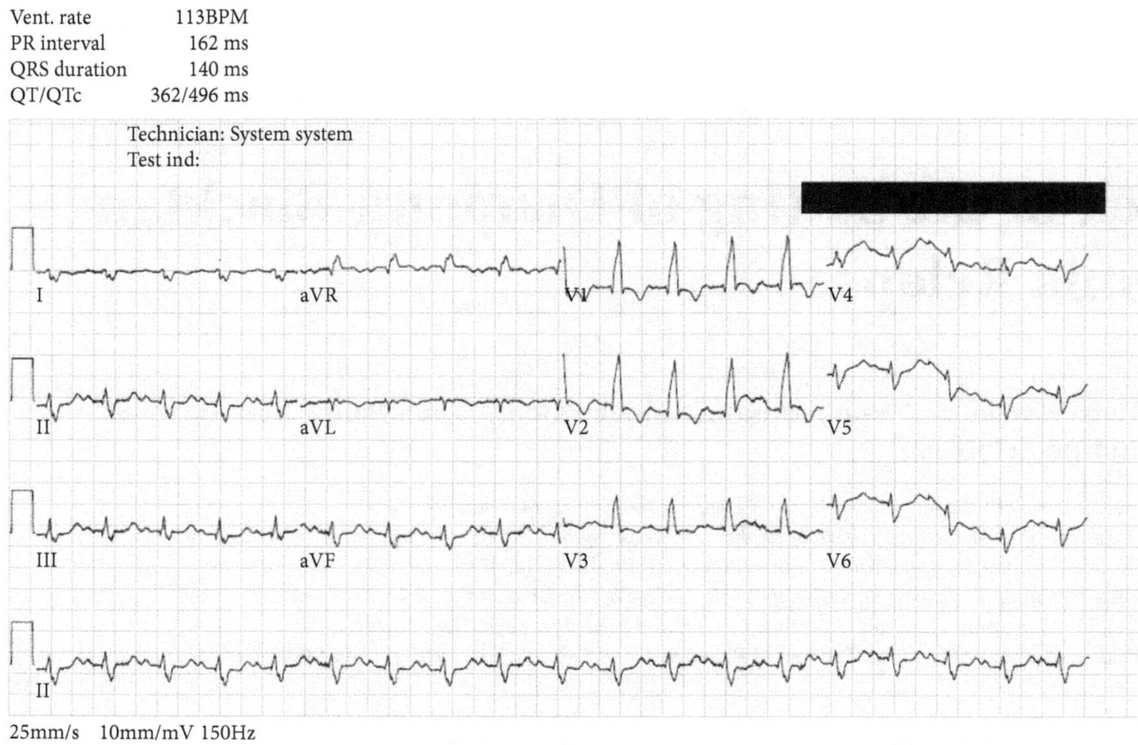

FIGURE 1: Initial electrocardiogram (EKG) demonstrating right bundle branch block, right axis deviation, and sinus tachycardia.

otherwise negative. His vital signs demonstrated a blood pressure of 138/90 mmHg, tachypnea (respiratory rate: 30 breaths/minute), tachycardia (pulse rate: 110 beats/minute), and a temperature of 36.4°C, and he was saturating 88% on a nonrebreather mask. He appeared in visible respiratory distress and pale and had evidence of a Klippel-Feil deformity, a triphalangeal thumb, and a harsh diastolic murmur over the left sternal border.

His labs demonstrated profound anemia with an hemoglobin of 2.5 g/dl, an elevated white blood cell count of 26.4 cells/mm^3, and a normal platelet count. His serum creatinine was 1.02 mg/dl, and his serum lactic acid was 6.3 mmol/L. Liver chemistries demonstrated elevated aspartate aminotransferase of 1072 U/L, alanine aminotransferase of 1568 U/L, and total bilirubin of 3.2 mg/dl. His international normalized ratio (INR) was 3.2, and his activated partial thromboplastin time (aPTT) was 49.5 seconds. A brain natriuretic peptide (BNP) was elevated at 2942 pg/ml. A thyroid stimulating hormone (TSH) level was normal. A chest X-ray (CXR) demonstrated cardiomegaly and pulmonary edema. An electrocardiogram (EKG) demonstrated a right bundle branch block (RBBB), a posterior left fascicular block, and sinus tachycardia (Figure 1).

Progressive worsening of clinical status with bilevel positive airway pressure (BiPAP) prompted intubation and mechanical ventilation. He was transfused 6 units of packed red blood cells (PRBC) with improvement of his hemoglobin to 8.8 g/dl. He received concomitant doses of furosemide to avoid further volume overload. He required norepinephrine for hemodynamic instability for 48 hours. A repeat echocardiogram demonstrated severe right ventricular enlargement

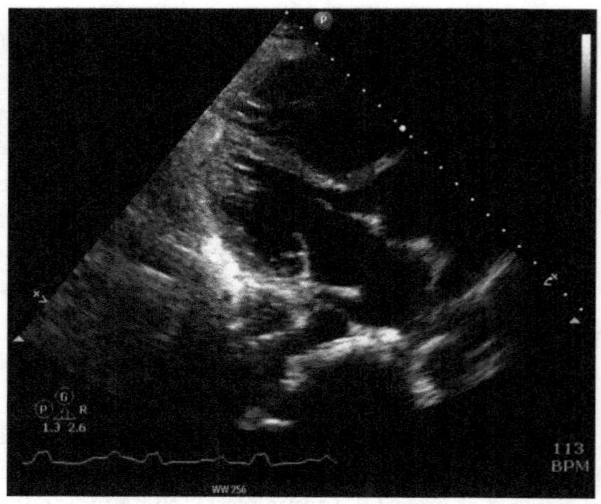

FIGURE 2: Transthoracic echocardiogram (TTE) demonstrating right sided ventricular hypertrophy.

(Figure 2). He was extubated after three days of optimizing his volume and respiratory status, and his liver chemistries, INR, and serum lactate normalized. Figure 3 compares an initial CXR and one performed at day 4. He was diuresed gently and discharged after 7 days of admission. A cardiac magnetic resonance image (MRI) showed a normal left ventricular ejection fraction (EF) of 55%, a severely enlarged right atrium and right ventricle (RV) with marked depression in right ventricular function (RV EF: 18%) (Figure 4), and severe bioprosthetic pulmonary regurgitation. His anemia was attributed to a relapse of his DBA, and he was restarted on prednisone. On 2 years of follow-up, he continues to

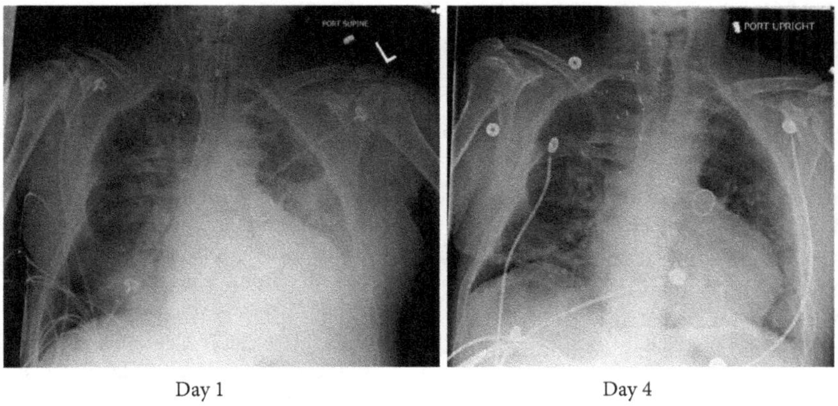

Figure 3: Initial plain chest film demonstrating acute pulmonary edema and repeat study at four days of hospitalization with improvement in volume overload. Congenital rib deformity and pulmonic valve ring are visible in both images.

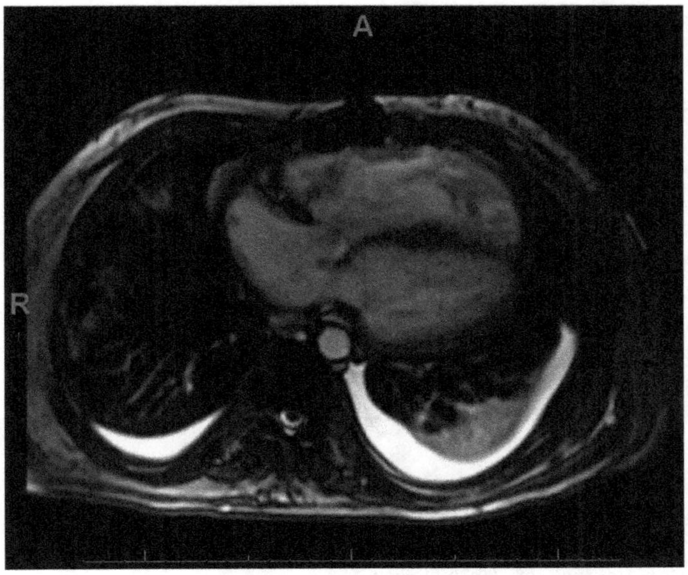

Figure 4: Cardiac magnetic resonance imaging demonstrating marked right ventricular enlargement.

refuse a bone marrow transplant, is transfusion-dependent, and is planned for a percutaneous pulmonary valve replacement. On evaluation of reasons for loss to follow-up, the patient reported a traumatic experience receiving a bone marrow aspiration in his adolescence.

3. Discussion

DBA diagnosis requires a correlation between examination findings and laboratory abnormalities demonstrating macrocytic anemia, elevated hemoglobin F levels, high erythrocyte deaminase activity, and confirmation with bone marrow biopsy and gene karyotyping. DBA is associated with congenital heart disease (CHD) in 30% of patients with atrial and ventricular septal defects constituting the majority of associated anomalies [1–3]. Associated Tetralogy of Fallot (TOF) accounts for only 3.5% of associated anomalies, and pulmonary hypertension following TOF repair occurs in around 1% of patients and often seen in patients with major aortopulmonary collateral arteries [1–3]. DBA management requires cooperation and coordination between multiple specialties given the complexity of the disorder and its effect on different organs. High dose followed by maintenance steroids and supportive transfusions represent initial lines of therapy with bone marrow transplantation utilized as definitive therapy in patients failing to achieve or maintain remission [8, 9]. Pregnancy and viral infections can cause relapse of the anemia with the latter being a possible trigger in the reported patient [8, 9].

Our patient presented with severe anemia resulting in high-output cardiac failure precipitating shock in the setting of severe pulmonary hypertension following a repaired TOF. This case represents several missed opportunities for earlier intervention that could have prevented the significant morbidity that our patient endured because of loss to follow-up. Firstly, early recognition of DBA relapse and reintroduction of steroids could have treated his anemia. Additionally, serial monitoring for development of pulmonary regurgitation, pulmonary hypertension, and subsequent right ventricular failure prompting early consideration for pulmonic valve replacement.

Multiple factors contribute to fractured transitions of care into adulthood including improper planning and coordination and low adult provider comfort levels and familiarity with chronic and complex pediatric diseases [10]. Patient factors include psychological effects of chronic disease on children and adolescents and lack of access to advanced healthcare and resources in rural populations [7, 11]. Efforts to create safer transitions of care for pediatric patients transitioning into adulthood are needed to prevent additional morbidity and mortality.

Additional Points

Article Guarantor. Zaid Imam, MBBS. *Presentation*. American Thoracic Society Conference 2018, San Diego, California, USA; poster presentation.

Consent

Informed consent obtained from the patient.

Authors' Contributions

All the authors were involved with manuscript preparation and draft revisions and have reviewed and approved the manuscript for submission. M. H and S. H have performed a review on the literature on similar reported cases.

References

[1] A. Vlachos, S. Ball, N. Dahl et al., "Diagnosing and treating Diamond Blackfan anaemia: results of an international clinical consensus conference," *British Journal of Haematology*, vol. 142, no. 6, pp. 859–876, 2008.

[2] A. Vlachos, L. Blanc, and J. M. Lipton, "Diamond Blackfan anemia: a model for the translational approach to understanding human disease," *Expert Review of Hematology*, vol. 7, no. 3, pp. 359–372, 2014.

[3] L. Da Costa, A. Narla, and N. Mohandas, "An update on the pathogenesis and diagnosis of diamond-blackfan anemia," *F1000Research*, vol. 7, 2018.

[4] American Academy of Pediatrics; American Academy of Family Physicians; American College of Physicians-American Society of Internal Medicine, "A consensus statement on health care transitions for young adults with special health care needs," *Pediatrics*, vol. 110, pp. 1304–1306, 2002.

[5] M. Mazzucato, L. Visonà Dalla Pozza, C. Minichiello et al., "The epidemiology of transition into adulthood of rare diseases patients: Results from a population-based registry," *International Journal of Environmental Research and Public Health*, vol. 15, no. 10, p. 2212, 2018.

[6] J. Yasuhara and H. Yamagishi, "Pulmonary arterial hypertension associated with tetralogy of Fallot," *International Heart Journal*, vol. 56, Supplement, pp. S17–S21, 2015.

[7] P. Touraine and M. Polak, "Challenges of the transition from pediatric care to care of adults: "say goodbye, say hello"," *Endocrine Development*, vol. 33, pp. 1–9, 2018.

[8] G. Engidaye, M. Melku, and B. Enawgaw, "Diamond blackfan anemia: genetics, pathogenesis, diagnosis and treatment," *Electronic Journal of the International Federation of Clinical Chemistry and Laboratory Medicine*, vol. 30, no. 1, pp. 67–81, 2019.

[9] A. Vlachos and E. Muir, "How I treat Diamond-Blackfan anemia," *Blood*, vol. 116, no. 19, pp. 3715–3723, 2010.

[10] M. J. Okumura, M. Heisler, M. M. Davis, M. D. Cabana, S. Demonner, and E. A. Kerr, "Comfort of general internists and general pediatricians in providing care for young adults with chronic illnesses of childhood," *Journal of General Internal Medicine*, vol. 23, no. 10, pp. 1621–1627, 2008.

[11] H. Li, S. Ge, B. Greene, and J. Dunbar-Jacob, "Depression in the context of chronic diseases in the United States and China," *Int J Nurs Sci.*, vol. 6, no. 1, pp. 117–122, 2019.

48

A Rare Case of MRSA Pericarditis with Expanding, Purulent Pericardial Effusion Leading to Uremic Kidney Failure from a Right, Necrotic Toe

Justin Brilliant, Diep Edwards, Ritu Yadav, Jana Lovell, and Lena Mathews

Johns Hopkins Hospital, Baltimore, MD, USA

Correspondence should be addressed to Justin Brilliant; jbrilli1@jh.edu

Academic Editor: Yigit Canga

Purulent pericarditis is an extremely rare entity with only a few reported cases so far. This condition deserves prompt diagnosis because of its significant mortality rate if left untreated. A 76-year-old man with a past medical history of coronary artery disease (CAD) with percutaneous coronary intervention (PCI) to the left anterior descending artery (LAD) and right circumflex artery (RCA), ischemic cardiomyopathy with moderately reduced ejection fraction (EF 45-50%), peripheral artery disease (PAD), COVID-19 pneumonia complicated by fibrotic lung disease (on 3 liters of home oxygen), type-2 diabetes mellitus (T2DM), hypertension (HTN), hyperlipidemia (HLD), and chronic kidney disease (CKD) stage III presented with complaints of pleuritic chest pain and shortness of breath. On hospital day 1, he was afebrile and hemodynamically stable with physical exam remarkable for bibasilar crackles and dry gangrene of his right first toe. He developed progressive altered mental status, hypotension, oliguric renal failure, and respiratory distress on hospital day 6. On exam at this time, he had an elevated jugular venous distension (JVD) of 12-14 cm water, pericardial friction rub with decreased heart sounds, and orthopnea; all were consistent with cardiac tamponade clinically. An electrocardiogram (EKG) showed new ST elevations in leads I, II, and aVL with ST depression in aVR and V1 with only mild elevation in troponin I to 0.07 ng/mL. A transthoracic echocardiogram (TTE) was done on hospital day 7 and showed a moderate sized pericardial effusion with inferior vena cava (IVC) enlargement but no atrial collapse, ventricular collapse, IVC collapse, or respiratory variation in the mitral and tricuspid inflow velocities. Blood cultures grew methicillin-resistant *Staphylococcus aureus* (MRSA) on hospital day 6, and he was started on intravenous (IV) vancomycin. The differential diagnosis for his enlarging pericardial effusion included purulent pericarditis, uremic pericarditis, or hemorrhagic effusion. He had urgent diagnostic and therapeutic pericardiocentesis with removal of 350 milliliters of fluid. The pericardial fluid was cloudy, tan-brown with a gram stain showing gram-positive cocci in clusters and cultures growing MRSA, which confirmed the diagnosis of purulent pericarditis secondary to MRSA infection. After the pericardiocentesis, his blood pressure, respiratory distress, and renal failure improved. The source of the bacteremia was from osteomyelitis of his gangrenous, right toe with bone biopsy growing both MRSA and *Streptococcus anginosus*. He underwent toe amputation for definitive source control. He was discharged on hospital day 24 with a plan to complete 6 weeks of IV vancomycin.

1. Introduction

Pericarditis is the most common disease of the pericardium worldwide, which can be a manifestation of an underlying systemic disease or an unrelated primary process. In developed countries, most pericarditis is idiopathic with a presumed viral etiology [1]. Purulent pericarditis, a localized bacterial infection of the pericardial space characterized by gross pus, only accounts for less than 1% of all cases with MRSA being the most commonly isolated organism [1]. This organism colonizes the nasopharynx, perineum, and skin, and it can migrate into the circulatory system and lead to hematogenous spread if the cutaneous barrier is disrupted or damaged. The diagnosis of purulent pericarditis from MRSA is extremely rare, with only a few case reports thus far [2–8]. However, the mortality rate for untreated patients can approach 100% but decreases to 40% in those patients who are appropriately treated with antibiotics and source control [9]. Furthermore, the coincidental diagnosis of uremia may lead to further pericardial injury to facilitate the accumulation of fluid. In this report, we present a case of MRSA pericarditis with purulent pericardial effusion and development of uremic renal injury complicated by a right necrotic toe.

2. Case Presentation

We present a 76-year-old man with a past medical history of CAD who had undergone multiple PCIs with drug-eluting stents to the LAD (18 and 12 years prior to admission) and RCA (2 years prior to admission) complicated by ischemic cardiomyopathy with moderately reduced ejection fraction (EF 45%), PAD, CKD stage III, T2DM, HTN, and HLD. Fifteen months prior to admission, he had developed viral pneumonia from SARS-CoV-2 complicated by chronic hypoxemic respiratory failure with fibrotic lung disease requiring supplemental oxygen of 3 liters since that time. Our patient presented with acute onset of substernal, pleuritic chest pain exacerbated by inspiration and accompanied by shortness of breath on the morning of presentation. The chest pain was noted to be very different from his prior myocardial infarctions and was not relieved by sublingual nitroglycerin. The patient described shortness of breath as if "someone threw a bucket of water" at him. His home pulse oximeter showed that at that time of pain, his oxygen saturation was in the 90 s, and his heart rate varied from 50 s to 130 s. The patient also reported right great toe gangrene that developed after a traumatic toenail clipping with worsening discoloration over the last month, but overall, he was able to bear weight and did not experience fevers, chills, or toe pain.

Vital signs on admission showed a temperature of 98.2°F, heart rate of 91/min, blood pressure of 147/81 mm of Hg, and respiratory rate of 18/min with oxygen saturation 98% on 3 L supplemental oxygen (home requirement). Physical exam was notable for bibasilar crackles, JVD 9 cm water, and dry gangrene of his right first toe. His chest pain subsided, and he remained chest pain free in the emergency department; serial troponins were negative. His initial labs were notable for white blood cell count (WBC) 11.31 K/μL, hemoglobin (Hb) 9.1 g/dL, platelets 289 K/μL, creatinine 1.6 mg/dL (baseline 1.3-1.4 mg/dL), blood urea nitrogen (BUN) 23 mg/dL, international normalized ratio (INR) 1.0, D-dimer 1.19 g/L, T4 1.25 nmol/L, *troponin I* < 0.04 *ng/mL*, negative urine toxicology, erythrocyte sedimentation rate (ESR) 87 mm/hr, C-reactive protein (CRP) 25.9 mg/L, lactate 1.2 mmol/L, negative testing for SARS-CoV-2 via nasopharyngeal swab (Labcorp PCR test), negative testing on a respiratory viral pathogen nasopharyngeal swab (Labcorp PCR test), and negative blood cultures. EKG showed normal sinus rhythm with no ST changes greater than 1 mm or T wave inversions. Computed tomography angiography (CTA) showed chronic fibrotic lung disease, new small pericardial effusion of 1.5 cm in its largest diameter, but no pulmonary embolism (Figure 1). Initial TTE showed an EF of 45-50%, with small, posterior pericardial effusion. There was mild concentric hypertrophy of the left ventricle (LV) with moderate hypokinesis of the mid and apical inferolateral, mid to distal anteroseptal, apical, apical lateral, and mid anterolateral segments along with akinesis of the basal inferoseptal segment; no significant valvular dysfunction or vegetation was seen. He was admitted for acute decompensated heart failure and underwent IV diuresis with furosemide. He developed new onset atrial fibrillation with rapid ventricular response on day 2 for which he was started on an IV heparin drip and an IV amiodarone drip. He converted to sinus rhythm on hospital day 5.

On day 6, our patient developed oliguric acute kidney injury with creatinine peaking at 4.4 mg/dL with BUN 102 mg/dL. He also became hypotensive with oliguria no longer responsive to diuresis at the time, which had required the initiation of continuous venovenous hemodialysis (CVVHD). However, our patient did not tolerate ultrafiltration because of low blood pressure. The administration of broad-spectrum antibiotics including IV vancomycin and IV cefepime was initiated due to concern for septic shock. However, with elevated JVD of 12-14 cm H20, hypotension, and evidence of ongoing renal failure, our team was concerned about obstructive shock in the setting of cardiac tamponade. He had persistent shortness of breath and developed worsening pleuritic chest pain, orthopnea, and a friction rub on exam. A repeat CT scan showed that the pericardial effusion enlarged from 1.5 cm to 2 cm in its greatest width (Figure 1). An EKG at the time showed normal sinus rhythm with new 2 mm ST elevations in leads I and II, 1 mm elevation in aVL, submillimeter elevations in V5-V6, and 1 mm ST depression in aVR (Figure 2). Troponin I was only mildly elevated to 0.07 ng/mL. On hospital day 7, an expanding pericardial effusion was seen on a limited TTE measuring 2.5 cm posteriorly in subcostal view with enlarged IVC but no evidence of tamponade without findings of atrial collapse, ventricular collapse, IVC collapse, or respiratory variation in mitral or tricuspid inflow (Figure 3). With concern for hemorrhagic effusion, anticoagulation for atrial fibrillation was held. Given the characteristics of his chest pain, pericardial friction rub on exam, EKG findings, and evidence of pericardial effusion on TTE, our patient met 4/4 criteria for acute pericarditis based on the most recent 2015 European Society of Cardiology (ESC) guidelines for diagnosis of pericardial disease [10].

Our patient's blood cultures from hospital day 6 returned positive for MRSA, for which the patient's antibiotics was narrowed to only vancomycin after two days of receiving cefepime. On day 8, he was transferred to the cardiac critical care unit for therapeutic pericardiocentesis; 350 mL of tan-brown cloudy thin fluid was drained under pressure, and a pericardial drain was left in place (Figure 4). He had immediate improvement in his hypotension and renal failure, and thus, did not require any additional dialysis. Postprocedure TTE confirmed complete drainage. Fluid pH was 6.9 with WBC 18,500/mm^3 with 95% neutrophilic predominance, red blood cells of 13000/mm^3, and gram stain showed gram positive cocci, raising concern for purulent pericarditis. Pericardial fluid cultures grew MRSA. The pericardial drain was left in place until hospital day 12 after no additional drainage for 48 hours and only a trace pericardial effusion seen on repeat TTE without echocardiographic evidence of tamponade. A

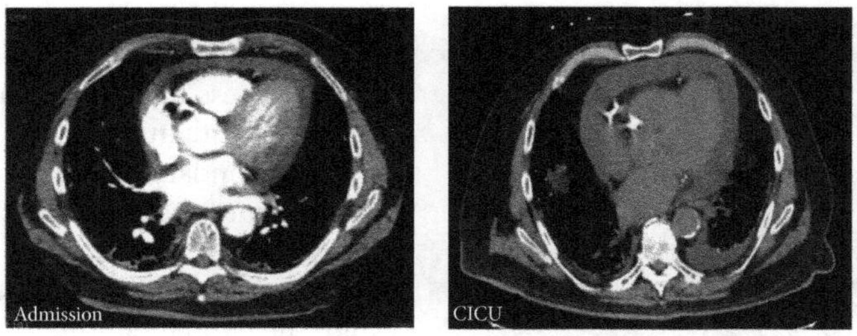

(a) (b)

FIGURE 1: CT chest on hospital day 1 (a) and hospital day 7 (b). The pericardial effusion had expanded from a largest diameter of 1.5 cm (a) to 2.0 cm (b) along with increase in left pleural effusion.

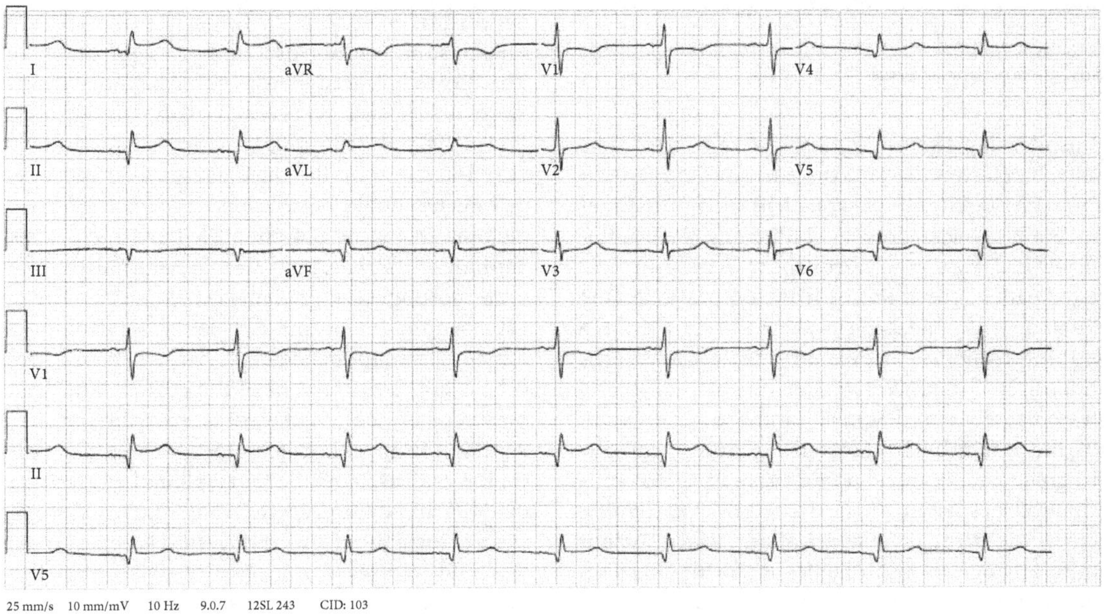

FIGURE 2: EKG on hospital day 7 with enlarging pericardial effusion. Normal sinus rhythm with new 2 mm ST elevations in leads I and II, 1 mm elevation in aVL, submillimeter elevations in V5-V6, and 1 mm ST depression in aVR and V1.

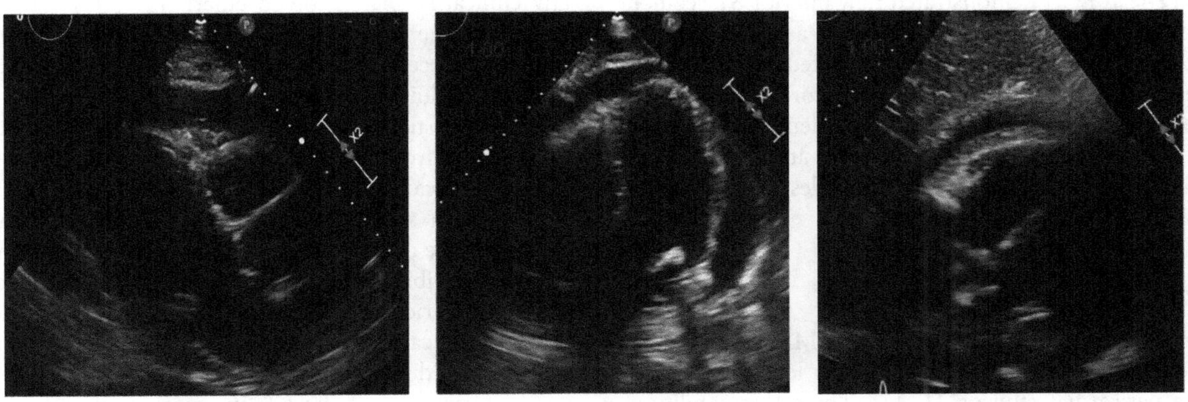

(a) (b) (c)

FIGURE 3: Parasternal long (a), apical 4-chamber view (b), and subxiphoid view (c) via echocardiography of expanding pericardial effusion on hospital day 7. No right atrial or right ventricular collapse or respiration variation in mitral or tricuspid inflow was seen. The inferior vena cava (IVC) was enlarged without collapse.

magnetic resonance imaging (MRI) scan of the right foot performed on hospital day 11 showed an increased T2 signal of the distal phalanx of the great toe with corresponding T1 hypointense signal in the bone marrow compatible with acute osteomyelitis. His right necrotic great toe up to the metatarsophalangeal joint was amputated by vascular

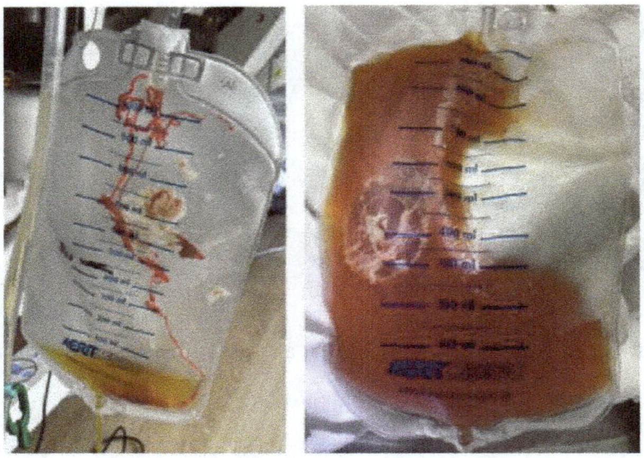

FIGURE 4: Pericardiocentesis with immediate removal of 350 cc cloudy, tan-brown, sanguinous fluid.

surgery on hospital day 18 for primary source control. The cultures from the resected toe and the surrounding margin of resection grew MRSA (and *Streptococcus anginosus*) that were both susceptible to vancomycin confirming the diagnosis of osteomyelitis. Given renal recovery to a creatinine of 1.3 (baseline for patient) with robust urine output following pericardial drainage, the decision was made to continue treatment with intravenous vancomycin (rather than daptomycin or linezolid) for 6-weeks after his repeat blood cultures became negative on day hospital day 8.

Regarding the patient's peripheral artery disease complicated by right great toe gangrene, noninvasive imaging demonstrated impaired perfusion to the right lower extremity. He was taken to the cardiac catheterization lab for a right lower extremity angiogram and diagnostic aortogram with long segment balloon angioplasty of the peroneal and anterior tibial arteries before amputation of necrotic right toe. As the patient was progressing towards medical readiness for discharge, he developed the acute onset of chest discomfort. A 12-lead ECG demonstrated new inferior ST segment elevations with reciprocal lateral changes as compared to a prior tracing. The patient was transported to the cardiac catheterization laboratory for emergent coronary angiography and possible primary PCI. The patient was found to have chronically occluded right coronary artery (RCA) and diffusely diseased distal left anterior descending (LAD) artery. PCI was not attempted.

3. Discussion

Both purulent pericarditis secondary to MRSA bacteremia and uremia are distinct entities that can lead to a rapidly evolving pericardial effusion [1, 11]. These two conditions can be difficult to differentiate because of similarly presenting symptoms such as acute chest pain, particularly in the recumbent position, pericardial friction rub on examination, and possibly wide-spread ST segment elevation [1, 12, 13]. Our patient met all of the criteria (4/4) for diagnosis of acute pericarditis given his history with physical examination, EKG, and echocardiography. However, early diagnosis and treatment of purulent pericarditis from MRSA with sufficient source control are critical because of the downstream complications of pericardial tamponade, septic shock, pericardial abscess formation, and constrictive pericarditis [10]. With greater than one-third of patients with purulent pericarditis secondary to MRSA initially presenting with a lack of bacteremia and a high risk of pericardial injury in the setting of uremia, identification of the etiology can be difficult, but pericardial drainage and source control is critical to avoid the aforementioned complications due to delay in intervention [14].

Purulent pericarditis from any bacterial organism is very rare and accounts for less than 1% of all cases of pericarditis with the majority being idiopathic from a presumed viral etiology [1]. The risk factors for development of purulent pericarditis include prior thoracic surgery, CKD, immunosuppression, alcohol use, and undiagnosed neoplasm [10]. The most commonly cited organisms include *Staphylococci*, *Streptococci*, and *Enterococci* with anaerobic species (e.g., *Prevotella* and *Peptostreptococcus*) seen more with concomitant infection in the mediastinum or neck [15]. Fungal pathogens should be considered for patients at risk for candidemia including parenteral hyperalimentation, prolonged antibiotic therapy, or steroid administration [16]. For immunosuppressed patients on chemotherapy or diagnosed with acquired immune deficiency syndrome (AIDS) from human immunodeficiency virus (HIV), *Mycobacterium tuberculosis* involvement of the pericardium has been documented [10, 15]. Purulent pericarditis most commonly develops from either hematogenous spread from a distant source or direct spread from a pleural empyema or pneumonia [10]. In addition, perforating injury, surgery, myocardial abscess formation, and endocarditis are less common etiologies [15]. However, for cases of purulent pericarditis from MRSA, hematogenous spread has been the most commonly cited means of seeding the pericardium with only a few cases reporting osteomyelitis as a documented source [17, 18]. An expedited TTE with pericardiocentesis should be done for any clinical suspicion for an enlarging pericardial effusion because of the high prevalence of cardiac tamponade (84%) noted in a recent systematic review [14]. Cultures from the pericardial fluid should be sent for bacterial, fungal, and tuberculosis studies to confirm the diagnosis [10]. Purulent pericarditis from MRSA has a 100% mortality rate if untreated because of resulting multiorgan failure from sepsis, but with adequate drainage and antibiotic treatment, mortality rate decreases to 30% [19]. Therefore, prompt initiation of antibiotics that target MRSA along with placement of either a pericardial drain (such as our patient), pericardial window, pericardiotomy, or even surgical pericardiectomy is recommended since the recurrence of effusion is common and had been noted to be 30% in reported cases [1, 10]. Even with attempted source control with the use of antibiotics and drainage of pus in the pericardial space, the feared complications of septic shock, reaccumulation of pus with potential abscess formation, and constrictive pericarditis can occur and have been reported in 15.4%, 30.8%, and 3.5% of reported cases, respectively [14, 19].

In addition to purulent pericarditis, uremia alone can lead to the accumulation of toxic metabolites and nitrogenous waste products that are highly toxic to the pericardium leading to inflammation, fibrin deposition, and adhesion [10]. In severe cases, a pericardial effusion can also develop; however, large volume fluid accumulation in the pericardial space may be partially related to platelet dysfunction in patients with renal failure. The diagnosis of uremic pericarditis requires a strong clinical suspicion. Aside from pleuritic chest pain, objective data include diffuse ST and T-wave elevation, elevated cardiac biomarkers, and confirmatory echocardiogram; however, those EKG findings may not always occur because epicardial injury can be uncommon [20]. Initial treatment includes prompt initiation of dialysis as most patients (87%) resolve rapidly with intensive dialysis [21]. Urgent pericardiocentesis is only recommended within 7-14 days or emergently if there is evidence of cardiac tamponade [22]. The precipitants of cardiac tamponade in uremic pericarditis include hypovolemia, paroxysmal tachyarrhythmia, and concomitant epicardial injury [23].

The prompt initiation of antibiotic treatment for suspicion of purulent pericarditis, in conjunction with drainage and source control with pericardiocentesis, is critical and should be directed against the most likely pathogens based on patient-specific factors. An empiric regimen includes a combination of an antistaphylococcal antibiotic (e.g., vancomycin) along with either an aminoglycoside (e.g., gentamicin) or cephalosporin (e.g., ceftriaxone and cefepime) for gram-negative coverage; the addition of a fluoroquinolone (e.g., ciprofloxacin and levofloxacin) can be considered if no rapid improvement in clinical signs of infection is seen to cover for atypical infections such as *Legionella* and *Mycoplasma* [15, 24]. Empiric therapy should be continued until signs and symptoms of infection are improving and then narrowed after the diagnosis is confirmed from the pericardial fluid with the specific pathogen isolated. There are no specific guidelines on the duration of treatment for purulent pericarditis, but treatment should last for at least 2-4 weeks contingent upon the adequacy of drainage with definitive source control and the antimicrobial susceptibilities of the isolated strain of microbe(s) [15]. The duration of antibiotics should also be based on additional sources of infection for which guideline-based courses of therapies exist such as concomitant osteomyelitis and endocarditis where antibiotic duration would be extended to 6 weeks. Finally, no current recommendation exists for serial monitoring of the pericardial effusion via echocardiography after completion of treatment unless new symptoms or lab abnormalities arise to suggest recurrence of infection.

In regard to the complications of purulent pericarditis, notably cardiac tamponade, and constrictive pericarditis, invasive procedures such as pericardiocentesis, subxiphoid pericardiotomy with fibrinolytic therapy, and pericardiectomy are considered depending on the degree of cardiac compression, chronicity, and recurrence [10]. Although urgent pericardiocentesis with effective drainage is a class I recommendation for diagnosis and treatment of purulent pericarditis, transcatheter intrapericardial fibrinolysis has been shown to decrease rate of constriction by 38.3% [25]. Furthermore, subxiphoid pericardiotomy with fibrinolytic therapy and even surgical pericardiectomy may be considered (class IIa recommendation) for more definitive management to allow for complete drainage of the effusion, manual lysis of adhesions, and decreased risk of developing constrictive pericarditis [10]. A subxiphoid pericardiotomy is preferred over a surgical pericardiectomy when surgery is too high of a risk (i.e., large, recurrent pericardial effusions or cardiac tamponade) or for a more palliative approach [10]. However, the communicating passage from the pericardial space may close off and repeated, and loculated effusions may occur. A pericardiectomy, therefore, allows for complete removal and can be the definitive therapy for either recurrent episodes of purulent pericarditis or constrictive pericarditis with the removal of each constricting pericardial layer [26]. Additional studies are needed to clarify the timing, delivery, and efficacy of transcatheter and intrapericardial fibrinolytic therapies in relation to surgical pericardiectomy in patients with purulent pericarditis.

Ultimately, our patient was discharged from the hospital without any complications on IV vancomycin to complete a 6-week duration of treatment for osteomyelitis of his right foot. Purulent pericarditis from MRSA was suspected early in our patient's admission because of an expanding pericardial effusion with clinical evidence of cardiac tamponade. The subsequent drainage of pus with pericardiocentesis and drain placement along with a source of the MRSA isolated from the right toe explained the hematogenous spread to the pericardium. Although our patient's uremic renal injury could have contributed to his worsening pericardial effusion, uremic pericarditis was not a consideration for his initial presentation given the presence of a small effusion before his clinical decompensation, lack of improvement following dialysis, and prompt resolution of symptoms following pericardial drainage and antibiotic treatment. With early initiation of antibiotics against MRSA and successful amputation of his right necrotic toe that grew MRSA confirming osteomyelitis, our patient was discharged on IV vancomycin to complete a total 6-week duration of therapy because of residual infected bone present after resection. However, our patient was transitioned from vancomycin to linezolid to complete the final 5 days of his treatment course given an increase in his creatinine from 1.3 to 2.6. Following his completed course of antibiotics, his right foot has healed without any complications, creatinine has improved close to baseline at 1.7, and a repeat TTE showed stable cardiac function with trace pericardial effusion similar in size prior to discharge.

4. Conclusion

MRSA purulent pericarditis is an extremely rare diagnosis. In this report, we present a case of MRSA pericarditis in a patient with type 2 diabetes mellitus and peripheral artery disease complicated by a right necrotic toe who developed acute, oliguric renal failure with an enlarging pericardial effusion. The patient underwent diagnosis and primary source control with pericardial drainage and toe amputation in addition to a total, six-week course of antibiotics with activity against MRSA. Given the significant morbidity and mortality of MRSA pericarditis, early recognition and treatment of bacterial pericarditis are critical. Further studies are warranted to guide diagnostics and optimize therapies in high-risk populations such as those with multiple cardiovascular and renal comorbidities.

Consent

I have received written informed consent from the patient to publish the details of this case report.

References

[1] M. Imazio, F. Gaita, and M. LeWinter, "Evaluation and treatment of pericarditis," *Journal of the American Medical Association*, vol. 314, no. 14, pp. 1498–1506, 2015.

[2] M. Ganji, J. Ruiz, W. Kogler, J. Lung, J. Hernandez, and C. Isache, "Methicillin-resistant _Staphylococcus aureus_ pericarditis causing cardiac tamponade," *IDCases.*, vol. 18, 2019.

[3] Y. Kurahara and T. Kawaguchi, "Cardiac tamponade with community-acquired methicillin-resistant Staphylococcus aureus pericarditis," *Internal medicine (Tokyo, Japan)*, vol. 52, no. 15, p. 1753, 2013.

[4] M. A. Hussam, M. F. Ragai, M. F. Iman, and A. Zakaria, "Community-acquired methicillin-resistant Staphylococcus aureus pericarditis presenting as cardiac tamponade," *Southern medical journal.*, vol. 103, no. 8, pp. 834–836, 2010.

[5] H. DeYoung, A. Bloom, and S. Tamayo, "Successful treatment of community-acquired methicillin-resistant Staphylococcus aureus purulent myopericarditis," *BMJ case reports*, vol. 2017, article bcr-2017-221931, 2017.

[6] M. Terada, H. Watanabe, Y. Kobukai et al., "Successful treatment of a patient with purulent pericarditis by daily intrapericardial washouts," *The Annals of thoracic surgery.*, vol. 98, no. 4, pp. 1451–1454, 2014.

[7] K. A. Rodvold and K. W. McConeghy, "Methicillin-resistant Staphylococcus aureus therapy: past, present, and future," *Clinical infectious diseases : an official publication of the Infectious Diseases Society of America.*, vol. 58, Supplement 1, pp. S20–S27, 2014.

[8] N. P. Arora, A. Kottam, N. Mahajan et al., "Purulent pericardial effusion from community-acquired methicillin-resistant _Staphylococcus aureus_," *The American journal of the medical sciences*, vol. 344, no. 2, pp. 160–162, 2012.

[9] J. Sagristà-Sauleda, J. A. Barrabés, G. Permanyer-Miralda, and J. Soler-Soler, "Purulent pericarditis: review of a 20-year experience in a general hospital," *Journal of the American College of Cardiology*, vol. 22, no. 6, pp. 1661–1665, 1993.

[10] Y. Adler, P. Charron, M. Imazio et al., "2015 ESC guidelines for the diagnosis and management of pericardial diseases: the task force for the diagnosis and management of pericardial diseases of the European Society of Cardiology (ESC)endorsed by: the European Association for Cardio-Thoracic Surgery (EACTS)," *European Heart Journal*, vol. 36, no. 42, pp. 2921–2964, 2015.

[11] S. Ben-Horin, I. Bank, V. Guetta, and A. Livneh, "Large symptomatic pericardial effusion as the presentation of unrecognized cancer: a study in 173 consecutive patients undergoing pericardiocentesis," *Medicine (Baltimore)*, vol. 85, no. 1, pp. 49–53, 2006.

[12] Y. Bentata, F. Hamdi, A. Chemlal, I. Haddiya, N. Ismaili, and N. El Ouafi, "Uremic pericarditis in patients with end stage renal disease: prevalence, symptoms and outcome in 2017," *The American Journal of Emergency Medicine*, vol. 36, no. 3, pp. 464–466, 2018.

[13] T. Dad and M. J. Sarnak, "Pericarditis and pericardial effusions in end-stage renal disease," *Seminars in Dialysis*, vol. 29, no. 5, pp. 366–373, 2016.

[14] M. Radovanovic, M. Petrovic, R. D. Hanna et al., "Clinical presentation and management of methicillin-resistant Staphylococcus aureus pericarditis—systematic review," *Journal of Cardiovascular Development and Disease.*, vol. 9, no. 4, p. 103, 2022.

[15] S. Pankuweit, A. D. Ristić, and P. M. Seferović, "Bacterial pericarditis," *American Journal of Cardiovascular Drugs*, vol. 5, no. 2, pp. 103–112, 2005.

[16] J. H. Schrank Jr. and D. P. Dooley, "Purulent pericarditis caused by Candida species: case report and review," *Clinical Infectious Diseases*, vol. 21, no. 1, pp. 182–187, 1995.

[17] P. A. Dherange, S. Patel, E. Enakpene, and P. Suryanarayana, "From bone to heart: a case of MRSA osteomyelitis with haematogenous spread to the pericardium," *BMJ case reports*, vol. 2015, article bcr2015211410, 2015.

[18] H. Khutan, R. Kaur, G. Singh, P. Singh, and A. Kaur, "Case of disseminated community-acquired methicillin-resistant Staphylococcus aureus: unique behavior of the organism in an immunocompetent adult," *Archives of Medicine and Health Sciences.*, vol. 6, no. 2, pp. 254–256, 2018.

[19] P. Augustin, M. Desmard, P. Mordant et al., "Clinical review: intrapericardial fibrinolysis in management of purulent pericarditis," *Critical Care*, vol. 15, no. 2, p. 220, 2011.

[20] E. A. Rutsky and S. G. Rostand, "Pericarditis in end-stage renal disease: clinical characteristics and management," in *Seminars in Dialysis*, vol. 2, pp. 25–30, Blackwell Publishing Ltd, Oxford, UK, 1989.

[21] E. A. Rutsky and S. G. Rostand, "Treatment of uremic pericarditis and pericardial effusion," *American Journal of Kidney Diseases*, vol. 10, no. 1, pp. 2–8, 1987.

[22] M. Kabukcu, F. Demircioglu, E. Yanik, I. Basarici, and F. Ersel, "Pericardial tamponade and large pericardial effusions: causal factors and efficacy of percutaneous catheter drainage in 50 patients," *Texas Heart Institute Journal*, vol. 31, no. 4, pp. 398–403, 2004.

[23] K. A. Rehman, J. Betancor, B. Xu et al., "Uremic pericarditis, pericardial effusion, and constrictive pericarditis in end-stage renal disease: Insights and pathophysiology," *Clinical Cardiology*, vol. 40, no. 10, pp. 839–846, 2017.

[24] L. J. Goodman, "Purulent Pericarditis," *Current Treatment Options in Cardiovascular Medicine*, vol. 2, no. 4, pp. 343–350, 2000.

[25] H. B. Cui, X. Y. Chen, C. C. Cui et al., "Prevention of pericardial constriction by transcatheter intrapericardial fibrinolysis with urokinase," *Chinese Medical Sciences Journal*, vol. 20, no. 1, pp. 5–10, 2005.

[26] Y. H. Cho, H. V. Schaff, J. A. Dearani et al., "Completion pericardiectomy for recurrent constrictive pericarditis: importance of timing of recurrence on late clinical outcome of operation," *The Annals of Thoracic Surgery*, vol. 93, no. 4, pp. 1236–1240, 2012.

49

A Rare Case of Gastrointestinal Stromal Tumor with a Liver Metastasis Infiltrating the Inferior Vena Cava and Extending to the Right Atrium with an Early Recurrence after Surgical Extraction

Dimitrios Siamkouris, Marc Schloesser, Amr Yousef, and Elmar Offers

Department of Cardiology, Dreifaltigkeits Hospital Lippstadt, Germany,
Academic Teaching Hospital of Westfaelische Wilhelms University Muenster, Germany

Correspondence should be addressed to Dimitrios Siamkouris; jimsiamkouris@yahoo.gr

Academic Editor: Ertugrul Ercan

Gastrointestinal stromal tumors (GISTs) are mesenchymal tumors of the gastrointestinal tract. The major cause of GIST is the presence of an abnormal form of tyrosine protein kinase (KIT) protein also known as CD117, which causes uncontrollable growth of the gastrointestinal cells. Most studies report incidences between 10 and 15 cases of GISTs per million. Metastases to the liver and peritoneum are the most frequent. We report a case of advanced GIST with a liver metastasis infiltrating the inferior vena cava (IVC) and extending to the right atrium in the form of a large, floating, isolated intracardiac liver metastasis with diastolic prolapsing through the tricuspid valve. This is a very rare manifestation. One week after heart surgery and removal of a 5 × 6 cm tumor mass from the right atrium and the IVC, echocardiography depicted an early recurrence.

1. Case

A 51-year-old female patient was admitted about 4 years ago to the emergency room for nausea, vomiting, dizziness, melena, and syncope. The patient's history indicated upper gastrointestinal bleeding, and immediate esophagogastroduodenoscopy (EGD) revealed an ulcerating tumor in the pyloric antrum with blood oozing, strongly suspected for a gastric GIST. Haemostasis was achieved after endoscopic injection of epinephrine and subsequent adequate blood transfusion due to haemorrhagic shock led to the stabilisation of the patient. The histological diagnosis was ulcerating epitheloid GIST (Figure 1). Immunohistochemically, tumor cells were strongly positive for CD117, platelet-derived growth factor receptor-alpha (PDGFRA), discovered on GIST-1 (DOG1), and Bcl-2. CD34 was not evident. The mitotic rate was 8/50 high-power fields (HPF), and the Ki67-index/proliferation rate was estimated at 5%. The molecular pathological examination showed duplication in exon 11 of the KIT gene. The abdominal computed tomography (CT) scan showed no lymph node, liver, or bone metastasis. The pT2 M0 R0 (TNM classification) staged tumor was operated successfully with an open 2/3 stomach resection with a Roux-en-Y anastomosis and jejunojejunostomy. The 3.5 cm tumor was completely excised with edges clear of infiltration and no tumor infiltration of the serosa. The postoperative course was very satisfactory with no sequelae, and no adjuvant imatinib therapy was administrated after multidisciplinary treatment planning. The patient could be discharged 3 weeks after admission with the recommendation for abdominal (CT) scan and EGD every 6 months for the next 5 years.

15 months later and in the scope of the follow-up examination, the patient complained for discomfort and slight pain in the right upper abdomen. The abdominal ultrasonography revealed multiple liver metastases, and the EGD

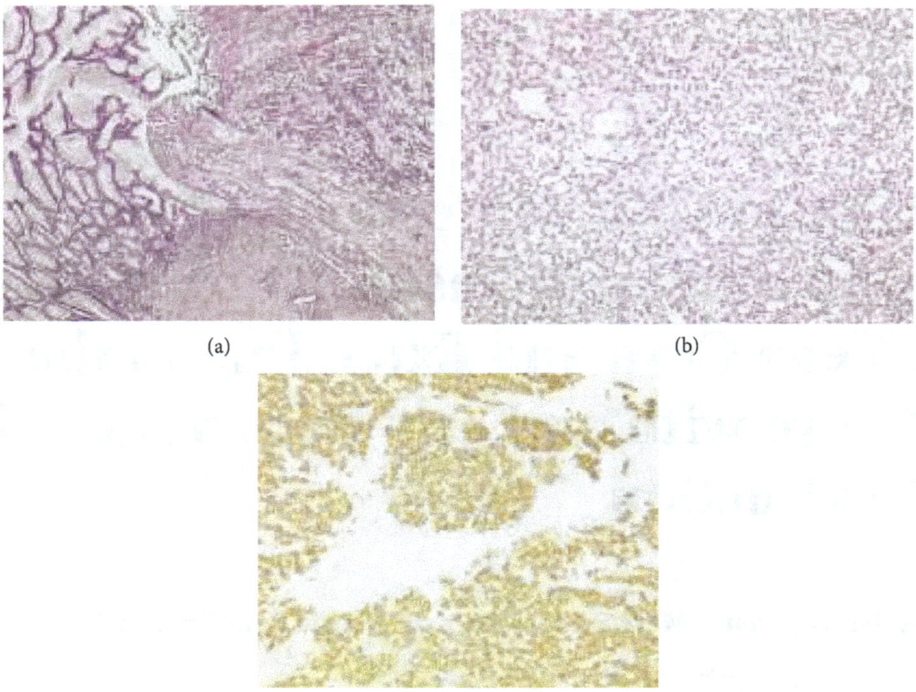

FIGURE 1: (a) Stomach ulcer with epithelioid GIST (50x, hematoxylin and eosin stain). (b) Gastric epithelioid GIST (100x, hematoxylin and eosin stain). (c) Membrane pattern of KIT immunostaining in epithelioid GIST (100x, CD117).

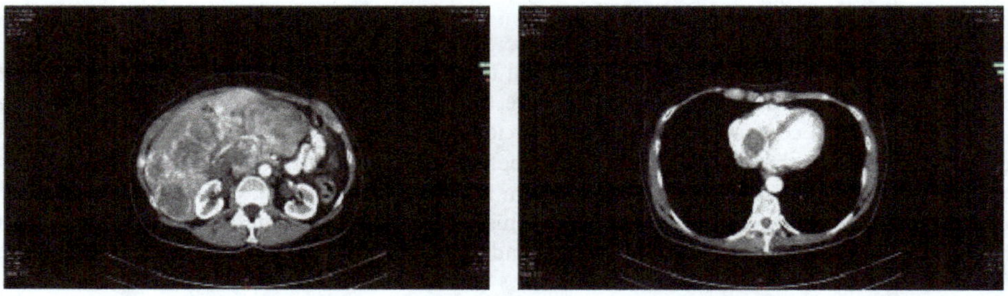

FIGURE 2: (a) Abdominal CT scan with IV contrast showing multiple liver metastases. (b) Chest CT scan showing a filling defect within the contrast-enhanced right atrium which was initially thought to be a large thrombus.

confirmed a recurrence of GIST in the anastomosis. The abdominal and chest CT scan (Figure 2) confirmed diffuse liver metastases and revealed an encircling wall architecture of the GIST around the hepatic hilum with a partial obstruction of the common bile duct and a shifting of the portal vein without signs of portal vein thrombosis. However, no icterus was present. The CT scan revealed furthermore a suspected large thrombus in the IVC and right atrium. There was no evidence of lymph node, bone, or lung metastasis. The transthoracic (TTE) and subsequent transoesophageal echocardiography (TEE) disclosed the presence of a 5.3×3.4 cm large mass in the right atrium with diastolic prolapsing through the tricuspid valve, without any clear attachment to the atrial wall, with an inhomogeneous appearance, and without vacuolisation (Figure 3), along with a similar 1.1 cm large mass in the IVC (Figure 4) with a suspected but no clear continuation between these two masses even after free style image acquisition. The patient denied any angina or dyspnoea. Anticoagulant therapy with low molecular weight heparin showed no improvement within few days, ruling out a thrombus formation and suggesting intracardiac metastasis. Due to recurrent electrocardiogram (ECG) alternations in the precordial leads suggestive of intermittent lung embolism, the imminent right ventricular diastolic flow obstruction with a resulting obstructive form of a cardiogenic shock, and because of the young age of the patient and the potential good response to imatinib therapy, she was referred to a cardiothoracic clinic.

The patient underwent cardiac catheterization which revealed no obstructive coronary atherosclerotic plaque. Prior to surgery, cardiac magnetic resonance imaging (Figure 5) verified the cardiac findings of echocardiography but also clearly exhibited a propagation of a liver metastasis

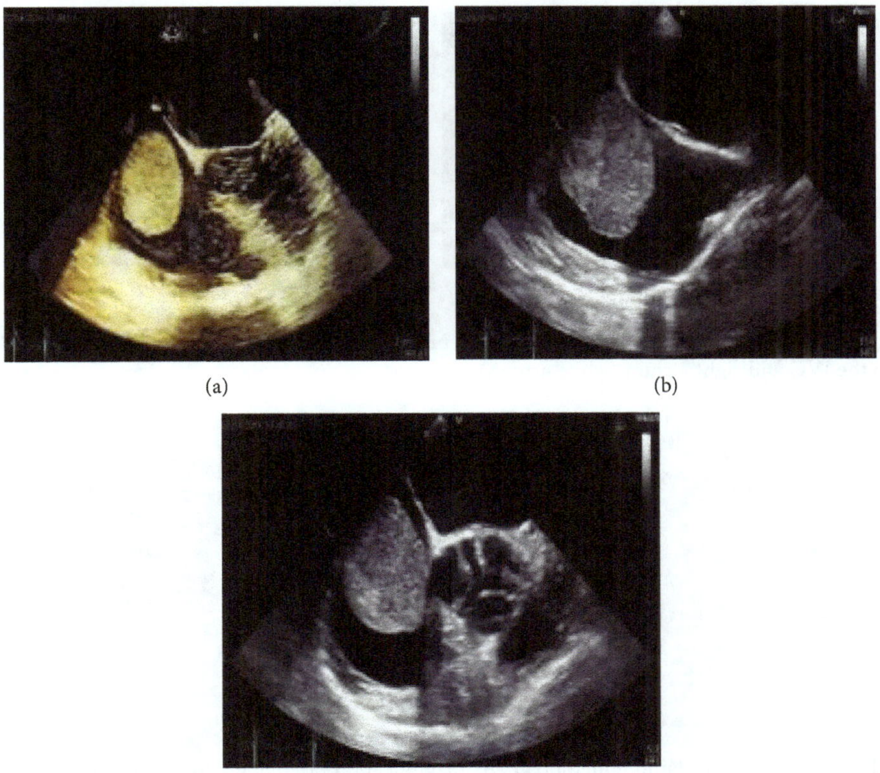

(a) (b) (c)

FIGURE 3: Large atrial mass in (a) the TEE 3D 4-chamber view, (b) the TEE 2D bicaval view, and (c) the TEE 2D short-axis view, conclusive for a mobile large atrial mass.

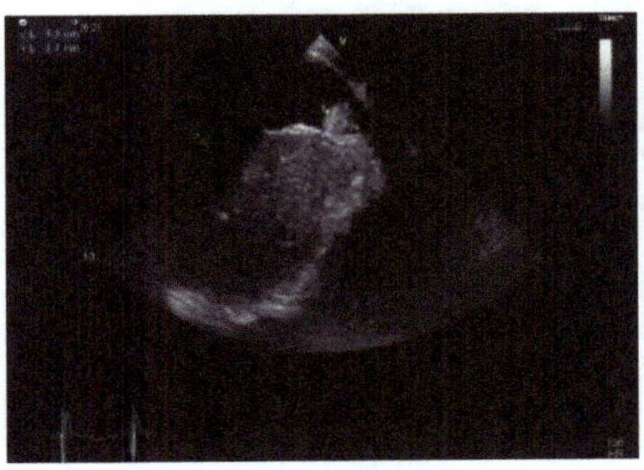

FIGURE 4: TEE reveals a similar mass in the IVC.

as a continuous mass to the IVC and right atrium with no adherence to the cardiac wall. Surgical resection of the tumor in the right atrium and IVC was performed using a minimally invasive anterior lateral access approach supplemented with video-assisted thoracoscopy. The 50 × 60 mm resected tumor with endothelial infiltration of the IVC, concomitant local thrombosis (Figure 6), and no endocardial and myocardial infiltration of the right atrium was histologically and immunohistologically identical to the prediagnosed GIST (Figure 7) and was a contiguous extension of a liver metastasis to the heart. The patient could recover from the operation and was treated with 400 mg imatinib daily. However, a week after surgery, transthoracic echocardiography (Figure 8) revealed a new mass in the right atrium indicative of early recurrence. The patient deteriorated over time due to a further progression of the GIST with icterus. The course was furthermore complicated by *Staphylococcus aureus* sepsis due to central venous catheter infection, and the patient finally died due to multiorgan failure.

2. Discussion

GISTs are rare, potentially aggressive forms of cancer that may develop anywhere in the GI tract [1]. Most studies report incidences between 10 and 15 cases of GISTs per million. Estimates suggest that the prevalence is over 10 times the incidence [2]. Surgical resection remains the aimed therapy of GIST. Complete resection of the tumor is the main predictor of the postoperative survival of the patient [1]. Despite successful surgical therapy, GISTs exhibit a high risk for metastatic relapse. The work of Hirota et al. and subsequently Heinrich et al. proved that most of the GISTs are caused by c-KIT somatic gain-of-function mutations followed by similar mutations in platelet-derived growth factor receptor-alpha (PDGFRA) [3, 4]. The initiation of KIT-selective tyrosine kinase inhibitor therapy such as imatinib and its successors improved the survival of these patients [5, 6]. However, the benefit in recurrence-free survival appears to be related to tumor size, with the most marked improvement in patients who had a large tumor (≥10 cm) [6]. In our case, the multidisciplinary tumor board conference involving pathologists, radiologists, surgeons, and medical oncologists as well as gastroenterologists, based on the positive surgical and clinical course of the patient and

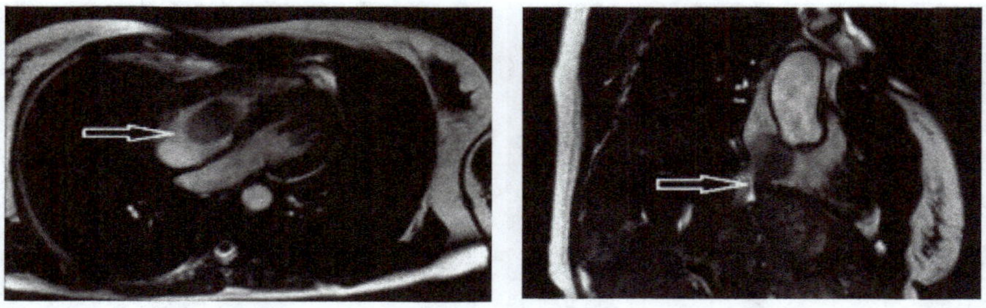

(a) (b)

FIGURE 5: Cardiac MRI confirms the mass in (a) the right atrium with prolapsing through the tricuspid valve and (b) the contiguous extension of the liver metastasis to the IVC and right atrium (white arrows).

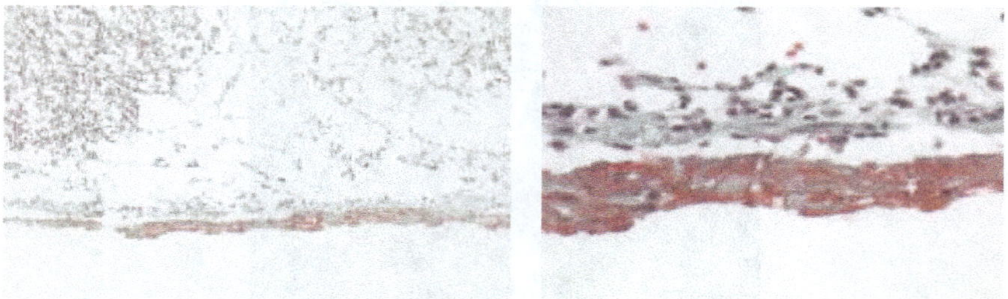

(a) (b)

FIGURE 6: Goldner's trichrome histological staining method at 20x magnification (a) and 80x magnification (b) exhibiting the tumor in the upper layer, fibrosis in the middle green layer, and thrombosis in the lower red layer. Between the fibrotic band and the thrombosis, there are identifiable gut endothelial cells from the VCI.

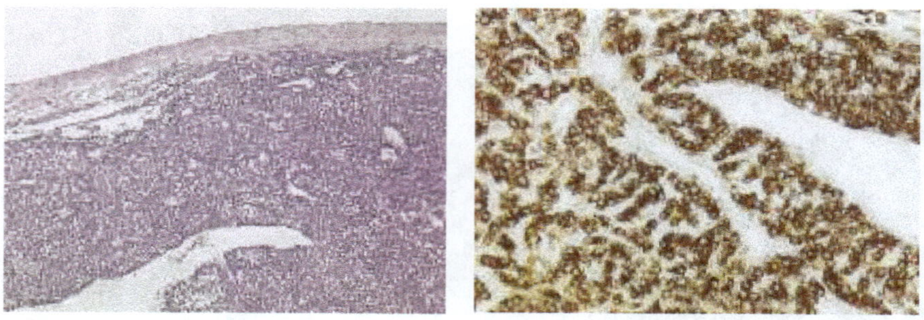

(a) (b)

FIGURE 7: (a) Metastasis of epithelioid GIST in the right atrium of the heart (50x, hematoxylin and eosin stain). (b) Strong cytoplasmic pattern of KIT immunostaining in epithelioid GIST in the right atrium of the heart (200x, CD117 antibody).

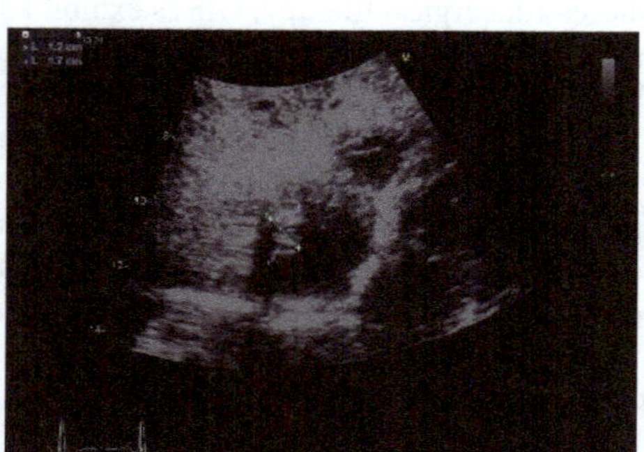

FIGURE 8: Tumor recurrence one week after surgical removal.

the so far scientific evidence at the time of treatment of our patient, which was not conclusive for adjuvant imatinib therapy in patients with locoregional GISTs and R0 surgery (i.e., an excision whose margins are clear of tumour cells) with no expected major sequelae, saw no clear indication for an adjuvant imatinib therapy taking also the size of the tumor into consideration. Gastric tumors have a more favourable prognosis than the intestinal ones, and according to risk stratification based on location, size, and mitotic activity, this GIST carried an intermediate risk for recurrence in the absence of tyrosine kinase inhibitor therapy [7].

Current consensus of the experts at that time was to recommend adjuvant imatinib for patients at high risk of relapse and not for those at low risk of relapse. But there was no consensus for patients at intermediate risk such as our patient [8, 9].

Metastatic GISTs are however associated with poor survival. GISTs most frequently metastasize within the abdominal cavity, especially to the liver and peritoneum, with bone and lung metastases being uncommon sites [1, 10]. Very rare metastasis to the skeletal muscle, adrenal gland [11], brain [12], and testicles [13] is also reported.

Cardiac metastasis after a traditional narrative review using PubMed is reported to our knowledge in only 3 cases so far: 2 cases of metastasis in the left ventricle [6] and one in the right atrium [11] which coincides with the localisation of our case. The initial recognition of the mass was always accidental in CT scan. The differentiation from a thrombus is difficult because intracardiac tumors appear in CT scan as a low-attenuation filling defect, similar to a thrombus [14]. In one report, the differentiation was established through positron emission tomography (PET). PET showed that the mass was metabolically active and a thrombus was by this means excluded. However, PET is certainly not always available and could require patient transportation which may not be possible as the patient may be unstable. In our case, failed improvement after anticoagulation, TEE, and cardiac MRI consolidated the suspected diagnosis of a GIST metastasis which was verified after surgery. In the 3 reported cases of cardiac metastasis so far, the masses diagnosed in the left ventricle and right atrium, respectively, appeared to be attached to the cardiac wall and were therefore consistent with metastatic GIST; however, there is neither histological evidence of GIST nor histological evidence of infiltration of the endocardium or myocardium as the patients underwent no surgical therapy due to very limited prognosis. In our patient, surgery was endorsed because of the high risk for an obstructive form of a cardiogenic shock which could lead to a sudden circulatory deterioration of the patient and because of the possibility for a good response to imatinib therapy. This is the only case reported with histological analysis of a suspected cardiac metastasis of GIST. In our case, because of the lack of endocardial and myocardial infiltration, there is no evidence of hematologous or lymphatic spread of the GIST to the heart in the form of a classic cardiac metastasis and the cardiac involvement of the GIST is due to a contiguous extension of a liver metastasis to the IVC and the right atrium.

Additionally, of clinical interest is the appearance of a new smaller cardiac mass in the right atrium only one week after surgical resection of the tumor. This is the first report of surgical removal of a GIST from the heart, and it shows that early recurrence of cardiac tumors involving GIST after surgery is possible. This experience should be taken into consideration for similar future decisions questioning the meaningfulness of a surgery in advanced cases before implementing KIT-selective tyrosine kinase inhibitor therapy (wait and see how the patient responds to KIT-selective tyrosine kinase inhibitor therapy before cardiac surgery).

The incidence of cardiac metastases is reported in literature, which is highly variable, ranging from 2.3% to 18.3% [15]. This case in addition to the so far published cases of cardiac metastasis involving GIST underlines the importance of considering GIST as a possible cause of cardiac metastasis or cardiac deterioration, associated with a very unfavourable prognosis and a possible high recurrence after surgery. GIST patients should therefore routinely undergo TTE by the time of diagnosis and in follow-up examinations, and cardiac surgery should be considered as the last resort in the battle against metastasized GIST.

Consent

Informed consent for publishing this case report has been obtained from the husband, the legal representative of the patient, as the patient has died.

Acknowledgments

The authors would like to acknowledge Henning Warnecke MD, Ph.D. (Cardiothoracic Surgery, Schuechtermann Clinic, Bad Rothenfelde, Germany), and Frank Henschke MD, Ph.D. (Institute of Pathology, Driburger Str. 34, 33100 Paderborn, Germany).

References

[1] A. El-Menyar, A. Mekkodathil, and H. Al-Thani, "Diagnosis and management of gastrointestinal stromal tumors: an up-to-date literature review," *Journal of Cancer Research and Therapeutics*, vol. 13, no. 6, pp. 889–900, 2017.

[2] K. Søreide, O. M. Sandvik, J. A. Søreide, V. Giljaca, A. Jureckova, and V. R. Bulusu, "Global epidemiology of gastrointestinal stromal tumours (GIST): a systematic review of population-based cohort studies," *Cancer Epidemiology*, vol. 40, pp. 39–46, 2016.

[3] S. Hirota, K. Isozaki, Y. Moriyama et al., "Gain-of-function mutations of *c-kit* in human gastrointestinal stromal tumors," *Science*, vol. 279, no. 5350, pp. 577–580, 1998.

[4] M. C. Heinrich, C. L. Corless, A. Duensing et al., "PDGFRA activating mutations in gastrointestinal stromal tumors," *Science*, vol. 299, no. 5607, pp. 708–710, 2003.

[5] H. Joensuu, M. Eriksson, K. Sundby Hall et al., "Adjuvant imatinib for high-risk GI stromal tumor: analysis of a randomized trial," *Journal of Clinical Oncology*, vol. 34, no. 3, pp. 244–250, 2016.

[6] R. P. Dematteo, K. V. Ballman, C. R. Antonescu et al., "Adjuvant imatinib mesylate after resection of localised, primary gastrointestinal stromal tumour: a randomised, double-blind, placebo-controlled trial," *The Lancet*, vol. 373, no. 9669, pp. 1097–1104, 2009.

[7] J. S. Gold, M. Gönen, A. Gutiérrez et al., "Development and validation of a prognostic nomogram for recurrence-free survival after complete surgical resection of localised primary gastrointestinal stromal tumour: a retrospective analysis," *The Lancet*, vol. 10, no. 11, pp. 1045–1052, 2009.

[8] M. Miettinen and J. Lasota, "Gastrointestinal stromal tumors: pathology and prognosis at different sites," *Seminars in Diagnostic Pathology*, vol. 23, no. 2, pp. 70–83, 2006.

[9] H. Joensuu, "Risk stratification of patients diagnosed with gastrointestinal stromal tumor," *Human Pathology*, vol. 39, no. 10, pp. 1411–1419, 2008.

[10] C. Cauchi, J. C. Trent, K. Edwards et al., "An unusual site of metastasis from gastrointestinal stromal tumor," *Rare Tumors*, vol. 2, no. 4, article e58, 2010.

[11] U. Bashir, A. Qureshi, H. A. Khan, and N. Uddin, "Gastrointestinal stromal tumor with skeletal muscle, adrenal and cardiac metastases: an unusual occurrence," *Indian Journal of Pathology & Microbiology*, vol. 54, no. 2, pp. 362–364, 2011.

[12] B. Hughes, D. Yip, D. Goldstein, P. Waring, V. Beshay, and G. Chong, "Cerebral relapse of metastatic gastrointestinal stromal tumor during treatment with imatinib mesylate: case report," *BMC Cancer*, vol. 4, no. 1, p. 74, 2004.

[13] M. Dorić, S. Radović, M. Babić et al., "Testicular metastasis of gastrointestinal stromal tumor of the jejunum," *Bosnian Journal of Basic Medical Sciences*, vol. 7, no. 2, pp. 176–179, 2007.

[14] D. Kassop, M. S. Donovan, M. K. Cheezum et al., "Cardiac masses on cardiac CT: a review," *Current Cardiovascular Imaging Reports*, vol. 7, p. 9281, 2014.

[15] R. Bussani, F. De-Giorgio, A. Abbate, and F. Silvestri, "Cardiac metastases," *Journal of Clinical Pathology*, vol. 60, no. 1, pp. 27–34, 2007.

Permissions

All chapters in this book were first published by Hindawi Publishing Corporation; hereby published with permission under the Creative Commons Attribution License or equivalent. Every chapter published in this book has been scrutinized by our experts. Their significance has been extensively debated. The topics covered herein carry significant findings which will fuel the growth of the discipline. They may even be implemented as practical applications or may be referred to as a beginning point for another development.

The contributors of this book come from diverse backgrounds, making this book a truly international effort. This book will bring forth new frontiers with its revolutionizing research information and detailed analysis of the nascent developments around the world.

We would like to thank all the contributing authors for lending their expertise to make the book truly unique. They have played a crucial role in the development of this book. Without their invaluable contributions this book wouldn't have been possible. They have made vital efforts to compile up to date information on the varied aspects of this subject to make this book a valuable addition to the collection of many professionals and students.

This book was conceptualized with the vision of imparting up-to-date information and advanced data in this field. To ensure the same, a matchless editorial board was set up. Every individual on the board went through rigorous rounds of assessment to prove their worth. After which they invested a large part of their time researching and compiling the most relevant data for our readers.

The editorial board has been involved in producing this book since its inception. They have spent rigorous hours researching and exploring the diverse topics which have resulted in the successful publishing of this book. They have passed on their knowledge of decades through this book. To expedite this challenging task, the publisher supported the team at every step. A small team of assistant editors was also appointed to further simplify the editing procedure and attain best results for the readers.

Apart from the editorial board, the designing team has also invested a significant amount of their time in understanding the subject and creating the most relevant covers. They scrutinized every image to scout for the most suitable representation of the subject and create an appropriate cover for the book.

The publishing team has been an ardent support to the editorial, designing and production team. Their endless efforts to recruit the best for this project, has resulted in the accomplishment of this book. They are a veteran in the field of academics and their pool of knowledge is as vast as their experience in printing. Their expertise and guidance has proved useful at every step. Their uncompromising quality standards have made this book an exceptional effort. Their encouragement from time to time has been an inspiration for everyone.

The publisher and the editorial board hope that this book will prove to be a valuable piece of knowledge for researchers, students, practitioners and scholars across the globe.

List of Contributors

Friedhelm Küthe
Ilmkreis-Kliniken, Clinic for Internal Medicine I, Bärwinkelstrasse 33, 99310 Arnstadt, Germany

Marcus Franz
Department of Internal Medicine I, University Hospital Jena, Am Klinikum 1, 07747 Jena, Germany

Sandesh Dinesh
Ilmkreis-Kliniken, Clinic for Internal Medicine I, Bärwinkelstrasse 33, 99310 Arnstadt, Germany
Department of Internal Medicine I, University Hospital Jena, Am Klinikum 1, 07747 Jena, Germany

Angelo Acitelli, Sabrina Bencivenga, Renata Petroni, Maria Penco and Silvio Romano
Cardiology, Department of Life, Health & Environmental Sciences, University of L'Aquila, Italy

Maria B. Giannico, Chiara Lanzillo, Luciano Maresca and Leonardo Calò
Division of Cardiology, Policlinico Casilino, Rome, Italy

Salem Badr, Daniel O. Johnsrud, Charnai D. Sherry and Eric S. Weiss
Aurora Cardiovascular and Thoracic Services, Aurora Sinai/Aurora St. Luke's Medical Centers, 2801 W. Kinnickinnic River Parkway, Ste. 880, Milwaukee, WI 53215, USA

Suhail Q. Allaqaband and Tanvir K. Bajwa
Aurora Cardiovascular and Thoracic Services, Aurora Sinai/Aurora St. Luke's Medical Centers, 2801 W. Kinnickinnic River Parkway, Ste. 880, Milwaukee, WI 53215, USA
University of Wisconsin School of Medicine and Public Health, 750 Highland Ave., Madison, WI 53726, USA

Jérémy Laïk, Anne Bellemain-Appaix, François Bernasconi and Laurent Jacq
Department of Cardiology, Antibes Juan-les-Pins Hospital, France

Virginie Fouilloux
Department of Cardiac Surgery, La Timone Children Hospital, France

Philippe Aldebert, Linda Koutbi and Jérôme Hourdain
Department of Cardiology, La Timone Children Hospital, France

Philippe De Swardt and Fabrice Tiger
Department of Reanimation, Antibes Juan-les-Pins Hospital, France

Srikala R. Gumireddy, Minako Katayama and Hari P. Chaliki
Division of Cardiovascular Diseases, Mayo Clinic, Scottsdale, Arizona, USA

Steen Reed
Department of Medicine, John Hunter Hospital, Australia

Michael McGee
Hunter Medical Research Institute, Australia
The University of Newcastle, Australia
The University of New England, Australia
Department of Medicine, Tamworth Hospital, Australia
Department of Cardiology, John Hunter Hospital, Australia

Shanathan Sritharan
Department of Medicine, Tamworth Hospital, Australia

Mohammad Hashim Jilani
Department of Medicine, Carle Foundation Hospital, Urbana IL, USA

Hina Khawar Jamali, Fahad Waqar and Mohamed Effat
Division of Cardiovascular Health and Disease, University of Cincinnati College of Medicine, Cincinnati OH, USA

Ali Abbood, Hareer Al Salihi, Jorge Parellada, Mario Madruga and S. J. Carlan
Department of Internal Medicine, Division of Academic Affairs and Research, Orlando Regional Healthcare, Orlando, Florida, USA

Cooper B. Kersey, Andrew M. Pattock and Linda Liu
University of Washington, Department of Medicine, USA

Fitsumberhan Medhane, Gary Huang and Younghoon Kwon
University of Washington, Division of Cardiology, USA

Abhijit V. Lele
University of Washington, Department of Anesthesiology and Pain Medicine, USA

Takafumi Terada, Yoshimori Araki, Akihiro Kobayashi and Osamu Kawaguchi
Department of Cardiac Surgery, JA Aichi Koseiren Toyota Kosei Hospital, Aichi, Japan

Osayi Lawani
HCA Houston Healthcare-Kingwood, USA

Jiries Ganim
University of Southern California, USA

Rick Ganim
Vital Heart & Vein, USA

Su Nam Lee, Gee-Hee Kim and Ki-Dong Yoo
Division of Cardiology, Department of Internal Medicine, St. Vincent's Hospital, The Catholic University of Korea, Seoul, Republic of Korea

Sotirios Mitsiadis, Nikolaos Miaris, Antonios Dimopoulos, Anastasios Theodosis-Georgilas, Spyridon Tsiamis, Nikolaos Patsourakos, Nikolaos Papakonstantinou and Evangelos Pisimisis
Department of Cardiology, "Tzaneio" General Hospital of Piraeus, Piraeus, Greece

Raghavendra Rao K, S. Reddy, J. R. Kashyap, K. Vikas and Hithesh Reddy
Department of Cardiology, Government Medical College and Hospital, Sector 32, Chandigarh 160030, India

Vadivelu Ramalingam
Department of Cardiology, Velammal Medical College Hospital and Research Institute, Madurai 625009, India

Vicken Zeitjian
Department of Cardiovascular Diseases, University of Texas San Antonio Health Science Center, 7703 Floyd Curl Dr. San Antonio, TX 78229, USA

Carmel Moazez
Department of Internal Medicine, Creighton University Maricopa Medical Center, 2601 E. Roosevelt St. Phoenix, AZ 85006, USA

Waqas Arslan
Department of Hematology and Oncology, Creighton University Maricopa Medical Center, 2601 E. Roosevelt St. Phoenix, AZ 85006, USA

Mehrdad Saririan
Department of Cardiovascular Diseases, Creighton University Maricopa Medical Center, 2601 E. Roosevelt St. Phoenix, AZ 85006, USA

Julián Alejandro Rivillas
Resident of Neurology, Universidad Icesi, Cali, Colombia

Juan David Lopez-Ponce de Leon, Noel Alberto Florez-Alarc6n , Pastor Olaya-Rojas and Juan Esteban Gomez-Mesa
Cardiology Department, Fundaci6n Valle del Lili Hospital Universitario, Cali, Colombia

Stephania Galindo-Coral
Cardiology Department, Fundaci6n Valle del Lili Hospital Universitario, Cali, Colombia
Clinical Research Center, Fundaci6n Valle del Lili Hospital Universitario, Cali, Colombia

Francisco Arias-Mora
Neurology Department, Fundaci6n Valle del Lili Hospital Universitario, Cali, Colombia

Karthik Seetharam, Ayesha Cheema, Gary Friedman and Roman Pachulski
Division of Cardiology, St. John's Episcopal Hospital-South Shore, New York, New York, USA

Daniel J. Chu
Cardiology Section, Department of Medicine, Baylor College of Medicine, Houston, TX 77030, USA

Wilson W. Lam
Cardiology Section, Department of Medicine, Baylor College of Medicine, Houston, TX 77030, USA
Texas Heart Institute, Baylor St. Luke's Medical Center, Houston. TX 77030, USA

Ramy Mando
Department of Internal Medicine, Beaumont Health System, Royal Oak, MI, USA

Daniel Tim, Anthony DeCicco, Justin Trivax and Ivan Hanson
Department of Cardiovascular Medicine, Beaumont Health System, Royal Oak, MI, USA
Oakland University William Beaumont School of Medicine, Auburn Hills, MI, USA

Safwan Gaznabi and Ashraf Abugroun
Department of Internal Medicine, Advocate Illinois Masonic Medical Center, 836 W Wellington Ave., Chicago, IL 60657, USA

Hasan Mahbub
Department of Internal Medicine, Flushing Hospital Medical Center, 4500 Parsons Blvd, Flushing, NY 11355, USA

Enrique Campos
Department of Cardiology, Advocate Illinois Masonic Medical Center, 836 W Wellington Ave, Chicago, IL 60657, USA

Caleb Norton
Department of Medicine, Vanderbilt University Medical Center, Nashville, TN, USA

Benjamin Holmes, Asad Al Aboud, Eun-Jeong Kim, Holly Gonzales, Christopher Ellis, Roy John, George H. Crossley III and Jay Montgomery
Division of Cardiovascular Medicine, Vanderbilt University Medical Center, Nashville, TN, USA

Alexandros P. Evangeliou, Evangelia Sotiroglou, Nikolaos Charitakis, Georgios Loufopoulos, Christos Varassas, Stergios Tzikas and Vassilios Vassilikos
3rd Department of Cardiology, Ippokratio Hospital, Aristotle University of Thessaloniki, Thessaloniki, Greece

Spiridon Papadopoulos
Department of Radiology, Ippokratio Hospital, Thessaloniki, Greece

Mohamed Magdi, Mahmood Mubasher, Hakam Alzaeem and Tahir Hamid
Hamad Medical Corporation, Qatar

Takanori Kono, Kazuyoshi Takagi, Shinya Negoto and Eiki Tayama
Department of Surgery, Division of Cardiovascular Surgery, Kurume University School of Medicine, 67 Asahi-machi, Kurume City, Fukuoka, Japan

Alisha Khan and Sana Riaz
Department of Medicine, SUNY Upstate Medical University, USA

Robert Carhart Jr.
Department of Cardiology, SUNY Upstate Medical University, USA

Catherine Champagne, Nicolas Dognin, Franck Molin, Christian Steinberg, François Philippon, Jean-François Sarrazin, Gilles O'hara, Isabelle Nault, Karine Roy, Benoit Plourde, Louis Blier and Jean Champagne
Department of Cardiology, Institut Universitaire de Cardiologie et de Pneumologie de Québec, Laval University, Quebec, Canada

Ahmed A. Hanfy, Nicholas T. Manasewitsch, Bryce D. Beutler, Daniel Antwi-Amoabeng, Mohamed Elnaggar, Munadel Awad and Gurpreet S. Chahal
Department of Internal Medicine, University of Nevada, Reno School of Medicine, Nevada, USA

Kritvikrom Durongpisitkul and Paweena Chungsomprasong
Division of Pediatric Cardiology, Department of Pediatrics, Faculty of Medicine Siriraj Hospital, Mahidol University, Bangkok, Thailand

Porntip Panjasamanvong
Siriraj Piyamaharajkarun Hospital, Mahidol University, Bangkok, Thailand

Somrach Thamtorawat
Division of Diagnostic Radiology, Department of Radiology, Faculty of Medicine Siriraj Hospital, Mahidol University, Bangkok, Thailand

Mohammed Alshaikh, Abdullah Muharib, Radhi Alshehri and Abdulaziz Alshoaibi
Medical Imaging, King Fahad Medical City, Central Second Health Cluster, Ministry of Health, Riyadh, Saudi Arabia

Mohammed Qattea
King Salman Heart Center, King Fahad Medical City, Central Second Health Cluster, Ministry of Health, Riyadh, Saudi Arabia

Shahad AlOtaiby
Research Center, King Fahad Medical City, Central Second Health Cluster, Ministry of Health, Riyadh, Saudi Arabia

Stephen J. Hankinson, Elliot A. Sultanik and Gautam V. Ramani
Department of Medicine, Division of Cardiovascular Medicine, University of Maryland School of Medicine, Baltimore, Maryland 21201, USA

João Pedro E. Sant'Ana, Amanda O. Vicente, Amanda S. Pereira and Pedro V. Bertozzi
Advanced Research Center in Medicine, School of Medicine, União das Faculdades dos Grandes Lagos (UNILAGO), São José do Rio Preto SP, Brazil

Rodrigo A. S. Sardenberg
Thoracic Surgeon Hospital Alemão Oswaldo Cruz, Thoracic Surgery Departament, São Paulo (SP), Brazil

Vivek D. Shah and Adeba Mohammad
1Department of Internal Medicine, Loma Linda University Medical Center, CA, USA

Shuktika Nandkeolyar, Liset Stoletniy and Tahmeed Contractor
Department of Internal Medicine, Division of Cardiology, Loma Linda University Medical Center, CA, USA

Ruchika Meel
Department of Internal Medicine, Division of Cardiology, Chris Hani Baragwanath Hospital, University of the Witwatersrand, Johannesburg, South Africa

Bongane Ngutshane and Shungu Mogaladi
Department of General Surgery, Division of Cardio-Thoracic Surgery, Charlotte Maxeke Hospital, University of the Witwatersrand, Johannesburg, South Africa

Ricardo Gonçalves
Olivedale Hospital, Johannesburg, South Africa

Valerie R. Ramiro, Donna Ricca M. Hornilla and Maria Teresa B. Abola
Section of Cardiology, University of the Philippines–Philippine General Hospital, Manila, Philippines

Carmegie C. Saliba
Department of Medicine, University of the Philippines–Philippine General Hospital, Manila, Philippines

John Anthony D. Tindoc
Department of Pathology, University of the Philippines–Philippine General Hospital, Manila, Philippines

Marinette R. Jambaro
Section of Rheumatology, University of the Philippines–Philippine General Hospital, Manila, Philippines

Enrique M. Chua III
Section of Thoracic Cardiovascular Surgery, University of the Philippines–Philippine General Hospital, Manila, Philippines

Edgar Stroppa Lamas
Department of Interventional Cardiology, Intercor, Hospital 13 de Maio, Sorriso, Brazil

Alan Vinicius Gamero Osti
Department of Interventional Cardiology, Intercor, Hospital Santo Antonio, Sinop, Brazil

Tania Ahuja
New York University Langone Health, Department of Pharmacy, 550 First Avenue, New York, NY 10016, USA

Scarlett Murphy and Daniel J. Sartori
New York University Langone Health, Department of Medicine, 550 First Avenue, New York, NY 10016, USA

Kanako Akamatsu, Takahide Ito, Kazushi Sakane, Yumiko Kanzaki, Koichi Sohmiya and Masaaki Hoshiga
Department of Cardiology, Osaka Medical College, Takatsuki, Osaka, Japan

Kevin Lee and Osman Rahimi
Department of Internal Medicine, University of Nevada, Las Vegas, 1707 W Charleston Blvd, Suite 100, Las Vegas, NV 89102, USA

Neelesh Gupta and Chowdhury Ahsan
Department of Cardiology, University of Nevada, Las Vegas, 1800 W Charleston Blvd, Las Vegas, NV 89102, USA

Ata Firouzi, Zahra Hosseini and Ehsan Khalilipur
Cardiovascular Intervention Research Center, Rajaie Cardiovascular Medical and Research Center, Iran University of Medical Sciences, Tehran, Iran

Prathap Kumar, Stalin Roy, Blessvin Jino, Manu Rajendran and Sandheep G. Villoth
Meditrina Hospital, Kollam, Kerala, India

Avik Ray, Ahmad Najmi and Balakrishnan Sadasivam
Department of Pharmacology, All India Institute of Medical Sciences Bhopal, Saket Nagar, Bhopal 462020, Madhya Pradesh, India

Gaurav Khandelwal
Department of Cardiology, All India Institute of Medical Sciences Bhopal, Saket Nagar, Bhopal 462020, Madhya Pradesh, India

Mingkui Zhang, Hui Xue, Lifu Miao, Xiujie Tang and Yanbin Shao
Heart Center, First Hospital of Tsinghua University, No. 6 1st Street, Jiuxianqiao, Chaoyang District, Beijing 100016, China

Justin Ugwu
Department of Hospital Medicine, Miami Valley Hospital, Dayton, Ohio, USA

Umbreen Hussein
Cardiovascular Disease Fellowship, Wright State University, Dayton, Ohio, USA

Sampson Alliu
Department of Cardiovascular Medicine, Maimonides Medical Center, Brooklyn, New York, USA

Ravi Gurujal
Department of Cardiology, Miami Valley Hospital, Dayton, Ohio, USA

Ruben Schleberger, Leon Dinshaw, Andreas Rillig and Andreas Metzner
Department of Cardiology, University Heart and Vascular Center, University Medical Center Hamburg -Eppendorf, Martinistraße 52, 20246 Hamburg, Germany

Moritz Nies
Department of Cardiology, University Heart and Vascular Center, University Medical Center Hamburg -Eppendorf, Martinistraße 52, 20246 Hamburg, Germany
DZHK (German Center for Cardiovascular Research), Partner Site Hamburg/Lübeck/Kiel, Berlin, Germany

Christian Meyer
Department of Cardiology, University Heart and Vascular Center, University Medical Center Hamburg -Eppendorf, Martinistraße 52, 20246 Hamburg, Germany
DZHK (German Center for Cardiovascular Research), Partner Site Hamburg/Lübeck/Kiel, Berlin, Germany
Division of Cardiology, EVK Düsseldorf, cNEP, Cardiac Neuro- and Electrophysiology Research Consortium, Kirchfeldstraße 40, 40217 Düsseldorf, Germany
4cNEP, Cardiac Neuro- and Electrophysiology Research Consortium, Institute for Neural and Sensory Physiology, Heinrich Heine University Düsseldorf, Medical Faculty, Düsseldorf, Germany

Constantin Mork, Luca Koechlin, Friedrich Eckstein and David Santer
Department of Cardiac Surgery, University Hospital Basel, Basel, Switzerland

Matthias Streif
Department of Radiology, University Hospital Basel, Basel, Switzerland

Alexa Hollinger and Martin Siegemund
Intensive Care Unit, University Hospital Basel, Basel, Switzerland
Department of Clinical Research, University of Basel, Basel, Switzerland

Metri Haddaden
MedStar Health, Department of Internal Medicine, Baltimore, Maryland, USA

Samir Husami
Department of Medicine, Division of Nephrology, Washington University School of Medicine, St. Louis, Missouri, USA

Modar Alom
National Cancer Institute, National Institutes of Health, Bethesda, Maryland, USA

Yifan Pang
Department of Medicine, University of Toledo-College of Medicine and life Sciences Toledo, OH, USA

Zaid Imam
William Beaumont Hospital, Department of Internal Medicine, Royal Oak, Michigan, USA

Daniel Keena
William Beaumont Hospital, Division of Pulmonary and Critical Care, Department of Internal Medicine, Royal Oak, Michigan, USA

Justin Brilliant, Diep Edwards, Ritu Yadav, Jana Lovell and Lena Mathews
Johns Hopkins Hospital, Baltimore, MD, USA

Dimitrios Siamkouris, Marc Schloesser, Amr Yousef and Elmar Offers
Department of Cardiology, Dreifaltigkeits Hospital Lippstadt, Germany
Academic Teaching Hospital of Westfaelische Wilhelms University Muenster, Germany

Index